Other monographs in the series, Major Problems in Clinical Surgery:

CHILD: The Liver and Portal Hypertension
WELCH and HEDBERG: Polypoid Lesions of the Gastrointestinal Tract, *2nd edition*
MADDING and KENNEDY: Trauma to the Liver, *2nd edition*
BARKER: Peripheral Arterial Disease, *2nd edition*
HALLER: Deep Thrombophlebitis
COLCOCK and BRAASCH: Surgery of the Small Intestine in the Adult
JACKMAN and BEAHRS: Tumors of the Large Bowel
BOTSFORD and WILSON: The Acute Abdomen
COLCOCK: Diverticular Disease of the Colon
SPRATT, BUTCHER and BRICKER: Exenterative Surgery of the Pelvis
CHILD: Portal Hypertension
SEDGWICK: Surgery of the Thyroid Gland
THORBJARNARSON: Surgery of the Biliary Tract
MENGUY: Surgery of Peptic Ulcer
SALISBURY AND PRUITT: Burns of the Upper Extremity
BUSHKIN and WOODWARD: Postgastrectomy Syndromes
BLAISDELL and LEWIS: Respiratory Distress Syndrome of Shock & Trauma
FOSTER and BERMAN: Solid Liver Tumors
MAY: Surgery of the Veins of the Leg and Pelvis
KRETSCHMER: Intestinal Stomas
WOLFE and SABISTON: Pulmonary Embolism
DONEGAN and SPRATT: Cancer of the Breast, *2nd edition*
MASON: Surgical Treatment of Obesity
LAWRENCE: Problems of the Pleural Space
ROSES, HARRIS and ACKERMAN: Diagnosis and Management of Cutaneous Malignant Melanoma
WACHTEL and FRANK: Burns of the Head & Neck
WILSON: Surgical Problems in Immuno-Depressed Patients

Ideal Cardiac Pacing

A-Hadi Hakki, M.D., F.R.C.S.

Assistant Professor of Surgery
Cardiothoracic Surgical Associates, Inc.
Hahnemann University Hospital
Philadelphia, Pennsylvania

Volume 31
in the Series
MAJOR PROBLEMS IN CLINICAL SURGERY

1984

W. B. SAUNDERS COMPANY

PHILADELPHIA / LONDON / TORONTO / MEXICO CITY / RIO DE JANEIRO / SYDNEY / TOKYO

W. B. Saunders Company: West Washington Square
Philadelphia, PA 19105

1 St. Anne's Road
Eastbourne, East Sussex BN21 3UN, England

1 Goldthorne Avenue
Toronto, Ontario M8Z 5T9, Canada

Apartado 26370—Cedro 512
Mexico 4, D.F., Mexico

Rua Coronel Cabrita, 8
São Cristovao Caixa Postal 21176
Rio de Janeiro, Brazil

9 Waltham Street
Artarmon, N.S.W. 2064, Australia

Ichibancho, Central Bldg., 22-1 Ichibancho
Chiyoda-Ku, Tokyo 102, Japan

Library of Congress Cataloging in Publication Data

Hakki, A-Hadi.

Ideal cardiac pacing.

(Major problems in clinical surgery; v. 31)

1. Pacemaker, Artificial (Heart)—Addresses, essays, lectures. I. Title. II. Series. [DNLM: 1. Cardiac pacing, Artificial. 2. Pacemaker, Artificial. W1 MA492R v. 31 / WG 168 H155i]

RC684.P3H35 1984 617'.412059 83–20050

ISBN 0–7216–1251–2

Ideal Cardiac Pacing ISBN 0-7216-1251-2

Last digit is the print number: 9 8 7 6 5 4 3 2 1

To the patient: The source of infinite knowledge

CONTRIBUTORS

JOSEPH R. CARVER, M.D.
Assistant Professor of Medicine, Hahnemann University; Staff Physician, Jeane's Hospital and American Oncologic Hospital, Philadelphia, Pennsylvania
Indications for Cardiac Pacing

JEFFREY M. DUNN, M.D.
Associate Professor, Department of Surgery, Temple University School of Medicine; Chief, Cardiovascular Surgery, St. Christopher's Hospital for Children, Philadelphia, Pennsylvania
Cardiac Pacing in Children

SUSAN J. FRYE, R.N., M.S.N.
Consultant, Critical Care Management, Education, and Development, Drexel Hill, Pennsylvania
Cardiac Pacing: A Nursing Perspective

LAWRENCE R. GOODMAN, M.D.
Professor and Head, Chest Radiology, Department of Radiology, Medical College of Wisconsin; Attending Radiologist, Milwaukee County Hospital, Froedtert Memorial Lutheran Hospital, Woods Veterans Administration Medical Center, Milwaukee, Wisconsin
Radiographic Evaluation of Cardiac Pacemakers

ALLAN M. GREENSPAN, M.D.
Associate Professor of Medicine, Hahnemann University; Associate Director, Clinical Cardiac Electrophysiology Laboratory, Likoff Cardiovascular Institute, Hahnemann University Hospital, Philadelphia, Pennsylvania
Electrophysiology of Pacing

A. HADI HAKKI, M.D., F.R.C.S.
Assistant Professor of Surgery, Hahnemann University; Attending Physician, Hahnemann University Hospital, Philadelphia; Assistant Attending Surgeon, Department of Surgery, Bryn Mawr Hospital, Bryn Mawr, Pennsylvania
Permanent Cardiac Pacing: Surgical Technique; Permanent Cardiac Pacing: Complications and Management

A-HAMID HAKKI, M.D.
Assistant Professor of Medicine, Hahnemann University; Attending Cardiologist, Hahnemann University Hospital, Philadelphia, Pennsylvania
Hemodynamics of Pacing

LEONARD N. HOROWITZ, M.D.
Associate Professor of Medicine, Hahnemann University; Director, Clinical Cardiac Electrophysiology Laboratory, Likoff Cardiovascular Institute, Hahnemann University Hospital, Philadelphia, Pennsylvania
Temporary Cardiac Pacing: Indications, Techniques, and Management

ABDULMASSIH S. ISKANDRIAN, M.D.
Professor of Medicine, Hahnemann University; Director, Nuclear Cardiology, Hahnemann University Hospital, Philadelphia, Pennsylvania
Hemodynamics of Pacing

MORRIS N. KOTLER, M.D.
Professor of Medicine, Hahnemann University; Director, Noninvasive Cardiac Laboratory, Likoff Cardiovascular Institute, Hahnemann University Hospital, Philadelphia, Pennsylvania
Cardiac Pacing Following Open-Heart Surgery

GEORGE LUMB, M.D., M.R.C.P., F.R.C.Path.
Professor of Pathology, Hahnemann University; Attending Pathologist, Hahnemann University Hospital, Philadelphia, Pennsylvania
The Conduction System: Anatomic and Pathologic Correlations

HANI S. MATLOUB, M.D.
Assistant Professor of Plastic Surgery, and Director, Microsurgery, Medical College of Wisconsin; Attending Physician, Woods Veterans Administration Medical Center, Milwaukee, Wisconsin
Flap Coverage for Exposed Pacemakers

ASHOK V. MEHTA, M.D.
Assistant Professor, Department of Pediatrics, Temple University School of Medicine; Director, Cardiac Electrophysiology and Pacing, St. Christopher's Hospital for Children; Philadelphia, Pennsylvania
Cardiac Pacing in Children

JOEL MORGANROTH, M.D.
Professor of Medicine and Pharmacology, Hahnemann University; Director, Sudden Death Prevention Program, Hahnemann University Hospital, Philadelphia, Pennsylvania
Commentary: Clinical Perspectives in Cardiac Pacing

ELDRED D. MUNDTH, M.D.
Professor of Surgery and Chairman, Department of Cardiothoracic Surgery, Hahnemann University Hospital, Philadelphia; Assistant Attending Surgeon, Department of Surgery, Bryn Mawr Hospital, Bryn Mawr, Pennsylvania
Foreword

IOANNIS P. PANIDIS, M.D.
Assistant Professor of Medicine, Hahnemann University; Attending Cardiologist, Noninvasive Cardiac Laboratory, Likoff Cardiovascular Institute, Hahnemann University Hospital, Philadelphia, Pennsylvania
Cardiac Pacing Following Open-Heart Surgery

RONALD S. PENNOCK, M.D.
Associate Professor of Medicine, Hahnemann University; Director, Department of Cardiology, St. Joseph's Hospital; Director, Department of Cardiology, Guiffrey Medical Center, Philadelphia, Pennsylvania
Pacemaker Follow-up

STUART SNYDER, M.D.
Assistant Professor of Medicine, Hahnemann University, Philadelphia, Pennsylvania
Pacemaker Follow-up

SCOTT R. SPIELMAN, M.D.
Associate Professor of Medicine, Hahnemann University; Director, Coronary Care Unit; Assistant Director, Clinical Cardiac Electrophysiology; Chairman, Critical Care Committee, Hahnemann University Hospital, Philadelphia, Pennsylvania
New Advances in Cardiac Pacemaking

LINDA A. YACONE, R.N., B.S., CCRN
Electrophysiology Nurse Clinician, Clinical Cardiac Electrophysiology Department, Hahnemann University Hospital, Philadelphia, Pennsylvania
Cardiac Pacing: A Nursing Perspective

PAUL M. ZOLL, M.D.
Clinical Professor of Medicine, Emeritus, Harvard Medical School; Physician, Beth Israel Hospital, Boston, Massachusetts
History of Cardiac Pacing

FOREWORD

Accelerating growth and technological advances have been commonplace in all areas of cardiology and cardiac surgery during the past two decades, but perhaps there has been no single specialized area that has continuously evolved so rapidly and effectively as has cardiac pacing. This particular field imposes a unique interdisciplinary interface between clinical cardiologists and surgeons and electrophysiologists and bioengineers. A whole new generation of cardiac pacing concepts has revolutionized both techniques of implantation and pacemaker hardware. It has been exciting to watch the rapid developments and gratifying to be able to effectively apply the many new concepts to clinical problems.

This book discusses many of the newer concepts in cardiac pacing and will be a helpful source of knowledge in all its aspects: electrophysiology, hemodynamics, indications and applications, surgical techniques, and complications. Current advances and potential future advances are exciting to contemplate. The contributing authors have researched their assignments well and presented their material in understandable form. This book will provide a valuable source of useful information for all physicians, nurses, students, and paramedical personnel interested in any aspect of cardiac pacing.

ELDRED D. MUNDTH, M.D.

PREFACE

Cardiac pacing has undergone a tremendous evolution in the last decade. Where applicable, ventricular pacing is presently being gradually replaced by atrioventricular pacing, triggering increased demand for new ideas in the development of the ideal pacemaker lead and generator. Although the change is a rapid one, the pacemaker has a long way to go before reaching perfection. Nevertheless, the dual chamber pacemaker battery (DDD) appears to be the most physiological unit to date. As with any new device, further studies are indicated, especially in terms of follow-up management.

This text is a result of a team approach of the surgeon and the cardiologist in order to deliver a simple message regarding the principles of artificial cardiac pacing, their applications, techniques, and complications. It provides a concise and up-to-date clinical picture of pacemaker eletrophysiology and hemodynamics, as well as a look into the future of cardiac pacing.

It is hoped that this book will be a source of useful information to physicians and nurses interested in any aspect of cardiac pacing, thereby helping to achieve improved patient care. It may also serve as a quick reference for other medical and paramedical staff.

I am sincerely grateful to all of the authors for their invaluable contributions. I wish to thank Tamara C. Komarow, who provided invaluable assistance at every stage of the creation of this manual. I would also like to thank Carroll C. Cann, Medical Editor at W. B. Saunders Company, for his support of this work.

A. Hadi Hakki, M.D., F.R.C.S.

CONTENTS

I
GENERAL PRINCIPLES

1
History of Cardiac Pacing 3
Paul M. Zoll, M.D.

2
The Conduction System: Anatomic and Pathologic Correlations 12
George Lumb, M.D., M.R.C.P., F.R.C.Path.

3
Electrophysiology of Pacing 29
Allan M. Greenspan, M.D.

4
Hemodynamics of Pacing 59
A-Hamid Hakki, M.D., and Abdulmassih S. Iskandrian, M.D.

II
CLINICAL APPLICATIONS

5
Indications for Cardiac Pacing 79
Joseph R. Carver, M.D.

6
Temporary Cardiac Pacing: Indications, Techniques, and Management ... 86
Leonard N. Horowitz, M.D.

7
Permanent Cardiac Pacing: Surgical Technique 106
A. Hadi Hakki, M.D.

8
Cardiac Pacing in Children 120
Jeffrey M. Dunn, M.D., and Ashok V. Mehta, M.D.

9
Cardiac Pacing Following Open-Heart Surgery 133
Ioannis P. Panidis, M.D., and Morris N. Kotler, M.D.

III
TROUBLESHOOTING

10
Radiographic Evaluation of Cardiac Pacemakers 145
Lawrence R. Goodman, M.D.

11
Permanent Cardiac Pacing: Complications and Management 160
A. Hadi Hakki, M.D.

12
Flap Coverage for Exposed Pacemakers 177
Hani S. Matloub, M.D.

13
Pacemaker Follow-up 182
Ronald Pennock, M.D., and Stuart Snyder, M.D.

14
Cardiac Pacing: A Nursing Perspective 195
Susan J. Frye, R.N., M.S.N., and Linda A. Yacone, R.N., B.S., CCRN

IV
NEW FRONTIERS

15
New Advances in Cardiac Pacemaking 219
Scott R. Spielman, M.D.

Appendix I
Commentary: Clinical Perspectives in Cardiac Pacing 263
Joel Morganroth, M.D.

Appendix II
Atlas of Pacemaker Generators and Leads 265
Biotronik 265
Cardiac Pacemakers, Inc. 271
Cardio-Pace Medical 275
Cook Pacemaker Corporation 277
Coratomic, Inc. 284
Cordis Corporation 288
Ela Medical 295
Intermedics, Inc. 299
Medtronic, Inc. 315
Pacesetter Systems, Inc. 315
Siemens-Elema 327
Telectronics 332
Index 339

I

GENERAL PRINCIPLES

1

History of Cardiac Pacing

PAUL M. ZOLL, M.D.

HISTORY OF CARDIAC PACING

The association between electricity and excitation of the heart and other organs was recognized more than two centuries ago when Galvani used muscle contractions to demonstrate the passage of an electric current.[1] During the next century **direct** stimulation of the exposed heart was studied extensively and was even performed in attempts at resuscitation.[2, 3] **External** noninvasive stimulation was also suggested as a clinically feasible and appropriate means of resuscitation from cardiac arrest.[4]

In 1930 Hyman presented a method of direct cardiac stimulation for emergency resuscitation from ventricular standstill.[5] Electric stimuli from an external pulse generator were transmitted by a long-needle electrode through the chest wall to the right atrium. He demonstrated effective atrial stimulation in rabbits and subsequently resuscitated several patients at least temporarily. Clinical success was limited, however, and Hyman's method was abandoned. It was difficult to maintain contact between the needle electrode and the cardiac muscle without displacement or injury, and atrial stimulation would not have been useful in the presence of atrioventricular (AV) block.

In 1950 Bigelow and Callaghan described a technique of direct atrial stimulation with an external electric pacemaker attached to a wire electrode passed down a dog's jugular vein to the area of the sinoatrial (SA) node.[6] This method was intended for use in open-heart surgery to accelerate hypothermic hearts in bradycardia or standstill. The effort to stimulate the atrium, particularly the SA node, was not appropriate for clinical resuscitation.

In 1952 Zoll reported the resuscitation of two patients from ventricular standstill with **external** stimuli provided by electrodes on the chest surface attached to an electric pulse generator.[7] Both patients suffered repeated Stokes-Adams attacks—that is, AV block with episodes of ventricular standstill, bradycardia, tachycardia, or fibrillation. The first patient died after circulation was maintained for 20 minutes by the artificially stimulated ventricular rhythm. The second patient survived after external stimulation was continued for 52 hours, until intrinsic ventricular rhythmicity finally returned. To provide a clinically useful means of stimulating effective ventricular beats in the emergency of ventricular standstill it is necessary that the technique be simple, reliable, and quick and easy to apply. The frequency of recurrent attacks also requires that resuscitation not involve a major, invasive procedure or other significant risk. This method met these requirements and was widely used for many years for ventricular standstill or bradycardia due to any cause.[8] It was, of course, ineffective in arrest due to ventricular tachycardia or fibrillation or in the presence of poor myocardial contractility. For example, electric stimulation rarely, if ever, arouses electrical or mechanical responses in ventricular standstill that follows prolonged anoxic arrest from ventricular fibrillation or circulatory collapse.

No untoward **cardiac** effects of external electric stimulation have been observed. Repetitive or multifocal ventricular beats, tachycardia, or fibrillation has not been observed at the rates and amplitudes of stimulation available in clinical units, even in the presence of competition between an intrinsic rhythm and the artificial pacemaker or in the circumstances of acute myocardial infarction or other serious cardiac disease. No evidence of damage from the electric impulses to the heart or surrounding tissue has been found at pathologic examinations. The only untoward effect of external electric stimulation is pain from stimulation of local cutaneous nerves and from skeletal muscle contractions. Although in the past stimulation was occasionally continued for hours or days (in desperate circumstances), it was usually limited to brief applications, primarily for emergency resuscitation in the unconscious patient. The procedure of intravenous infusion of dilute solutions of epinephrine or isoproterenol at carefully controlled rates was developed for the temporary management of persistent or recurrent ventricular bradycardia or standstill, problems that often follow the initial restoration of circulation with electric stimulation of ventricular beats.[9] With these agents, intrinsic ventricular rhythmicity could usually be aroused within a few minutes. The ventricular rate could be accelerated to any level desired and maintained for hours or even weeks. It was observed very early that electric or pharmacologic cardiac stimulation at rates higher than the intrinsic ventricular rhythm prevented manifestations of abnormal ventricular irritability, such as multifocal and repetitive ectopic ventricular beats, tachycardia, and fibrillation. This regularization of ventricular rhythmicity by relatively rapid artificial stimulation was subsequently expanded, in the principle of overdrive suppression, to the termination and prevention of many arrhythmias.[10]

Beginning in 1947, the emergency of cardiac arrest due to ventricular fibrillation had been generally managed according to the precepts of Beck—by immediate thoracotomy, direct cardiac massage, and countershock defibrillation with electrodes on each side of the exposed heart.[11] This heroic procedure was widely practiced for many years and did save many lives, but it met none of the requirements posed for external cardiac stimulation and was often clinically unacceptable. A technique of noninvasive, external electric countershock defibrillation was developed and was first used successfully in 1955.[12] External electric countershock was then demonstrated to terminate other rapid arrhythmias as well. In 1962 Lown reported the elective termination of many arrhythmias with external countershock.[13] His modified technique of direct-current shocks synchronized to the QRS complex has become generally accepted and constitutes another advance in the electric control of cardiac arrhythmias.

The rapid progression of irreversible cerebral and cardiac ischemia following cardiac arrest mandates prompt recognition of the onset of arrest, identification of the arrhythmia, and evaluation of cardiac response to treatment. The unpredictability of arrest, especially in patients with Stokes-Adams disease, together with the stringent time limit led Zoll to the development of cardiac monitors in 1954. They provided an audible signal of each beat, continuous visual display of the electrocardiogram, an alarm signal upon preselected change in rate, and prompt, even automatic availability of electric stimulation.[14] In response to clinical needs many refinements and extensions of this apparatus were developed, such as prolonged cardiac monitoring with continuous recording for many hours or selected recording of arrhythmia intervals and computerized compilation and analysis of irregularities. The many new, primarily noninvasive, techniques for resuscitation (continuous cardiac monitoring; external and direct electric and mechanical cardiac stimulation; external electric countershock defibrillation; external cardiac massage introduced by Kouwenhoven in 1960;[15] prolonged, carefully regulated intravenous drug administration; and artificial respiration with mouth-to-mouth breathing or endotracheal intubation) together with personnel expert in their use were combined by Day in 1963.[16] His demonstration of a major reduction of mortality from arrhythmias in acute myocardial infarction led to the establishment of coronary care units throughout the world. These same techniques were also applied generally for cardiac arrest under any circumstances and led to the abandonment of the previous, invasive program of emergency thoracotomy with cardiac massage and countershock defibrillation of the exposed heart.

DIRECT CARDIAC STIMULATION

The frequent recurrence of cardiac arrest due to any cause made the provision of reliable long-term cardiac stimulation necessary, to prevent ventricular bradycardia and standstill and also to suppress tachycardia and fibrillation. Attempts at long-term cardiac pacing were frustrated for many years, however, by an unexpected problem—a continued rise in the threshold for stimulation. In 1958, for example, Weirich attempted direct cardiac stimulation in patients with Stokes-Adams disease with a stainless steel electrode placed in the myocardium at thoracotomy and connected to an externally carried pulse generator.[17] Stimulation failed uniformly within 8 weeks, however, as the threshold for cardiac response increased. The difficulty was finally recognized as a foreign body tissue reaction to minute, sterile contaminants on the electrode. The problem was ultimately solved by meticulous cleansing, as well as by use of inert metals for the active electrode (platinum, stainless steel, Elgiloy). Senning[18] in 1958 and Hunter[19] in 1959 were the first to achieve long-term cardiac pacing. In 1960 Chardack,[20] Kantrowitz,[21] and Zoll and Frank[22] all began series of implantations of myocardial electrodes with attached subcutaneous pulse generators by way of thoracotomy. The long-term management of Stokes-Adams disease was thus finally realized.

The early indications for implantation of a long-term cardiac pacemaker were, first, the appearance of a Stokes-Adams attack and, second, manifestations of inadequate cardiac output due to bradycardia. During the years, with improved techniques and lessened morbidity from implantation and improved performance of pacemaker systems, the indications have been expanded. Now they include high-degree AV block (even before an initial syncopal episode), multifascicular block, ventricular standstill or bradycardia in the absence of any conduction defect (as with SA depression in the sick sinus syndrome), and the prevention or termination of some arrhythmias under certain special circumstances.

Electrodes

After the initial problem of a continually rising threshold for stimulation was solved, many problems appeared in every aspect of direct electric cardiac stimulation, and many modifications have been made in every component of the pacemaker-electrode system. The threshold for response was found to vary inversely with the size of the exposed electrode and its distance from the excitable tissue. As a result, electrodes now generally have a small exposed surface area, and many configurations have been devised to obtain close, secure contact with myocardium.

A major modification of the technique of direct cardiac stimulation is the pervenous placement of an endocardial "catheter" electrode in the right ventricle under fluoroscopy rather than in the myocardium under direct vision by thoracotomy. In this approach, introduced clinically by Furman in 1959, the electrode was initially passed through an antecubital vein and was connected to an externally carried pulse generator.[23] Other veins were subsequently used in an effort to reduce displacement, perforation of the right ventricle, and breakage of the pervenous electrode.

In many institutions across the country the right cephalic vein is the most common first choice for long-term use. Its small size and aberrant anatomy not infrequently make catheterization difficult, so an external jugular or subclavian vein is occasionally used instead. The latter is increasingly chosen now because its large size permits easy placement of even two electrodes, an attractive feature for combined atrial and ventricular pacing. This large vein, however, should be approached only by very experienced operators, since some serious complications are being reported with its use. The pulse generator is connected to the distal end of the electrode and is placed subcutaneously in the subclavicular area so that the whole system is inside the body. The entire procedure can usually be performed under local anesthesia and carried little morbidity and mortality in comparison with thoracotomy for myocardial implantation. Consequently, the fluoroscopic placement of a pervenous right ventricular endocardial electrode has become the most widely used method for direct cardiac stimulation.

This approach is not entirely satisfactory, however, because electrode placement and fixation are occasionally very difficult and even unsuccessful, especially in large hearts. Furthermore, electrode displacement, myocardial perforation, high thresholds for stimulation or sensing, and wire breakage occur with significant frequency, even in the best of circumstances. Although the active electrode usually is of platinum-iridium, many variations have been developed in the material and configuration of the electrode, conducting wire, insulation, and terminal pin. These improvements increase the ease of placement and fixation, and long-term, stable, trouble-free performance of the electrodes.

Recent interest in long-term atrial as well as ventricular pacing has uncovered even more difficulties in electrode placement and fixation. The problems have largely been met by the development of new atrial electrodes[24] (some with features promoting active fixation), improved techniques and equipment for catheterization, use of the larger subclavian or jugular veins, and thinner polyurethane electrodes. In addition, small, self-retaining electrodes have been developed that can be inserted into atrial and ventricular myocardium through parasternal, subxiphoid, or subcostal routes to gain the advantage of quick, secure placement under direct vision with a minor, well-tolerated procedure.[25]

Temporary Cardiac Pacing

The procedure of direct cardiac stimulation with an endocardial catheter electrode attached to an externally carried pacemaker came to be used for temporary as well as long-term pacing. External, noninvasive stimulation generally fell into disuse, even for emergency resuscitation from standstill, for several reasons: the usual severe discomfort from stimulation in a conscious patient, the difficulty of recognizing EKG and pressure responses obscured by large stimulus artifacts and muscular contractions, and the erroneous belief that external stimulation is effective only in Stokes-Adams disease. This misconception may actually have resulted from ineffective stimulation after loss of myocardial contractility during ventricular fibrillation or prolonged arrest. Placement of an endocardial electrode during cardiac arrest is difficult and even inappropriate in the hectic, desperate circumstances of the emergency: It takes attention and space away from the more immediate needs for restoration of circulation and respiratory exchange. The time required for endocardial electrode placement in the most favorable circumstances is clearly much longer than that required for simple application of an external pacemaker. In 1981 Zoll introduced a modified, external pacemaker with which temporary, comfortable stimulation of the conscious patient and recognition of cardiac responses to stimulation are achieved.[26]

Energy Sources

Early techniques of long-term stimulation with endocardial electrodes connected to externally carried pulse generators[23] by long lead wires traversing the skin have been discarded because of wire fractures, disconnections, and infection. Other systems with inductively coupled[27] or radio-frequency[28] signals transmitted from external pulse generators across the chest wall also provided easy external replacement of the batteries. In addition, the small number and simplicity of the internal components led to their high reliability,[27] and the complete external control of the generator provided great flexibility of stimulation. These systems, however, suffered unacceptable interruptions of function from breakage, disconnection, displacement, and other electric or mechanical interference through accident, human error, or carelessness.

The major problems with long-term implantable pulse generators have centered on the provision of a long-lasting, reliable power source. A zinc-mercuric oxide electrochemical cell[29] was generally used from 1960 to 1973 and provided pacemaker life spans of usually about 2 to 3 years. The semipermeable encapsulation required to permit escape of the hydrogen gas formed in the electrochemical reaction allowed fluid seepage into the pulse generator, leading to frequent pacemaker malfunction and premature failure.

Cells of lithium iodide and other salts introduced in 1973[30] led to major improvements in pacemakers. The absence of gas formation in the chemical reactions and the high energy yield permit hermetic sealing and long life span (typically 8 years) of small units. Other sources of energy, such as radioactive isotope power cells,[31] externally rechargeable electrochemical cells,[32] and bioelectric energy from internal biologic processes,[33] were all studied intensively but have been supplanted by lithium cells in modern pacemakers. The lithium cells, together with major advances in electronic technology (large-scale integration with silicon chips, digital circuitry), have led to remarkable reliability, reduction in size, increased life span, and multiplication in complexity and variability in function of pacemakers. Noninvasive external programming now offers wide ranges of choice of many of the parameters and modes of function and even telemetric reporting of many aspects of the internal environment of the pacemaker.

Pacemaker Rhythmicity

Internal cardiac pacemakers were initially designed to provide regular stimulation of the ventricles at a preselected constant rate—that is, a "fixed-rate mode." It was soon found that cardiac output varied little with rates between 60 and 90 per minute, so that rates of about 70 per minute are still usually selected. In some early models, stimulation rates were changed by external manipulation (external magnetic change of an internal switch or mechanical adjustment of an internal potentiometer by a percutaneous needle), but these variations were not widely used. Of course, the external pacemakers with inductive coupling or radio-frequency transmission allowed easy variation of rate, which was occasionally useful for special circumstances. Subsequently, some special-purpose pacemakers were also devised to produce very rapid, brief bursts of stimuli by external activation of an otherwise dormant pacemaker whenever required to interrupt and terminate tachycardia.

Fixed-rate pacemakers had the major advantages of simplicity and fewer components. This feature meant greater reliability, significantly smaller size, and a lower energy requirement with a consequently longer life span.

Subsequently, many types of pacemakers were developed with modes other than fixed-rate stimulation. In these, the electrical activity from atrial or ventricular beats was sensed by the pulse generator and used to inhibit or trigger atrial or ventricular stimulation. The earliest and most widely used was the R-wave or ventricular-inhibited "demand" pacemaker,[34, 35] which reduced competition between pacemaker-stimulated and intrinsic beats conducted from the AV node or arising in an ectopic ventricular focus. In some special circumstances, particularly the placement of an electrode in an area of recent acute infarction, such competition may produce tachycardia or fibrillation.[36, 37]

Since 1980, several types of "physiologic pacemakers" have been developed, made possible by complex circuitry that provides external choice of multiple modes of function with variable values—that is, multiprogrammable capability. Reliable atrial excitation at any desired rate may be provided in patients with sick sinus syndrome. In addition, normal AV sequence may be restored, providing two important physiologic advantages: ventricular responses are allowed by the physiologically varying atrial rates, and the contribution of atrial systole to ventricular filling is restored in patients with AV block and cardiac decompensation.[38]

An important recent development in cardiac pacemakers has been their application to the temporary or long-term termination and prevention of atrial and ventricular tachycardias. Overdrive suppression of serious ventricular arrhythmias was observed in the first experiences with external stimulation in 1952. The efficacy of this principle has been amply confirmed in the long-term prevention of ventricular tachycardia and fibrillation with implanted pacemakers, both in Stokes-Adams disease and also in the absence of AV block.

Interruption and termination of paroxysmal atrial and ventricular tachycardias have also been accomplished by special-purpose pacemakers that may provide a competing rhythm slower than the tachycardia rate (underdrive suppression), short bursts of rapid stimulation, or single beats timed early after the refractory period and at carefully programmed intervals thereafter.[39, 40] The programs are usually designed after electrophysiologic studies of the tachycardias (often after their deliberate provocation) and of the temporal relationships critical for their interruption. The pacemaker may be activated manually (by an external signal provided by the patient) or automatically (by special circuitry with which the pacemaker senses and recognizes the arrhythmia and activates preprogrammed sequences of stimulation until termination is achieved).

Severe, recurrent arrhythmias that are refractory to usual drug and electrical control are also subjected to electrophysiologic evaluation of the effects of varying regimes of antiarrhythmic drugs in preventing their provocation.[41] In some circumstances, electrophysiologic studies are performed during cardiac surgery to enable surgical control of otherwise refractory arrhythmias.[42, 43]

By these varied developments in the field of cardiac pacing, the prevention and treatment of cardiac arrest have been greatly improved, many difficult arrhythmias have been brought under control, and the understanding of disturbances of cardiac rhythmicity and conduction has been extended.

REFERENCES

1. Schechter DC: Origins of electrotherapy. Part I. NY State J Med 71:997, 1971.
2. Schechter DC: Background of clinical cardiac electrostimulation. NY State J Med 71:1114, 2575, 2794, 1971; 72:270, 395, 605, 953, 1166, 1972.
3. Ziemssen H von: Studien über die Bewegungsvorgänge am menschlichen Herzen, sowie über die mechanische und elektrische Erregbarkeit des Herzens und des Nervus phrenicus, angestellt an dem freiliegenden Herzen der Catherine Serafin. Arch Klin Med 30:270, 1882.
4. Duchenne G: De l'Electrisation Localisée et de son Application á la Pathologie et á le Therapeutique. 3rd ed. Paris, JB Baulliere, 1872.
5. Hyman AS: Resuscitation of the stopped heart by intracardial therapy. Arch Intern Med 46:553, 1930.
6. Bigelow WA, Callaghan JC, Hopps JA: General hypothermia for experimental intracardiac surgery. The use of electrophrenic respiration, an artifical pacemaker for cardiac standstill, and radiofrequency rewarming in general hypothermia. Ann Surg 132:531, 1950.
7. Zoll PM: Resuscitation of the heart in ventricular standstill by external electric stimulation. NEJM 247:768, 1952.
8. Zoll PM, Linenthal AJ, Norman LR, et al: External electric stimulation of the heart in cardiac arrest: Stokes-Adams disease, reflex vagal standstill, drug-induced standstill, and unexpected transpositioncirculatory arrest. Arch Intern Med 96:639, 1955.
9. Zoll PM, Linenthal AJ, Gibson W, et al: Intravenous drug therapy of Stokes-Adams disease. Effects of sympathomimetic amines on ventricular rhythmicity and atrioventricular conduction. Circulation 17:325, 1958.
10. Sowton E, Leatham A, and Carson P: Suppression of arrhythmias by artificial pacemaker. Lancet 2:1098, 1964.
11. Beck CS, Pritchard WH, and Feil HS: Ventricular fibrillation of long duration abolished by electric shock. JAMA 135:985, 1947.
12. Zoll PM, Linenthal AJ, Gibson W, et al: Termination of ventricular fibrillation in man by externally applied electric countershock. NEJM 254:727, 1956.
13. Lown B, Amarasingham R, and Neuman J: New method for terminating cardiac arrhythmias. Use of synchronized capacitor discharge. JAMA 182:548, 1962.
14. Zoll PM, Linenthal AJ, Norman LR, et al: Treatment of unexpected cardiac arrest by external electric stimulation of the heart. NEJM 254:541, 1956.
15. Kouwenhoven WB, Jude JR, and Knickerbocker GG: Closed-chest cardiac massage. JAMA 173:1064, 1960.
16. Day HW: An intensive coronary care area. Dis Chest 44:423, 1963.
17. Weirich WL, Paneth M, Gott VL, and Lillehei CW: Control of complete heart block by use of an artificial pacemaker and a myocardial electrode. Cir Res 6:410, 1958.
18. Senning A: Discussion of paper by Stephenson SE Jr, Edwards WH, Jolly PD, and Scott HW Jr. Physiologic P-wave cardiac stimulator. J Thorac Cardiovasc Surg 38:639, 1959.
19. Hunter SW, Roth NA, Bernardez D, and Noble JL: A bipolar myocardial electrode for complete heart block. Lancet 79:506, 1959.

20. Chardack WM, Gage AA, and Greatbatch W: A transistorized, self-contained, implantable pacemaker for the long-term correction of complete heart block. Surgery 48:643, 1960.
21. Kantrowitz A, Cohen R, Raillard H, et al.: The treatment of complete heart block with an implanted controllable pacemaker. Surg Gynecol Obstet 115:415, 1962.
22. Zoll PM, Frank HA, Zarsky LR, et al: Long-term electric stimulation of the heart for Stokes-Adams disease. Ann Surg 154:330, 1961.
23. Furman S, and Schwedel JB: An intracardiac pacemaker for Stokes-Adams seizures. NEJM 261:943, 1959.
24. Smyth MPD, Vasarhelyi, I, McNamara W, and Kakoscik GE: A permanent transvenous atrial electrode catheter. J Thorac Cardiovasc Surg 58:773, 1969.
25. Ott DA, Gillette PC, and Cooley DA: Atrial pacing via the subxiphoid approach. Texas Heart Institute J 9:149, 1982.
26. Zoll PM, Zoll RH, and Belgard AH: External noninvasive electric stimulation of the heart. Critical Care Med 9:393, 1981.
27. Abrams LD, and Williams DO: Experience with the inductively coupled cardiac pacemaker between February 1960 and February 1972. *In* Thalen JJ Th (ed): Cardiac Pacing. Gronigen, VanGorcum and Co., 1973, p. 221.
28. Cammilli L, Pozzi R, Fantini F, and Grassi GR: R. F. impulses transmission: Clinical results and current status. *In* Thalen JJ Th (ed): Cardiac Pacing, Groningen, VanGorcum and Co., 1973, p. 225.
29. Ruben S: Sealed zinc-mercuric oxide cells for implantable cardiac pacemakers. Ann NY Acad Sci 167:627, 1969.
30. Lillehei RC, Romero LH, Beckman CB, et al: New solid-state, long-life, lithium-powered pulse generator. Ann Thorac Surg 18:479, 1974.
31. Laurens P, Alais M, Berger R, et al: Stimulateur cardiaque á énergie nucléaire. Ann Cardiol Angéiol 20:395, 1971.
32. Lewis KB, Criley JM, Nelson RJ, and Love JW: Early clinical experience with the rechargeable cardiac pacemaker. Ann Thorac Surg 18:490, 1974.
33. Roy OZ, and Wehnert R: Keeping the heart alive with a biological battery. Electronics 39:105, 1966.
34. Goetz RH, Dormandy JA, and Berkovitz BV: Pacing on demand in the treatment of atrioventricular conduction disturbances of the heart. Lancet 2:599, 1966.
35. Neville J, Millar K, Keller W, and Abildskov JA: An implantable demand pacemaker. Clin Res 14:256, 1966.
36. Wiggers CJ, and Wégria R: Ventricular fibrillation due to single localized induction and condenser shocks applied during the vulnerable phase of ventricular systole. Am J Physiol 128:500, 1939.
37. Chardack WM: Pacing and ventricular fibrillation. Ann NY Acad Sci 167:919, 1969.
38. Samet P, Costillo C, and Bernstein WH: Hemodynamic consequences of sequential atrio-ventricular pacing. Am J Cardiol 21:207, 1968.
39. Spurrell RAJ, and Sowton E: Pacing techniques in the management of supraventricular tachycardias. J Electrocardiol 8:287, 1975.
40. Fisher JD, Mehra R, and Furman S: Termination of ventricular tachycardia with bursts of rapid ventricular pacing. Am J Cardiol 41:94, 1978.
41. Fisher JD, Cohen HL, Mehra R, et al: Cardiac pacing and pacemakers. II. Serial electrophysiologic-pharmacologic testing for control of recurrent tachyarrhythmias. Am Heart J 93:658, 1977.
42. Josephson ME, Harken AH, and Horowitz LN: Endocardial excision: A new surgical technique for the treatment of recurrent ventricular tachycardia. Circulation 60:1430, 1979.
43. Gallagher JJ, Kasell J, Sealy WC, et al: Epicardial mapping in the Wolff-Parkinson-White Syndrome. Circúlation 57:854, 1978.

2

The Conduction System: Anatomic and Pathologic Correlations

GEORGE LUMB, M.D., M.R.C.P., F.R.C. Path.

THE CONDUCTION SYSTEM

The concept of a conduction system in the heart, as we know it, was not finally established until after its existence was suggested by Tawara in 1906.[1] He described the atrioventricular AV node leading into a bundle (later known as the bundle of His), which divides into left and right branches and finally communicates with the Purkinje fibers, which had been identified previously. Later the suggestion was made that a pacemaker existed in the mammalian heart. This pacemaker was identified as the sinoatrial (SA) node by Keith and Flack in 1907.[2]

Sinoatrial Node

The SA node lies between the superior vena cava and the right atrial appendage, in the sulcus terminalis. It partially consists of a thick portion, which extends from the epicardium to the endocardium and is usually known as the head of the SA node. This structure continues downward, tapering as it goes, forming a body and ending as a fine cord known as the tail, which lies adjacent to the intercaval band.

The SA node is not discernible by gross inspection in the human heart, and it is not possible to dissect it. Histologically, however, it can be identified quite easily if the correct portion of the heart is cut. The easiest way to find the SA node is by dissecting out its blood supply, which will be described in detail later. It consists of a plexiform mass of muscle cells with the fibers arranged longitudinally, with the exception of those that surround the artery to the sinus node. The fibers can be distinguished from the surrounding myocardial fibers of the atrium by their more slender appearance and smaller nuclei. There are very few myofibrils with cross striations, and even those that can be identified are less evident than the cross striations in the surrounding muscle fibers. Another feature is the lack of evidence of intercalated discs. Two types of cells, pale (P) cells and transitional (T) cells, have been described.[3–5]

The cardiac impulse probably arises in the P cells. These cells are the smallest in the heart. They stain poorly with hematoxylin and eosin. This phenomenon is explained by electron microscopic studies, which show the cells to have few mitochondria and a poorly developed sarcoplasmic reticulum. The cells tend to be found together in clusters surrounded by connective tissue. They have few intercellular attachments and contain few desmosomes, in striking contrast to the complex intercalated discs in contracting myocardial cells and Purkinje cells. It is usually accepted that the small number of intercellular connections associated with both P and T cells explains the slow conduction in the SA node.

T cells, which are found in the node in larger numbers than P cells, are intermediate in size and structure, between the P cells and the contracting myocardial cells. It is thought that they serve to organize the distribution of the impulses that originate from the P cells and probably also diminish access to any premature or ectopic atrial impulses.[6]

The fibers of the SA node merge into the surrounding myocardial fibers in the region of the superior vena cava, the interatrial band, and the anterior and posterior crests. This merging takes place by gradual transition from the smaller nodal cells with their indistinct cross striations into the more usual myofibrils of the atrial cells. A similar merging with the normal atrial fibers occurs between the tail of the SA node and the AV node. It is not absolutely certain whether there is a distinct junction between these nodes, but the evidence strongly supports the presence of three internodal tracts known as anterior, middle (Wenckebach), and posterior (Thorel) bundles.[7-9]

The anterior internodal tract arises from the anterior part of the SA node, passes around the anterior margin of the superior vena cava, and merges with the interatrial bundle of Bachmann. This bundle is a large group of muscle fibers connecting the right and left atria.[7-12] The middle internodal tract arises from the superior part of the SA node, passes around the posterior aspect of the superior vena cava, and enters the interatrial septum. It then traverses the middle part of the septum and joins the superior aspect of the AV node. The posterior internodal tract emerges from the posterior part of the SA node, passes posterior to the superior vena cava and down the crista terminalis to the interatrial septum, just above the coronary sinus, and terminates in the posterior part of the AV node. Although describing these tracts in this way makes it sound as though they are easy to dissect and find, this is not the case. It has only been by studying multiple serial sections that the concept of these three tracts has emerged. In normal practice, therefore, all that one finds in sections between the SA and AV nodes are groups of cells that are large and elongated and usually pale staining, thus resembling Purkinje cells.

Nerve fibers can be seen in the head of the node, but nerve cells can only be found around the periphery. With increasing age elastic tissue in the SA node is present in larger quantities, and the reticulin fibers increase in thickness and in number. Evidently some of the muscle fibers are lost, and there is usually infiltration of fat into both the node and the surrounding tissues.

Atrioventricular Node

The AV node lies in the floor of the right atrium, between the orifice of the coronary sinus and the medial leaflet of the tricuspid valve. There is almost invariably a pad of fat lying over it, and it is immediately adjacent to the central fibrous body and the base of the atrial septum. Once its position has been identified by cutting appropriate sections through this area, careful dissection can quite frequently render the node visible on gross examination. It is paler than the surrounding myocardium in most cases and is continuous with the so-called AV bundle, or bundle of His. It penetrates the central fibrous body and then lies in the lower part of the membranous septum (pars membranacea). A number of portions of the left bundle branch are then formed, and they continue to proliferate from the main bundle of His until it forms the right bundle branch and the remaining fibers of the left bundle branch.

The right branch is usually distinct and passes along the lower margin of the crista supraventricularis. It divides into three parts. Two of these are subendocardial, with the third penetrating directly into the myocardium. These branches become continuous with the network of Purkinje cells on the inferior and anterior walls of the lower part of the interventricular septum. The left bundle branch, passing down the interventricular septum on the left side, radiates into a number of fine branches, and these also merge with Purkinje fibers throughout the subendocardial region in the distal half of the septum. These groups of Purkinje cells usually terminate on the anterior and posterior papillary muscles.

Histologically, the node, the bundle, and the branches can be recognized quite easily unless they have been destroyed by pathologic processes. They consist of a network of muscle fibers that are smaller than atrial or ventricular fibers. In contrast with the fibers seen in the SA nodes, striations can readily be seen, and intercalated discs can also be identified. The node is very cellular and mixed with paler cells resembling endothelial cells, and these interlace with the muscle cells. As in the case of the SA node, the number of elastic fibers is greater than in the surrounding myocardium, and the reticular fibers are more delicate. As the fibers enter the bundle and its branches, they tend to be arranged in longitudinal fasciculi.

The appearance of the fibers of the left and right bundle branches when they first arise is essentially similar to that of the bundle itself, but as the branches proceed, the cells become larger and paler. They have relatively few myofibrils, and the nuclei are quite round. They merge into the appearance of Purkinje cells, and it is sometimes believed that these terminal cells in the bundle branches are of the same nature and should be called Purkinje cells. Purkinje fibers and accumulations of Purkinje cells merge into the cells of the left and right ventricles so as to become indistinguishable from them. There are still differences of opinion as to whether any Purkinje fibers are present in the myocardium.

As in the case of the SA node, nerve cells can be found in the immediate vicinity of the AV node, but they are not found within it or in the bundle or bundle branches. Nerve fibers, however, can be found in the node and usually in the proximal part of the bundle of His, but very few can be identified in the bundle branches.

Blood Supply

It is generally accepted that the SA node is supplied in approximately 60 per cent of human hearts from the first branch of the right main coronary artery (ramus ostii cavae superioris). In the remaining human hearts (approximately 40 per cent) this vessel arises from the left circumflex coronary artery and winds around the base of the heart to reach the same position as the more usual first branch of the right coronary artery. In either case, the vessel proceeds, as described previously in this discussion, directly into the SA node. By dissecting the artery, the position of the node can be identified. Sections then prepared from this area will show the vessel lying in the middle of the fibers.

The AV node, the bundle of His, and the bundle branches are supplied by the blood to the upper part of the interventricular septum. Dissection and perfusion experiments in human subjects showed that two principal arteries supply blood to the upper part of the interventricular septum in the region of the AV node and bundle of His.[13] One is a posterior vessel (the posterior septal artery or ramus septi fibrosi).[14–16] The other is an anterior vessel (the anterior septal artery or first anterior perforating vessel). In 93 per cent of 327 human heart dissections the posterior vessel arose from the terminal part of the right coronary artery just before, at, or after formation of the posterior descending artery. It passed anteriorly, to the left and inferior to the termination of the coronary sinus, lying on a flat plateau formed by the upper surface of the muscular interventricular septum. It continued anteriorly beneath the muscle of the floor of the right atrium, gave branches to the wall of the left and right atrium, and ended in capillaries near the root of the aorta. It passed inferior to the AV node and closely followed the course of the bundle of His. It was from this vessel that the blood supply to the AV node and bundle originated. Along its course it gave off arterial twigs, which passed through the annulus fibrosus to end in the upper portion of the interventricular septum. A branch to the upper part of the right ventricular wall frequently arose from the posterior septal artery and anastomosed with the first lateral division of the posterior descending artery. Blood supply to the first part of both bundle branches and the posterior radiations of the left bundle branch comes from these terminal branches.

Spalteholz[17] reported similar observations, demonstrating that in 85 to 97 percent of adult human hearts the posterior descending artery (ramus sulci longitudinalis posterioris) and the posterior septal artery (ramus septi fibrosi) arose from the terminal part of the right coronary artery. In 80 percent of cases the right coronary and left circumflex arteries terminated just to the left of the midline posteriorly; the right coronary artery was the significantly larger vessel in its distal part. In 5 to 17 percent of cases the right coronary artery continued all the way to the left lateral border of the heart, where the left circumflex also terminated. In 10 percent the reverse was true, and the left circumflex artery continued to the right lateral border, where the right coronary artery terminated. In our series 7 percent of cases were in this last group, and in these the posterior septal artery arose from the left circumflex artery.[13]

The origin and course of the anterior septal artery (first anterior perforating branch of the left anterior descending artery) were remarkably constant. It arose from the posterior surface of the anterior descending branch of the left coronary artery at approximately 4 cm from the origin of the left coronary artery from the aorta. It pursued a course across the posterior wall of the infundibulum of the right ventricle 4 to 5 mm deep to the endocardium. In the interventricular septum it divided into an inferior branch, which supplied branches to the upper two-thirds of the septum and to the papillary muscle, which is usually regarded as the equivalent of the moderator band in lower animals,[1] and a superior branch, which ended in capillaries near the aortic root. In human subjects, the anterior septal artery was the uppermost anterior branch to the interventricular septum and was always significantly larger than the vessels immediately inferior to it.

This anterior septal artery, together with the second perforating branch, provides blood supply to the terminal part of the bundle of His and the midpart of the right and the anterior radiations of the left bundle branches.

METHODS FOR OBTAINING MATERIAL FOR EXAMINATION

Sinoatrial Node

The SA node lies in the sulcus terminalis between the superior vena cava and the right atrial appendage. The best way to obtain material from this structure, which cannot be visualized, is to dissect the artery that supplies it. (This procedure has already been described in this discussion.) It arises either as the first branch from the right coronary artery or as a branch from the left circumflex. This vessel should be dissected up to the point where it reaches the sulcus terminalis, and then the piece of tissue between the superior vena cava and the atrium and adjacent material to this should be removed and sectioned. The blocks should be made so that the artery, as far as possible, is lying in the central part, as this will inevitably pass through the SA node.

Atrioventricular Node

With both atria and ventricles opened, a vertical cut should be made through the interventricular septum at the opening of the coronary sinus into the right atrium.[18] This forms the posterior extent of the area to be examined. The anterior boundary is made with a cut parallel to the former through the anterior limit of the membranous septum. The upper margin of the block should include the lower part of the interatrial septum and pass through the root of the aorta. The lower margin should be parallel to this and include the upper third of the interventricular septum (Fig. 2–1). The medial cusp of the right tricuspid valve will then be on the right side, and portions of the noncoronary cusp of the aortic valve and the aortic cusp of the mitral valve will be included on the left side. The tissue so removed includes the AV node, the bundle of His, and the upper portions of the right and left bundle branches. According to its size it can then be subdivided into varying numbers of blocks. Four are normally taken from an average size heart. Hypertrophic hearts sometimes require more sectioning than this, and the material from children can usually be divided adequately into three blocks. The histologic sections produced from these blocks appear as seen in Figures 2–2 to 2–5. The most posterior sections show the AV node usually lying under fat and against the underlying annulus fibrosus. Proceeding forward the bundle can be visualized, and the most anterior blocks show the division into the right and left bundle branches.

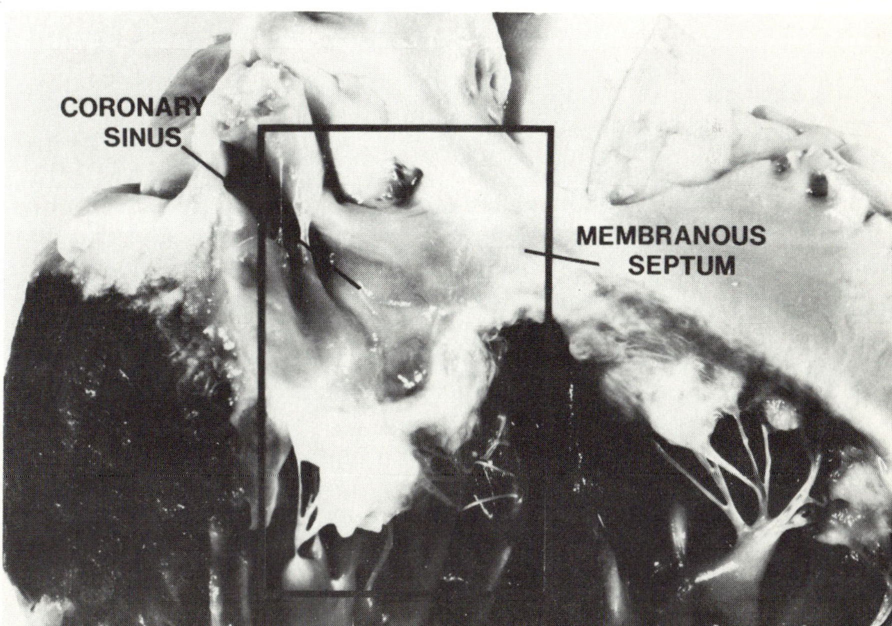

Figure 2–1. A heart opened from the right side. The rectangular block indicates the area that is removed in order to examine the AV node, the bundle of His, and the proximal parts of the bundle branches.

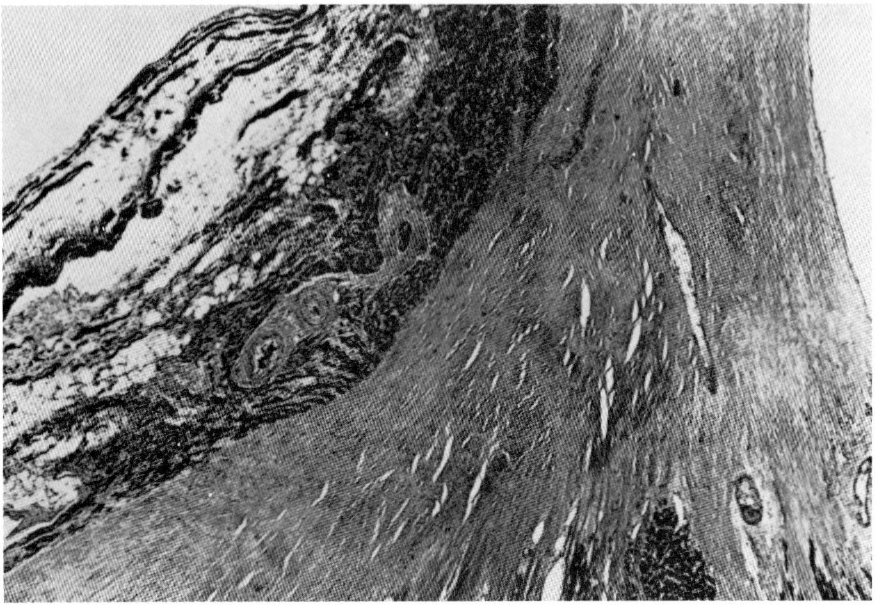

Figure 2–2. Anterior view of the posterior segment of the interventricular septum, showing the commencement of the bundle of His above the annulus fibrosus and to the right. ×21.

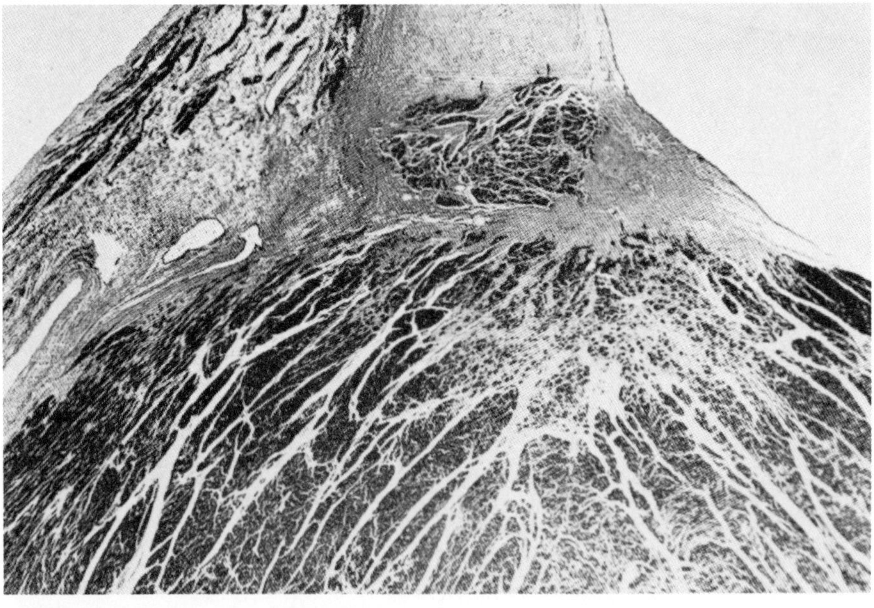

Figure 2–3. Anterior view of the posterocentral segment of the interventricular septum, showing the bundle of His in the annulus fibrosus. ×21.

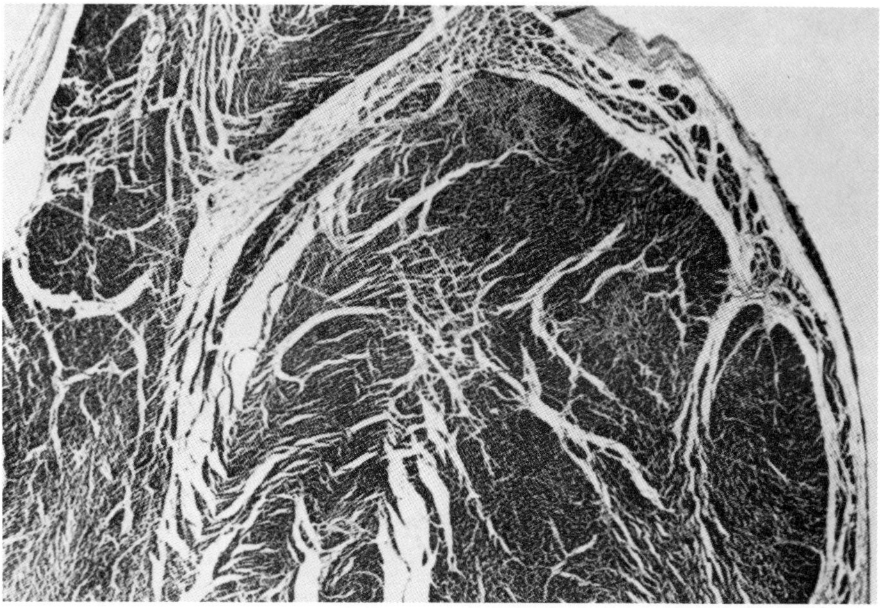

Figure 2–4. Anterior view of the anterocentral segment of the interventricular septum, showing the bundle of His dividing into right and left bundle branches below the annulus fibrosus and to the left. ×21.

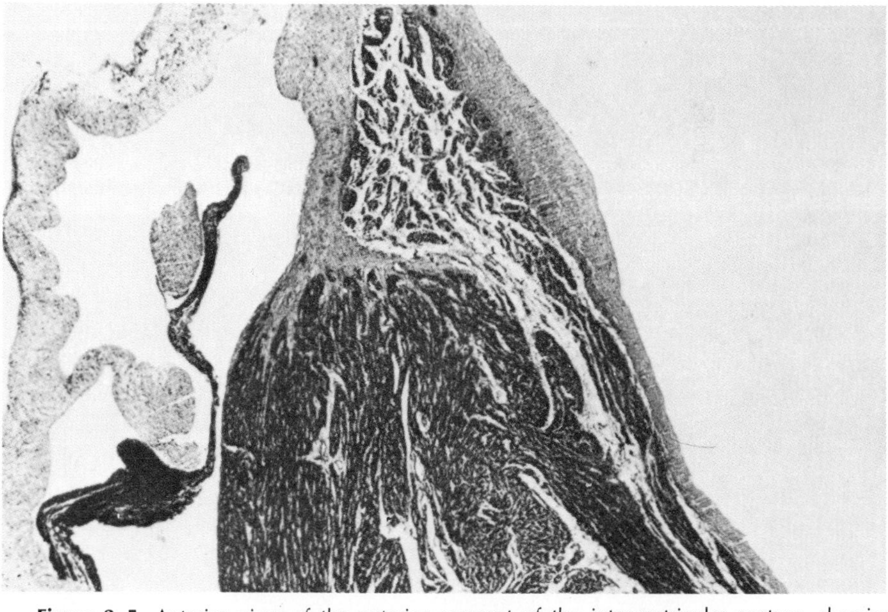

Figure 2–5. Anterior view of the anterior segment of the interventricular septum, showing termination of the bundle of His in the left bundle branch below the annulus fibrosus and to the left. ×21.

It is difficult to make practical suggestions as to how many sections should be cut when examining the conduction system. It is obvious that if a serious attempt is to be made to correlate pathologic appearance with EKG changes, then serial sections are necessary. This is not a reasonable approach for routine examinations. We have found that if two or three levels are examined from the blocks described above, considerable useful information is revealed.

PATHOLOGIC CHANGES

Any disease process or congenital abnormality that affects the heart may involve the conduction tissue.

Congenital Disorders

Congenital disorders may result in changes or abnormalities of position, interference with continuity, or augmentation of accessory communications in order to supplement or provide alternate pathways for normal structures.

The congenital lesions vary so greatly that individual cases present many diverse features, and each must be considered as a separate entity. It is very difficult to define any general principles. Even a condition as frequent as tetralogy of Fallot may have many variations in the positioning of the various components of the conduction system. No detailed discussion will be attempted here therefore. The importance of an awareness of the problems for a cardiac surgeon is obvious.

Disease Processes Associated with Conduction Tissue Damage

Frequent Occurrence

The conditions that are most likely to present a problem in causing pathologic changes in the conduction system are hypertensive and atherosclerotic heart disease with or without overt infarcts, including the general aging process involving calcific changes and degenerative changes around the base of the heart.

As has been described, the right coronary artery and its branches provide the blood supply, in the majority of cases, for the SA and AV nodes, the bundle of His, and the first portions of both bundle branches, including the posterior radiations of the left bundle branch. The anterior descending branch of the left coronary artery through its first (anterior septal) and penetrating branches supplies the midportion of the right bundle branch and the anterior radiations of the left bundle branch. Probably some blood reaches the distal part of the bundle in most cases.

Because of this arrangement, it is clear that AV block will occur much more frequently as a result of posterior infarcts, and because these are much less common than anterior infarcts the condition is infrequent. AV block, when it does occur as a result of infarction, frequently recovers after a few days, presumably as a result of collateralization. Complete AV block can occur as a result of coronary ischemia or may be associated with lesions of the AV bundle. More frequently, however, it is preceded by bundle branch block, and in these cases lesions are found at the origin of the branches and at the bifurcation.

Lev[19] has described a condition of "sclerosis of the left side of the cardiac skeleton" to account for cases of chronic AV or right and left bundle branch block when no vessel obstruction can be demonstrated. In these patients, who are usually in the sixth or seventh decade of life, extreme fibrosis and calcification are found. Lev believes that the pull of the left ventricle and the aortic and mitral valves, particularly in hypertrophic or hypertensive hearts, can lead to damage and disruption of the conduction tissues.

Less Frequent Occurrence

With the increasing number of open-heart surgical procedures, there has been a great advance in accuracy. It is therefore very unusual nowadays to see surgical injury involving the conduction system. It is obvious that the SA node and related structures are at risk when the right atrium is being opened or otherwise manipulated. The AV node could be involved in sutures, and more particularly the bundle branches may be involved in repair processes or interferences with the interventricular septum.

Occasionally, inflammatory disorders, including acute viral infections and rheumatic heart disease, may involve the system. Rare instances of traumatic injury[20] to the pericardium,[21] hemochromatosis,[22, 23] myxedema,[24] lead poisoning,[25] and myotonia dystrophica[26] involving the system have been cited.

Neoplasms are relatively unimportant in discussions of the conduction tissue. Primary tumors have not been described; therefore, only tumors that might compress or infringe upon various parts of the conduction system present any problem. Any tumors in the heart are quite uncommon; therefore this is not an area of great importance.

In an attempt to put these matters into some sort of perspective we examined a series of 260 human hearts obtained from necropsies randomly performed on all age groups. They included 176 males and 84 females. Seventy were white and 190 were black patients. Thirty-five specimens showed lesions that were considered to have affected the conduction tissue to a significant degree. No cases of congenital cardiac defects were included.[27] The cases are discussed in the remainder of the chapter.

Calcification and Fibrosis (12 Cases)

Calcification. There were seven specimens. All of these patients were old, and all except one had significant ventricular hypertrophy. Diastolic blood pressure was at hypertensive levels in only two patients. Four of the patients showed clinical evidence of cerebrovascular accidents, and an additional one had been admitted to a mental hospital with a diagnosis of senile psychosis. Four patients had a history of dizziness and falling, and consequently three of these had sustained hip fractures. Although examination of the brain in all of these patients revealed a moderate degree of cerebral atherosclerosis, there was no evidence of hemorrhage, thrombosis, or infarction except in one, in whom a small infarct was found in the external capsule. Varying degrees of congestive cardiac failure were exhibited by all the patients in this group. Three died suddenly, and all had brief terminal episodes. In four, significant calcification of the aortic valves was noted grossly at necropsy. EKGs were available on six patients. All showed bundle branch block, and four had AV dissociation.

Microscopic examination of the interventricular septum in the four cases with AV dissociation showed extensive deposits of calcium in the septum membranaceum, annulus fibrosus, and upper part of the muscular septum, with direct involvement of the conduction tissue in all blocks examined (Fig. 2–6). The two cases with only bundle branch block showed smaller deposits of calcium in this region, predominantly affecting the conduction tissue in the more anterior blocks. Examination of the remainder of the hearts revealed only a mild degree of coronary artery atherosclerosis. It is difficult to explain the calcium deposition, therefore, entirely on the basis of ischemia.

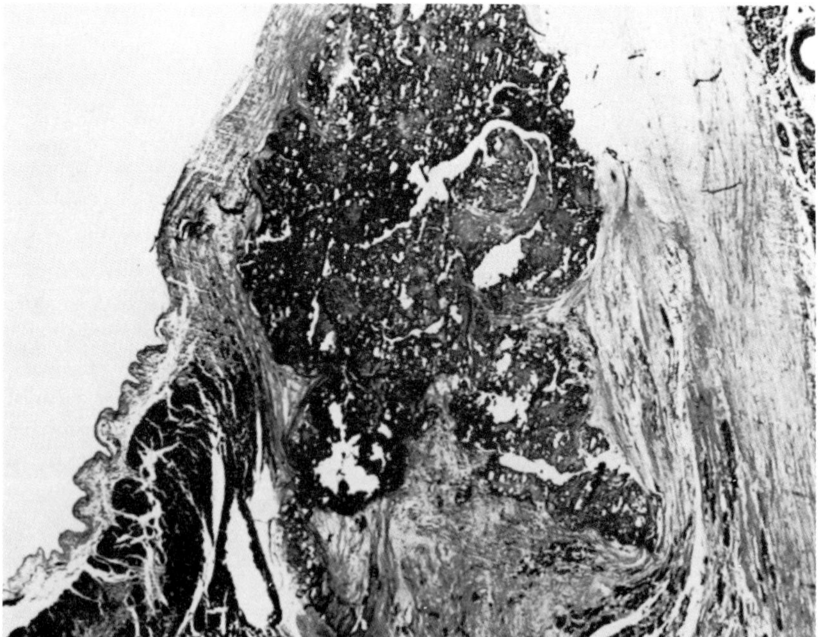

Figure 2–6. Massive calcification of the upper part of the interventricular septum, with destruction of the conduction tissue. ×21.

Fibrosis. Considerable care was exercised in selecting the five cases in this group. A large number of hearts, particularly from elderly patients, showed varying amounts of scattered fibrous tissue in the interventricular septum[28]—a finding that might have been related to degenerative changes in the conduction tissue. Occasionally, small flecks of calcium were mingled with the fibrous tissue.[29] The cases described here were those in which fibrosis was excessive, in which it was largely confined to the upper part of the muscular interventricular septum and the septum membranaceum, and in which the conduction tissue appeared to be unequivocally damaged.

In all of these cases the manner of death was abrupt. One patient had a cerebrovascular accident; the conduction tissue defect and EKG abnormality were considered coincidental. In three there was terminal acute coronary occlusion, and the conduction tissue damage was considered a factor that probably contributed to death. The fifth patient developed sudden cardiac arrest and died during a prostatectomy. In the absence of any other significant alteration at necropsy, the conduction tissue damage was considered to be a major factor in causing the death of this individual, and calcification was the major finding.

In contradistinction to the cases in which calcification was the major finding, the pathologic lesions in this group were characterized by widespread atherosclerosis, including coronary atherosclerosis. It is considered that the extensive septal fibrosis and degeneration and fibrous replacement of portions of the conduction tissue represented the results of ischemia. Two patients had AV block or dissociation, and they showed greater conduction tissue replacement posteriorly, involving the region of the main bundle and the AV node. On the other hand, the major damage in three cases that had left bundle branch block occurred anteriorly, principally in the distal part of the bundle of His and the origins of the bundle branches.

These cases of calcification and fibrosis were reviewed, particularly in the light of the observations regarding so-called sclerosis of the left side of the cardiac skeleton. In our series the cases in which calcification was the predominant feature seemed to fit the concept of sclerosis of the left side of the cardiac skeleton suggested by Lev.[19] The cases in which calcification was not predominant and fibrosis prevailed seemed to be examples of ischemia with coronary artery narrowing.

Myocardial Infarct (5 Cases)

In all five cases, diffuse generalized coronary atherosclerosis was present, but there was no demonstrable complete occlusion of any artery. Infarcts were found in all instances, however. In each there was good correlation between EKG findings and histologic alterations. One patient died in the terminal stages of bronchogenic carcinoma, but a healing posterior infarct was demonstrated. Evidence of this had been noted in EKGs. The lesion affected the upper part of the posterior wall of the heart and the posterior portion of the interventricular septum. Damage led to partial destruction of the AV node and the proximal part of the bundle of His. Two patients died within a few hours of admission, and one patient was dead on arrival. In all three of these patients there were recent

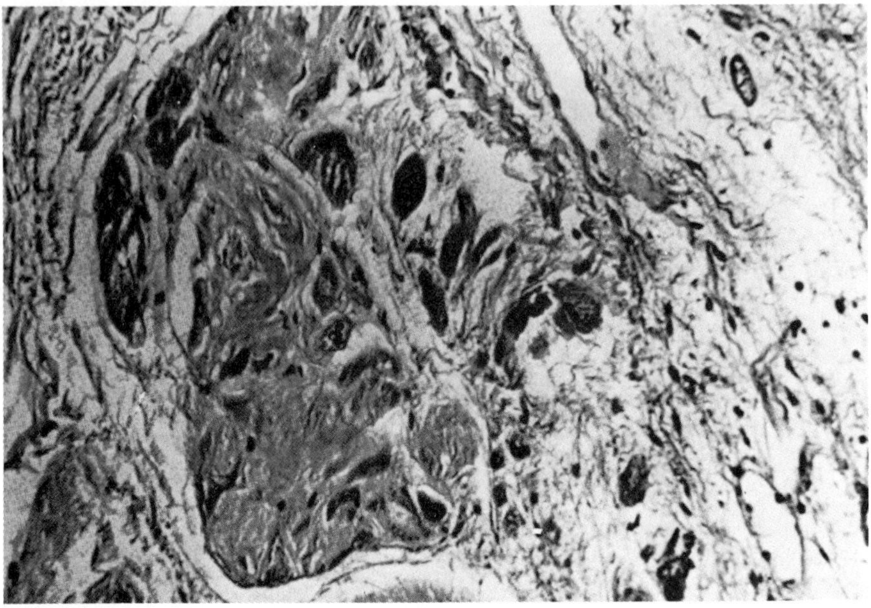

Figure 2–7. A recent infarct causing partial destruction of the left bundle branch as it lies under the endocardium. ×280.

infarcts confined to the upper part of the septum, affecting principally its anterior portion. There was destruction of the distal part of the bundle of His and the origin of the bundle branches (Fig. 2–7).

Hemorrhage (5 Cases)

There were five cases in this group, and they all showed hemorrhage into the conduction tissue and destruction of fibers. In one case this was associated with a dissecting aneurysm of the ascending aorta; the patient survived three days after the initial attack and then collapsed suddenly and died. EKG evidence of right bundle branch block had been present beforehand, but at necropsy a recent hemorrhage had destroyed the AV node and main bundle in addition to the origin of the bundle branches. In two cases there was cerebral hemorrhage. In both, also, subendocardial bleeding affected the distal part of the bundle of His and the commencement of the left bundle branch. One case was characterized by subendocardial hemorrhage and destruction of the terminal part of the bundle of His and the origin of the left bundle branch. The lesion was presumably traumatic in origin; the patient had chloral hydrate poisoning and unsuccessful cardiac massage. One case was a 75-year-old white woman who had sustained a fractured femur after a fall. She had apparently improved until three days after the bone was pinned, when a sudden drop in blood pressure occurred and she died immediately. No significant cause of death could be found other than a recent hemorrhage localized to the upper part of the interventricular septum, with destruction of the AV node and the proximal part of the bundle of His (Fig. 2–8). The cause of this hemorrhage remains undetermined, although the possi-

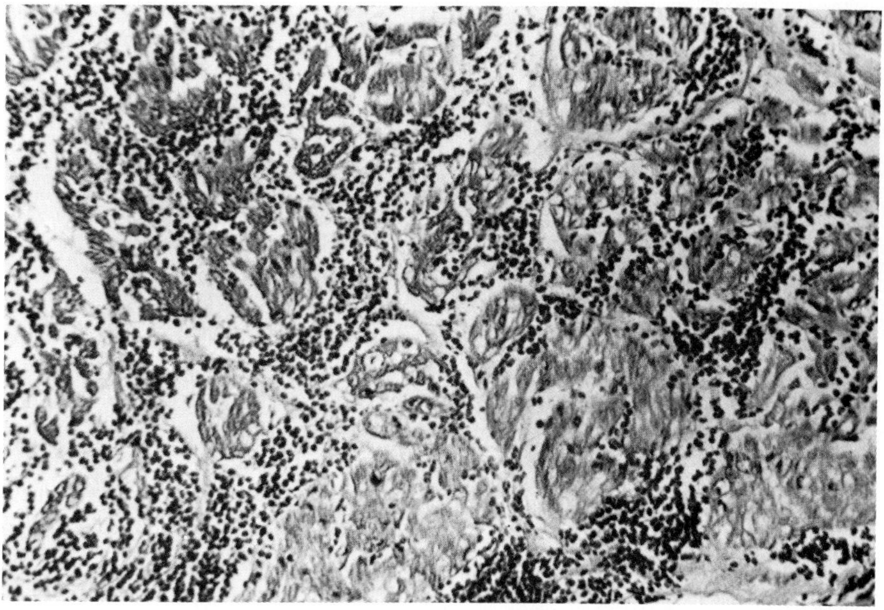

Figure 2–8. Hemorrhage into the bundle of His. ×280.

bility of fat embolization causing rupture of small vessels might be considered. It seems reasonable, however, to regard the hemorrhage as the mechanism of death in this case.

Myocarditis (4 Cases)

Three of these cases were young children, whose hearts displayed a typical diffuse myocardial round cell infiltration probably of viral origin. It was of interest to note that the cellular infiltration was more intense in the upper part of the interventricular septum than in other areas of the heart. In each instance diffuse involvement of the AV node area, bundle of His, and origin of the bundle branches was found. Interstitial pneumonia of very mild degree was thought to be present in two cases, but no pulmonary lesions could be found in the others. All of the children died suddenly. One patient survived 4 hours after admission, and EKGs showed very irregular complexes, which were difficult to interpret, but AV dissociation was considered probable. Two patients were dead on arrival at the hospital. It seems reasonable to suppose that interference with conduction may have played a major role in causing death.

The fourth case was of particular interest because the patient walked into the hospital complaining only of mild dyspnea and some chest pain. He had not been examined before. He was sent to the ward, and while a clinical history was being taken, he sat up, coughed, and died immediately. At necropsy there was rheumatic pancarditis with mild fibrinous pericarditis and early endocarditis with small vegetations on the mitral valves but no apparent valvular stenosis or incompetence. A diffuse myocarditis was most marked in the interventricular septum. Vasculitis was marked in the AV node region and typical Aschoff's bodies were found, directly involving the AV node, bundle of His, and left bundle branch.

Miscellaneous (9 Cases)

Amyloidosis. These were two patients who died suddenly. One died 4 hours after admission to the hospital, and the other was dead on arrival. The only significant findings at autopsy were large masses of amyloid, which were confirmed by special stains and identified as primary amyloidosis in the heart (Fig. 2–9). In both cases there was complete replacement of many portions of the bundle of His and partial destruction of the AV node. Elsewhere in the heart there was typical generalized distribution of amyloid, with particular involvement of the right atrial wall. It seemed in these two cases that the cause of death was related to the amyloid destruction of the conduction system.

Endocardial Fibroelastosis. There were four patients showing this disease, each with extensive involvement of the left bundle branch. One patient was somewhat older than usual but presented an atypical history and clinical course. The others were typical examples. Although the cause of death could not be attributed to the involvement of the bundle branch, the correlation with the EKG findings was good in two of the three cases, for whom EKGs were available. Although there was considerable damage to the left bundle branch in the third, left bundle branch block was not, at any time, shown in the EKGs.

Abscesses. Three patients developed acute bacterial endocarditis following surgical operations, and in each case abscesses were found involving the bundle

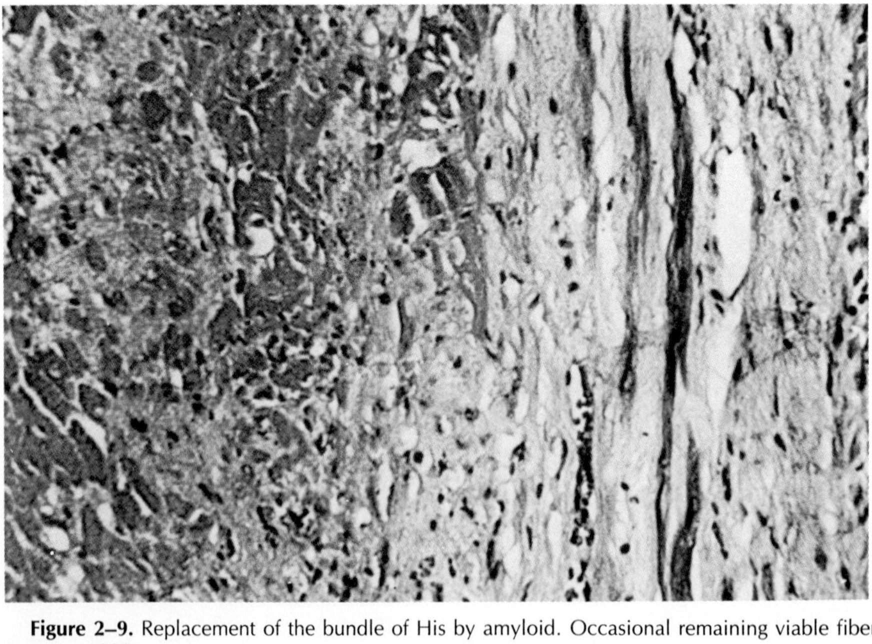

Figure 2–9. Replacement of the bundle of His by amyloid. Occasional remaining viable fibers are seen. ×280.

of His and the origin of the bundle branches. This involvement was not considered to be the cause of death in these cases, although correlation with EKG findings was good.

Summary

The 35 cases discussed here were selected on the basis of significant involvement of the conduction system in a random selection from autopsy material. When the cases were reviewed in terms of mechanism of death and correlation with EKG findings, the following conclusions were drawn:

Twenty-five of the cases had died suddenly, including 5 who were dead on arrival at the hospital. Sudden death is defined as exitus within 5 to 6 hours of arrival at the hospital or death occurring abruptly or unexpectedly when in the hospital. In 13 of these 25 cases there were pathologic processes other than those in the conduction tissue that might have led to sudden death. It was therefore impossible to assess the significance, if any, of the conduction tissue abnormalities in the final phase. The remaining 12 cases, however, showed considerable evidence that the conduction tissue lesion was the precipitating factor in the sudden death. Three were examples of massive myocardial calcification; 3 were examples of massive myocarditis; 2 were cases of primary cardiac amyloidosis; 1 showed an unexplained hemorrhage in the AV node and the bundle of His; 1 showed a recent infarct confined to the upper part of the interventricular septum involving the conduction mechanism; 1 developed cardiac arrest during an operation, and the fibrotic lesion in the conduction tissue was the only apparent cause of death; and 1 (the twelfth) case showed Aschoff's bodies with destruction of the bundle of His, which seemed to be the major cause of death.

Twenty-six of the 35 cases had EKGs available for investigation. Nineteen showed either bundle branch block or some degree of AV dissociation, and evidence of correlation between the EKGs and the morphologic alterations was good.

It was our conclusion, therefore, that there are advantages in making a reasonably complete examination of the conduction tissue a routine part of the examination of the heart at autopsy. An accurate correlation with EKG findings can be achieved in most cases. In a significant number of cases it becomes possible to determine more precisely the mechanism of death.

REFERENCES

1. Tawara S: Das Reizleitungssystem des Säugetierherzens. Eine anatomischhistologische Studie über das Atrioventrikularbündel und die purkinjeschen Fäden. Jena, G. Fischer. 1906, 200 pp.
2. Keith A, and Flack MW: The form and nature of the muscular connections between the primary divisions of the vertebrate heart. J Anat Physiol 41:172, 1907.
3. Truex RC: The sinoatrial node and its connections with atrial tissues. *In* Wellens HJJ, Lie KI, and Janse MJ (eds): The Conduction System of the Heart: Structure, Function, and Clinical Implications. Philadelphia, Lea and Febiger, 1976, p. 209.

4. James TN, Sherf L, Fine G, and Morales AR: Comparative ultrastructure of the sinus node in man and dog. Circulation 34:139, 1966.
5. Tranum-Jensen J: The fine structure of the atrial and atrioventricular (AV) junctional specialized tissues of the rabbit heart. *In* Wellens HJJ, Lie KI, and Janse MJ (eds): The Conduction System of the Heart: Structure, Function, and Clinical Implications. Philadelphia, Lea and Febiger, 1976, p. 55.
6. Strauss HC, and Bigger JT Jr: Electrophysiological properties of the rabbit sinoatrial perinodal fibers. Circ Res 31:490, 1972.
7. Robb JS, and Petri R: Expansions of the atrioventricular system in the atria. *In* Paes de Carvalho A, deMello WC, and Hoffman FB (eds): The Specialized Tissues of the Heart. New York, Elsevier, 1961, p. 1.
8. James TN: The connecting pathways between the sinus node and the A-V node and between the right and left atrium in the human heart. Circulation 53:609, 1963.
9. James TN, and Sherf L.: Specialized tissues and preferential conduction in the atria of the heart. Am J Cardiol 28:414, 1971.
10. de Mello WC, and Hoffman BF: Potassium ions and electrical activity of specialized cardiac fibers. Am J Physiol 199:1125, 1960.
11. Vassalle M, Greenspan K, Jomain S, and Hoffman BF: Effects of potassium on automaticity and conduction of canine hearts. Am J Physiol 207:334, 1964.
12. Bachmann G: The inter-auricular time interval. Am J Physiol 41:309, 1916.
13. Lumb G, and Singletary H: Blood supply to the atrioventricular node and bundle of His: A comparative study in pig, dog, and man. Am J Pathol 41:65, 1962.
14. Gross L: The Blood Supply to the Heart. New York, Paul B Hoeber Inc, 1921, p. 48.
15. Mahaim I: Nouvelles recherchés sur le lésions du faisceau de His-Tawara; le bloc de branche gauche et sa pathogénie; la septite mitrale. Ann Med, 38:185, 1935.
16. Lascano EF: Irrigacion normal del nodulo de Tawara, haz de His y sus ramas. Rev Argent de Cardiol 10:23, 1943.
17. Spalteholz KW: Die Arterien der Herzwand; anatomische Untersuchungen an Menschen- und Tierherzen, nebst Erorterund der Voraussetzunger für die Herstellung eines Kollateralkreislaufes. Leipzig, S Hirzel, 165 pp. 1924.
18. Lumb G, Hardy L: Technique for dissection and perfusion of heart. Arch Path 77:233, 1964.
19. Lev M: Anatomic basis for atrioventricular block (symposium on cardiac arrhythmias), Am J Med 37:742, 1964.
20. Rosenthal SR: Branch arborization and complete heart block. Arch Intern Med 50:730, 1932.
21. Coffen TH: Complete heart-block of seven years' duration in a child resulting from an injury. Am Heart J 5:667, 1930.
22. Petit DW: Hemochromatosis with complete heart block with a discussion of the cardiac complications. Am Heart J 29:253, 1945.
23. James TN: Pathology of the cardiac conduction system in hemochromatosis. NEJM 271:92, 1964.
24. Lee JK, and Lewis JA: Myxoedema with complete A-V block and Adams-Stokes disease abolished with thyroid medication. Br Heart J 24:253, 1962.
25. Myerson RM, and Eisenhauer JH: Atrioventricular conduction defects in lead poisoning. Am J Cardiol 11:409, 1963.
26. Soffer A: Delayed conduction in dystrophica myotonia. Dis Chest 40:594, 1961.
27. Lumb G, and Shacklett RS: Human cardiac conduction tissue lesions. Am J Pathol 36:411, 1960.
28. Erickson EE, and Lev M: Aging changes in the human atrioventricular node, bundle, and bundle branches. J Gerontol 7:1, 1952.
29. Yater WM, and Cornell VH: Heart block due to calcareous lesions of the bundle of His. Review and report of a case with detailed histopathologic study. Ann Intern Med 8:777, 1934–1935.

3

Electrophysiology of Pacing

ALLAN M. GREENSPAN, M.D.

A thorough understanding of the complexities of artificial pacing systems requires an appreciation of certain aspects of cellular electrophysiology and electrical circuitry. This chapter will examine both basic electrophysiologic and electrical engineering considerations in artificial pacing and will highlight the clinical implications of their application to the pacing and sensing functions of modern pacemaker systems.

BASIC ELECTROPHYSIOLOGIC CONSIDERATIONS

Excitability

Excitability may be defined as the ability of nerve and muscle tissue to respond to stimulation by developing a propagated electrical wave front;[1] the more excitable a tissue, the less intense the stimulus necessary to induce the response. A number of factors have been found to be required for the generation of a propagated electrical response in excitable tissue: (1) reduction of the resting membrane potential to threshold level, where the active membrane properties are brought into play,[2] (2) generation of a normal local regenerative response by the active membrane properties (local action potential),[3] and (3) conduction of the local regenerative response to adjacent tissue (local action potential induces sequential depolarization of the adjacent resting membrane).[4] The factors that affect excitability are the factors that influence the foregoing chain of events and include (1) the level of threshold potential—primarily the voltage dependence of resting ionic permeabilities,[5] (2) the amount and rate of charge transfer required to discharge the membrane capacitance to threshold,[6] which is dependent on passive electrical properties of the resting membrane (i.e., the membrane resistance and capacitance, the extracellular series resistance, the intramyoplasmic axial resistance),[7] (3) the configuration of the local regenerative response (i.e., the action potential upstroke velocity, and overshoot amplitude), which is dependent on the active membrane properties, and (4) tissue-membrane conduction characteristics related to the passive membrane cable properties (i.e., membrane resistance, extracellular resistance, intramyoplasmic axial resistance, membrane capacitance, cell-to-cell coupling).[8] Thus a number of factors affect excitability at a cellular level and make detailed quantification of excitability difficult.

The ideal measurement of excitability would include a complete description of the minimum electrical energy required to evoke a typical propagated response and its rate of delivery. In practical terms, measurement of threshold electrical characteristics, particularly threshold current, has become the basic standard for determining excitability. However, this gives an incomplete description of tissue excitability, and thus additional boundary conditions that affect excitability must simultaneously be defined.

Threshold Current

Threshold voltage is the membrane potential at which a series of changes in the membrane's ionic permeabilities occur, producing a regenerative electrical response (i.e., the action potential). The simplified equivalent circuit of the membrane is given by a resistance and capacitance in parallel with a variable voltage source at resting potential level (Fig. 3–1). The key factor in raising the membrane potential to threshold level is the transfer of adequate charge per unit time to the membrane capacitor to discharge it toward threshold. The current amplitude required to do so would be expected to vary with the duration of current flow, since total charge transferred is equal to current amplitude times pulse duration. Thus, threshold current amplitude (I_{th}) alone is an incomplete measurement of excitability and must be reported in association with the current pulse width. This can be more fully quantified as the strength-duration curve (Fig. 3–2), which shows that increased stimulus duration is associated with a decrease in threshold current amplitude.

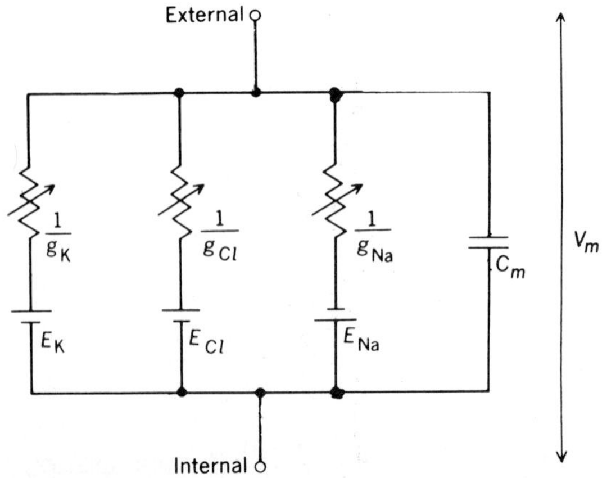

Figure 3–1. Equivalent circuit (RC circuit) of the membrane. The myocardial membrane can be modeled electrically as the parallel combination of the membrane capacitance (C) and three or more ionic conductances (g), each in series with a battery. The battery voltage for each ion is its equilibrium potential. (Reproduced from Katz B: Nerve, Muscle, Synapse. New York, McGraw Hill, 1966.)

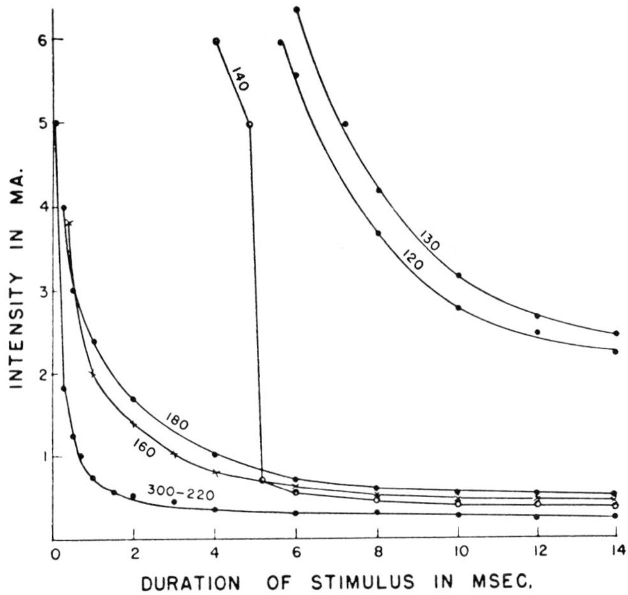

Figure 3–2. Strength-duration curve. Current amplitude or intensity for threshold stimulus duration is shown by the family of curves generated in canine myocardium. Stimulus intensity (in milliamperes) is plotted on the ordinate, and stimulus duration or pulse width (in milliseconds) is plotted on the abscissa. (Reprinted from Orias et al: Am J Physiol 163:272, 1950.)

Two other factors that influence threshold current are the size and position of the stimulating electrodes. The percentage of the applied current that actually traverses the membrane, or the effective stimulus current, varies inversely with electrode size and directly with the proximity of the electrodes to the tissue.[1] Electrodes with a smaller surface area, more closely applied, minimize shunting of the applied current through the extracellular space. In addition, by distributing the same current over a smaller membrane surface area, smaller electrodes transfer more charge per unit time per unit of cross-sectional area to discharge the membrane capacitor, and therefore less current is required to generate a propagated response. Current threshold is linearly and directly related to electrode surface area, but current density threshold is essentially independent of electrode surface area (i.e., is constant throughout a wide range of electrode surface area) (Fig. 3–3). Thus an electrode with a smaller surface area can maintain the same current density at a lower current threshold.[10] This is confirmed by Hoffman and Cranefield's finding that a reduction in electrode size of 3.0 mm^2 to 0.5 mm^2 results in a 100-fold decrease in threshold current.[1]

The direction of applied current, when stimulating with extracellular electrodes, influences current threshold. Unipolar stimulation involves passing current between two widely spaced electrodes, one close to and the other remote from the excitable tissue. Current flows from the close electrode through the excitable tissue and then through adjacent conductive tissues (e.g., blood or subcutaneous tissue) to the remote electrode. If the close electrode is negatively

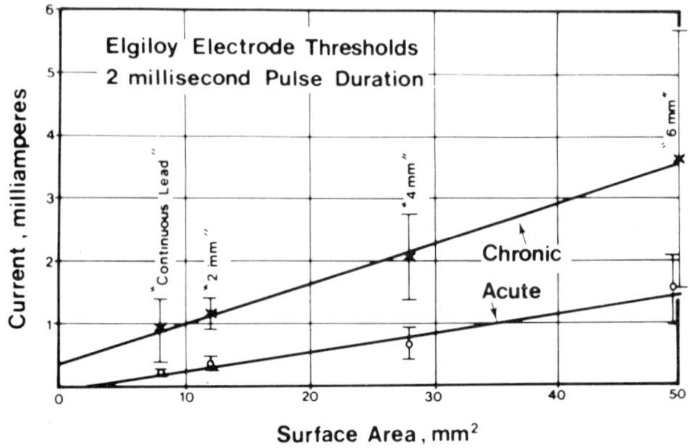

Figure 3–3. Relation between threshold current and electrode surface area. Threshold current (in milliamperes) for four Elgiloy electrodes of different surface area are plotted on the ordinate, and the electrode surface area (in square millimeters) is plotted on the abscissa for both acute (lower line) and chronic (upper line) human implant. (Reprinted from Furman et al: J Surg Res 19:149, 1975.)

charged and passes negative (real) current, unipolar cathodal stimulation occurs. If the close electrode is positively charged, it passes positively charged (conventional) current, and unipolar anodal stimulation takes place. Cathodal current depolarizes the membrane by discharging the membrane capacitor and directly reduces the membrane potential toward threshold (Fig. 3–4). Anodal current hyperpolarizes the membrane, causing an increase in resting membrane potential away from threshold but also increasing membrane excitability. On sudden termination of the anodal pulse, the membrane potential returns toward resting level, overshoots to threshold, and a propagated response occurs. Cathodal current, by directly reducing the resting membrane potential toward threshold, has a one-half to one-third lower threshold current in late diastole than does anodal current.[1]

Another factor that affects current threshold is the timing of current delivery during the excitability cycle. The generation of a normal action potential, particularly with respect to the amplitude and rate of rise of the upstroke, was shown by Weidmann to be dependent on the level of the membrane potential just prior to depolarization.[11] A decrease in resting membrane potential increases the percentage of fast sodium channels in the inactivated state, thus reducing the dV/dt and overshoot of the subsequently generated action potential. Indeed, at some reduced levels of resting potential, early in the cycle, late diastolic threshold current generates feeble, nonpropagative action potentials or none at all (Fig. 3–5). At these times, larger current strengths are required to induce a regenerative response. The effect of the timing of the stimulus delivery on threshold current may be quantified by measuring the relation between minimum current strength required to induce a propagated response at a given time interval from the previous response, or the so-called strength-interval relation (Fig. 3–6).[9]

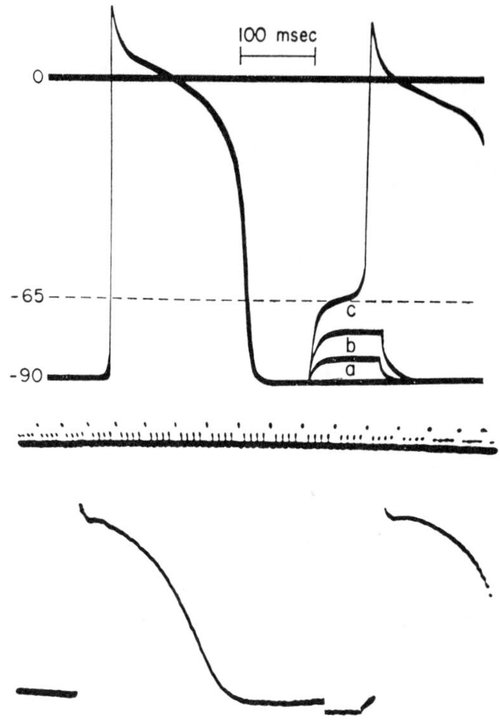

Figure 3–4. Effect of cathodal and anodal stimulation on induction of the action potential. The upper panel shows the effect of progressively larger cathodal stimuli (a-c) on the canine myocardial membrane potential, culminating in induction of a propagated action potential (C). Note that each cathodal stimulus decreases the resting potential. The lower panel demonstrates the effect of an anodal stimulus, which increases the resting potential and then induces an action potential when the pulse terminates and the membrane potential rapidly returns toward resting level and overshoots it. The membrane potential is plotted (in millivolts) on the ordinate, and time (in milliseconds) is plotted on the abscissa. (Reprinted from Hoffman BF, and Cranefiel PF: Electrophysiology of the Heart. Mt Kisco, Futura, 1976, pp. 214 and 221.)

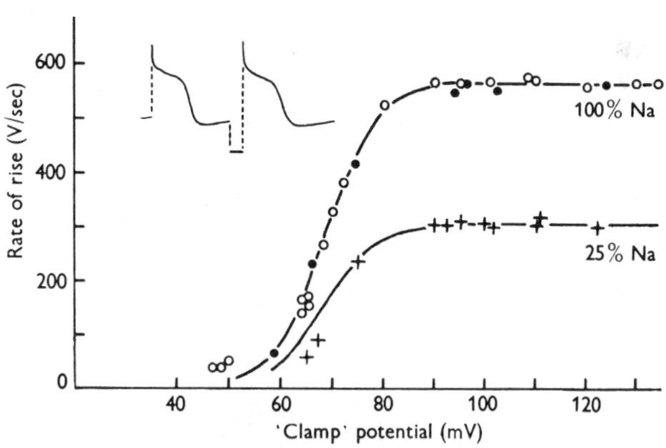

Figure 3–5. The relation between membrane potential and action potential upstroke velocity. The effect of the level of resting membrane potential on the action potential upstroke velocity just prior to stimulation is shown. The prestimulus membrane potential is controlled to a series of clamped potentials, and the resultant action potential upstroke velocity (dV/dt) is measured. The clamped membrane potential (in millivolts) is plotted on the abscissa, and the rate of rise of the action potential (in volts per second) is plotted on the ordinate. The curves through the circles were generated in calf Purkinje's fibers exposed to normal sodium Tyrodes solution, and the curve through the crosses in Purkinje fibers exposed to low (25% normal) sodium Tyrodes solution. (Reprinted from Weidmann S: J Physiol (London) 129:568, 1955.)

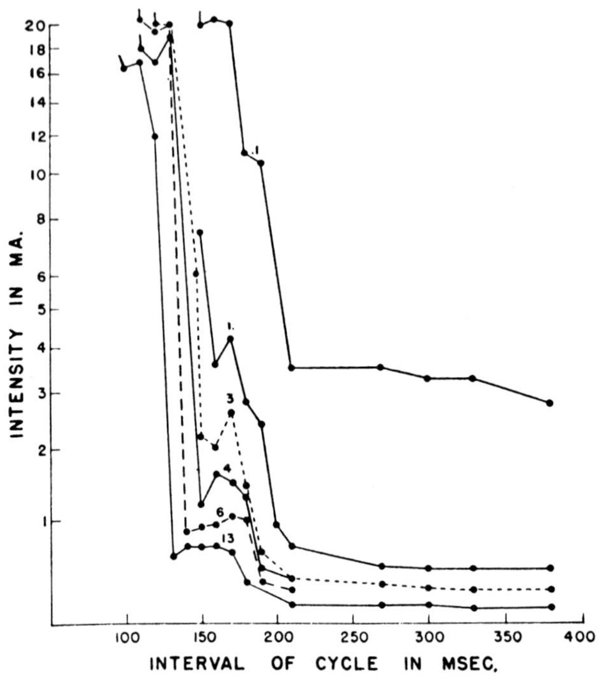

Figure 3–6. Strength-interval relations in canine myocardium. The stimulus intensity, or amplitude (in milliamperes), required to produce a propagated response at a specific coupling interval is plotted compared to that coupling interval (in milliseconds) for stimuli of varying durations (0.1 to 13.0 msec) as indicated. This generates a family of strength-interval curves. (Reprinted from Orias et al: Am J Physiol (London) 163:272, 1950.)

Current threshold assessment is the most practical direct method of measuring membrane excitability despite its somewhat incomplete characterization of excitability. Current threshold should optimally be measured when using a constant-current source.

Other Threshold Parameters

Voltage threshold, (V_{th}), the minimum change in membrane voltage necessary to induce a propagated response, is a function of membrane impedance but is less dependent than current threshold on external factors that influence current delivery. Voltage threshold, like current threshold, is dependent on electrode surface area. However, the effect of electrode surface area on voltage threshold is much less pronounced then it is on current threshold (Fig. 3–7). Voltage threshold is, however, dependent on pulse width and on timing of pulse delivery during the cardiac cycle. Voltage threshold is best measured when using a constant-voltage source, and since many implantable pulse generators are constant-voltage sources, voltage threshold is an appropriate parameter for evaluating these generators.

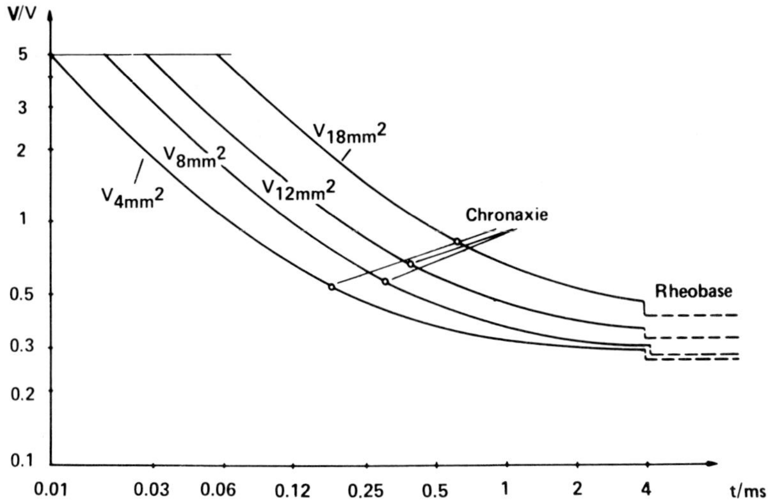

Figure 3–7. Effect of electrode surface area on voltage threshold. Threshold voltage (in volts) for a given stimulus duration is plotted on the ordinate, and stimulus duration (in milliseconds) is plotted on the abscissa for each of four electrodes of differing surface area (4, 8, 12, and 18 mm^2). Note that the effect of surface area on voltage threshold is not as pronounced as that on current threshold (see Figure 3–3). (Reprinted from Irnich et al: PACE 2:88, 1979.)

Charge threshold (C_{th}) is the amount of microcoulombs of change necessary to stimulate an evoked response. As such it incorporates the effects of current amplitude and pulse width on induction of a propagated response (charge threshold = current threshold × pulse width) and is independent of pulse width.

Energy threshold (E_{th}) is a measure of the minimum electrical energy required to induce a propagated response. It is related to current and voltage and pulse width as follows: $E_{th} = V_{th} \times I_{th} \times$ pulse width or $E_{th} = I_{th}^2 R_{th} T$, where T is the pulse width. Again the energy threshold incorporates the effect of pulse width on threshold and is therefore independent of it. Note that energy threshold varies geometrically with current threshold and is therefore highly dependent on current threshold.

Factors Influencing Threshold

Although initially thought to be constant, threshold has been found to vary even on a minute-to-minute basis. A number of investigators have shown that in humans, threshold measured as voltage threshold or energy threshold varies with alterations in physical activity, eating, sleeping, serum electrolytes, and a number of pharmacologic agents. Sowton and Barr[12] have shown that physical exercise may reduce voltage threshold by 20 to 30 per cent in both acutely and chronically implanted endocardial leads, presumably related to exercise-induced increases in catecholamine levels. Preston and colleagues[13] noted similar reductions in energy threshold with exercise and found increases in threshold during eating and sleeping, which they attributed to decreased sympathetic tone.

Support for the role of sympathetic tone in variation of threshold was provided by the finding that epinephrine infusions reduce the energy threshold in persons with chronically implanted electrodes.[13] However, isoproterenol infusion was found by the same investigators to increase energy threshold. Other pharmacologic agents noted to alter energy threshold include glucocorticoids, which raise threshold, and mineralocorticoids, which have the opposite effect.[13]

Alterations in intracellular ion concentration would be expected to influence threshold measurement. It was found that the infusion of potassium chloride and insulin increases energy threshold,[13] as might be predicted from the increase in intracellular potassium concentration that would increase resting membrane potential, drawing it further away from threshold. The effects of various electrolyte infusions on chronic thresholds are somewhat inconsistent, as shown by Sowton and Barr,[12] and may reflect more complex interactions with other pharmacologic factors.

Threshold measurements vary not only with physiologic activities, electrolyte changes, and administration of pharmacologic agents, but also with site of stimulation. Davies and Sowton[14] demonstrated that voltage threshold is consistently lower by 75 per cent for endocardial pacing sites compared with epicardial pacing sites, with both acutely and chronically implanted electrodes. In addition, stimulation threshold varies on the epicardium from site to site in both the right and left ventricle.

Thus threshold measurements are dynamic and vary with physiologic and pharmacologic factors as well as site of stimulation. The ability to deliver adequate electrical energy to the excitable tissue to generate a propagated response is dependent in part on tissue characteristics that determine threshold and excitability, as just discussed. In addition, it also depends on the interaction of the tissue and the components of the pacemaker system, which delivers energy to the myocardium (output circuit) and sense an incoming electrical signal from the myocardium (input circuit).

ELECTRICAL ENGINEERING CONSIDERATIONS

Pacing (Output) Circuit Characteristics

The circuit diagram that models a typical pacemaker output circuit is shown in Figure 3–8. The components of the circuit include the pulse generator itself and multiple sites of impedance—that is, the impedance generated by the lead, the electrode, the electrode-tissue interface, and in the case of unipolar pacing, the tissue bridge (myocardium, blood, extracellular fluid, and muscle and connective tissue) between the cathode and remote anode. The pulse generator may be a constant-current source, constant-voltage source or a current-limited modified constant-voltage source, and these variations will have implications for

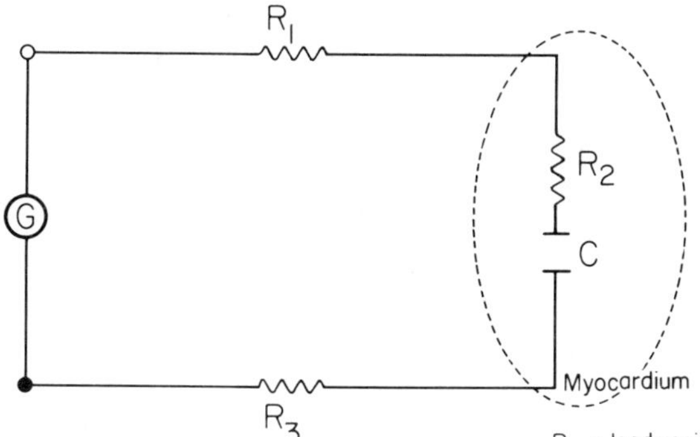

$$Z_o = R_l + R_2 + C\,(+R_3)$$

R_l = lead resistance
R_2 = myocardial resistance
R_3 = tissue bridge impedance (cathode to anode)
C = tissue-electrode interface capacitance
G = pulse generator
Z_o = pulse generator output impedance

Figure 3–8. The output circuit. The schematic of the pacing or output circuit shows the pulse generator (G), the lead impedance (R_1), the tissue-bridge impedance in the case of a unipolar system (R_3), the series combination of the myocardial impedance (R_2), and the tissue-electrode interface capacitance (C) as the net tissue-electrode impedance.

the functional characteristics of the circuit. The contributions of the different impedance sources to the total circuit impedance vary and may be manipulated to maximize the efficiency of energy transfer from the pulse generator to the myocardium. In addition, measurement of threshold values for current, voltage, and impedance give important information about the integrity and functional capability of the system.

Types of Pulse Generators

A constant-current source generates a constant current output by increasing its voltage output appropriately as the load impedance increases, up to the limit of its maximum voltage output (usually about 15 volts). The current-voltage characteristic of such a constant-current source is shown in Figure 3–9. Throughout the physiologic range of output circuit impedances (300 to 1000 ohms), the current output is essentially independent of load impedance. As load impedance exceeds 1000 ohms, the limits of the voltage output are reached and current output begins to fall. The smaller the current value the generator is set to function at, the less rapid is the falloff, such that at a setting of 1 ma, the pulse generator can function as almost a perfect constant-current source over an extended range of impedances.

The advantage of a constant-current source as a pulse generator is that transient increases in output impedance due to changes in polarization effects

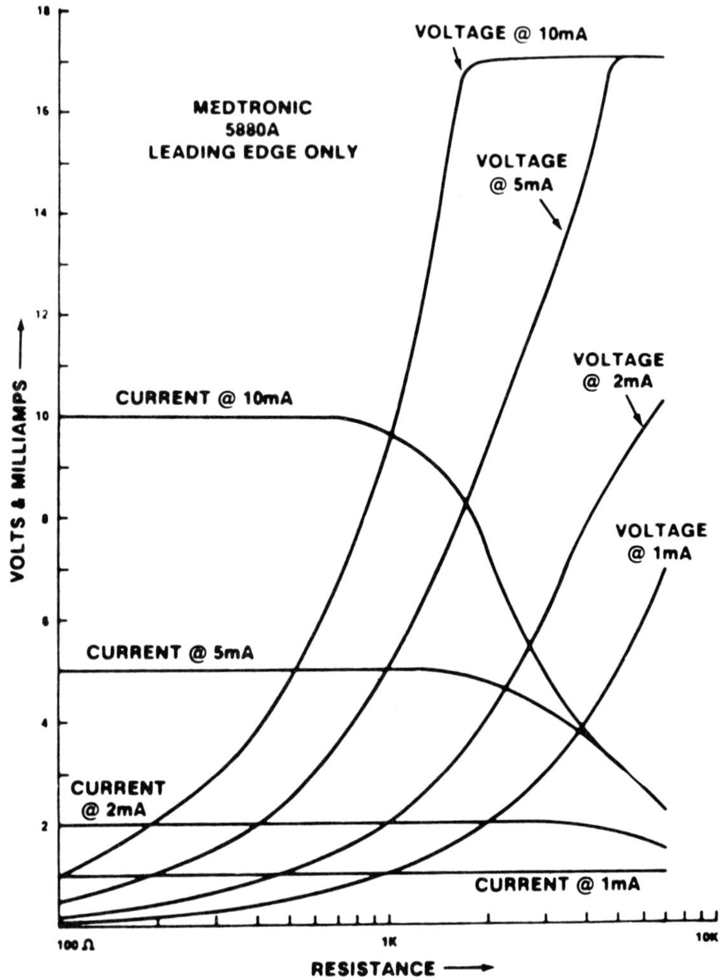

Figure 3–9. Current and voltage characteristics of a constant-current-source generator. The voltage output (in volts) and current output (in milliamperes) are both plotted on the ordinate, and various load impedances are plotted (in ohms) on a log scale on the abscissa. The current output is set at four different levels (1, 2, 5, and 10 ma), generating four different curves for voltage and current. Note that at higher impedances (>1 Kilohm), voltage output becomes limited and current output falls off. (Reprinted from Barold et al: Prog Cardiovasc Dis 24:1, 1981.)

at the electrode-tissue interface, or lead position, will not reduce delivered current to the myocardium and therefore will not interrupt pacing. Thus the constant-current source has a built-in compensatory mechanism. However, this is achieved at the expense of high battery current drain and consequent decreased pulse generator longevity.

Another drawback to a constant-current source as a pulse generator is the limitation on the maximum voltage output that can be generated. The maximum voltage output is a function of the load impedance seen by the pulse generator.

In some normally functioning chronically implanted endocardial and intramyocardial lead systems, the lead impedance can be as low as 250 to 300 ohms. If the maximum current output that a constant-current source can be set at is 10 ma, the maximum output voltage of the system is limited to 3 volts. An increase in threshold voltage beyond 3 volts is not unusual in a chronically implanted lead system and could lead to pacer failure. Thus constant-current sources as pulse generators are particularly suited for external temporary pacing devices, when transient changes in stimulation impedance are not uncommon and would otherwise reduce delivered current, but when there are minimal short-term changes in voltage threshold and when pulse generator longevity is not a real consideration.

Constant-voltage pulse generators supply a constant voltage output throughout a wide range of load impedances by increasing current output as load impedance falls (Fig. 3–10). At very low load impedances (<200 ohms), design limitations prevent continued increases in output current, and voltage output begins falling off. However, these lower impedances generally are outside the physiologic range for most chronically implanted lead systems. Because current output falls with increasing load impedance, battery drain is minimized in a constant-voltage pulse generator. A refinement of the design, the constant-voltage–constant-current pulse generator, further reduces battery drain by limiting the maximum current generated at low load impedances, thus giving the generator a constant-current source current-voltage characteristic at low impedances and a constant-voltage source current-voltage characteristic at high load impedances (Fig. 3–11).

One of the theoretical advantages of the constant-voltage source configuration for chronic pacer implants is that any reduction in load impedance that

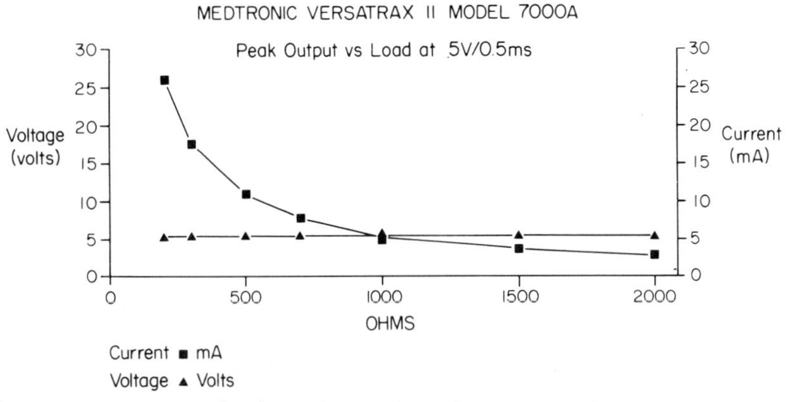

Figure 3–10. Current and voltage characteristic of a constant-voltage-source generator. The voltage output (in volts) is plotted on the left ordinate scale, and the current output (in milliamperes) is plotted on the right ordinate scale; the load impedance (in ohms) is plotted on the abscissa. Note that although voltage output remains constant over a wide range of output impedances at low impedances (<500 ohms), the increase in current output is limited, causing voltage output to fall off.

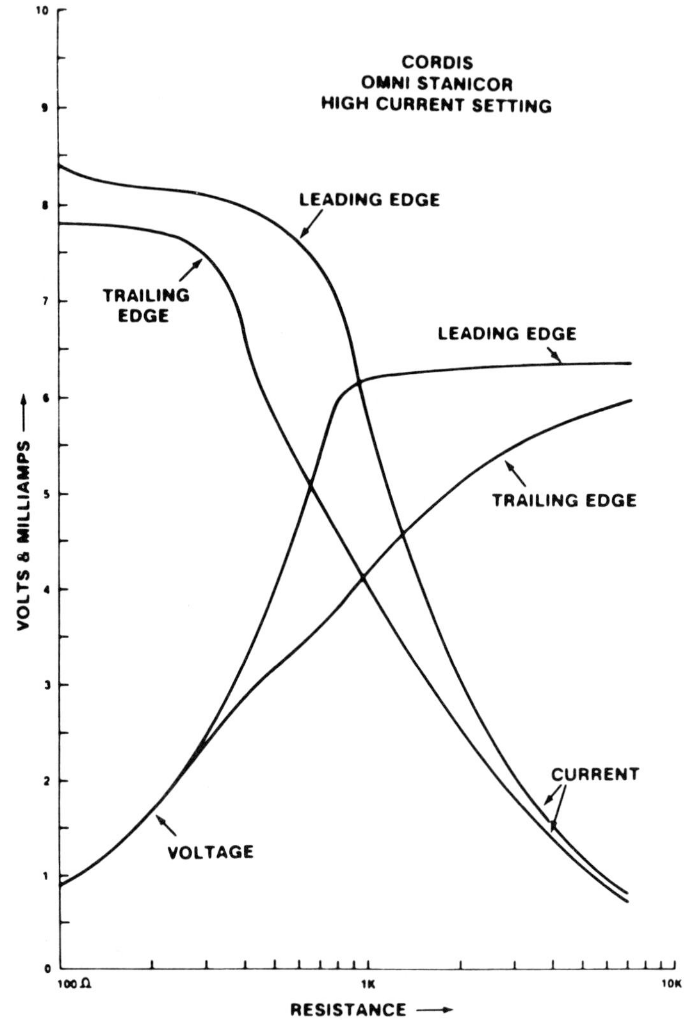

Figure 3–11. Current and voltage characteristic of a constant-current–constant-voltage generator. The voltage output (in volts) and current output (in milliamperes) are both plotted on the ordinate, and load impedance (in ohms) is plotted on the abscissa (log scale). In the lower impedance range (0 to 600 ohms) current output is fixed, and voltage output decreases with increasing impedance compatible with the characteristic of a constant-current source. In the higher impedance range (>1000 ohms) voltage output becomes fixed, and current output declines with increasing impedance. (Reprinted from Barold et al: Prog Cardiovasc Dis 24:1, 1981.)

might occur will not incur a loss of output voltage, and therefore voltage output will not fall below threshold.

The other major advantage is a lower battery drain and therefore longer pulse generator life. The drawback to the constant-voltage source is that it cannot compensate for small changes in current threshold at high load impedances. For example at a load impedance of 500 ohms, a 5.0-volt source can generate a maximum current output of 10.0 ma, which is well in excess of the measured acute current threshold of 0.8 to 1.2 ma and the projected increased current threshold with lead maturation. With a high load impedance of 2000.0 ohms, the 5.0-volt source can generate a maximum current output of only 2.5 ma. If threshold current increases beyond 2.5 ma as the lead matures, the pacer will fail.

This example also points out the importance of measuring lead impedance as well as current and voltage threshold for a constant-voltage generator at implantation. The calculation of maximal current output using the rated voltage output of the generator and lead impedance compared with the measured current threshold gives an idea of the safety margin for pacing. However, most currently available implantable pulse generators are of the constant-voltage source or constant-current–constant-voltage source configuration, as they frequently provide good safety margins for current delivery and can compensate for changes in load impedance vis-à-vis voltage threshold, and they do so at an acceptable level of battery drain.

Output Impedance

The circuit diagram in Figure 3–8 outlines the sources of impedance to current flow in the pacemaker circuit. The net output impedance is the sum of contributions from the pacemaker lead and electrode, the myocardial tissue, the electrode-electrolyte interface, the electrolyte-tissue interface, and the tissue bridge from the myocardium to the remote anode (blood, skeletal muscle, connective tissue).[15] The electrical behavior of the various impedances can be classified as resistive or ohmic (i.e., follows Ohm's law and therefore gives a linear current-voltage characteristic) or polarization type (i.e., has a time-dependent, nonlinear current-voltage characteristic). Potentials generated by ohmic impedances do not vary with time and are a linear function of current flow, whereas polarization impedances, which result from charge separation at various element interfaces, generate potentials that are time varying, develop slowly with current flow, are dependent on the current pulse width, and are nonlinear with respect to current flow.[16]

The ohmic impedances (Z_o) include the electrode and lead wire impedance, which are negligible with respect to the other impedances, and the electrolyte-tissue impedance (including the myocardial tissue impedance), which contributes a large electrochemical impedance to the total. The major polarization impedances (Z_p) include those at the electrode-electrolyte interface and are the activation impedance due to the potential necessary to provide activation energy to the electrochemical reactions that occur at the electrode-solution interface (e.g., $Ag - e^- \rightarrow Ag^+$) and the concentration impedance due to the potential required to replace ions lost during generation of electron flow at the electrode-solution interface (e.g., $Na^+ + e^- \rightarrow Na^o$).[16]

As indicated, the two major impedances, ohmic and polarization, and the overpotentials generated by these impedances (i.e., the excess potential that must be overcome to drive threshold current) vary with respect to current, current density, pulse width, and polarity of the electrode. As shown in Figures 3–12 and 3–13, the ohmic overpotential generated by Z_o varies linearly and directly with current (if surface area is held constant) and with current density, whereas the polarization overpotentials due to activation (Z_a) and concentration (Z_c) impedances vary directly but nonlinearly with current (when electrode surface area is held constant) and current density. At each current, and current density, the polarization impedances at the anode exceed those at the cathode.

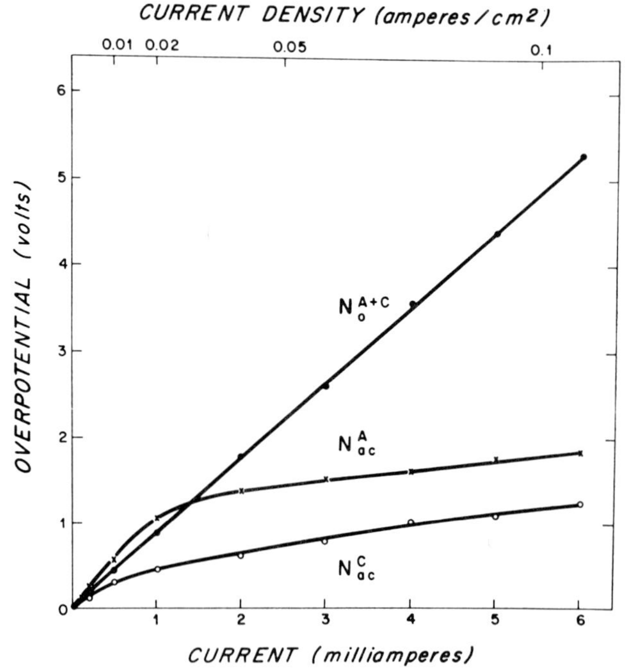

Figure 3–12. Relation between overpotential amplitude and current amplitude. The overpotentials generated during a stimulus pulse are plotted (in volts) on the ordinate as a function of the stimulus-current amplitude (in milliamperes) on the abscissa. N_o^{A+C} is the net ohmic overpotential generated at the anode plus cathode; N^A_{ac} is the net polarization overpotential generated by activation energy of the chemical reaction in charge of transfer at the anode plus the chemical energy due to the concentration gradient resulting from the charge transfer at the anode. N^C_{ac} is the net polarization overpotential generated at the cathode. Note that the net ohmic overpotential varies linearly with current amplitude, and the two polarization overpotentials vary nonlinearly with current amplitude. (Reprinted from Mansfield PB: Myocardial stimulation: The electrochemistry of electrode-tissue coupling. Am J Physiol 212:1475, 1967.)

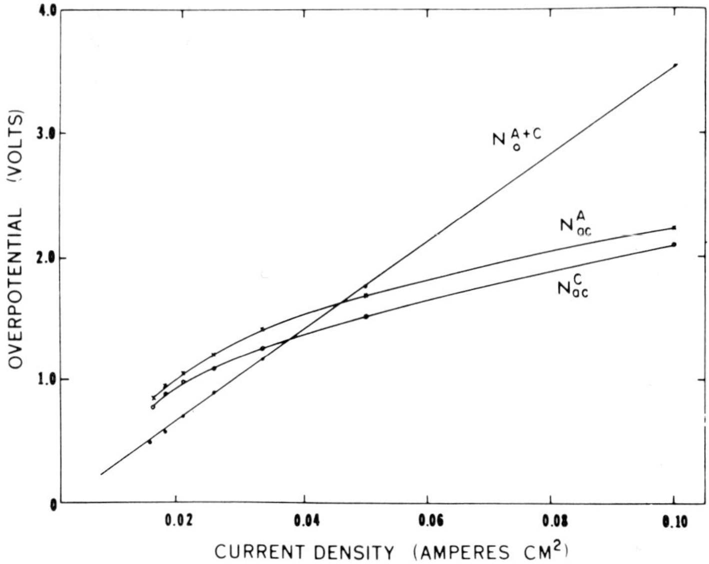

Figure 3–13. Relation between overpotential amplitude and current density. The net ohmic overpotential (N_o^{A+C}) and the anodal (N^A_{ac}) and cathodal (N^C_{ac}) net polarization overpotentials are plotted (in volts) on the ordinate, and the current density (in amperes per square centimeter) is plotted on the abscissa. Again the ohmic overpotential varies linearly, whereas the polarization overpotentials vary nonlinearly with current density. Note also that each current density the anodal polarization overpotential exceeds the cathodal polarization overpotential. (Reprinted from Mansfield PB: Myocardial stimulation: The electrochemistry of electrode-tissue coupling. Am J Physiol 212:1475, 1967.)

In addition, the polarization overpotentials and impedances exceed the ohmic overpotentials at low current and low current density but become significantly less than the ohmic overpotentials at high current and high current density. This implies that at low currents and low current densities, the polarization impedances provide a relatively large percentage of the total impedance, and that changes in the total overpotential are primarily caused by changes in the polarization overpotentials. On the other hand, at high currents ohmic impedance contributes the major percentage of the total impedance, and changes in total overpotential will primarily be attributable to changes in ohmic impedance. In addition, since the ohmic impedance is a constant with respect to current flow, although polarization impedances increase with increasing current, current flow can be more easily increased and requires less of a voltage increment at high initial current flows, when the ohmic impedance contributes most to total impedance, than at low initial current flows, when polarization impedances are the major component of the total impedance.[16]

The total impedance also varies with the type of electrode material, primarily because of differences in the polarization impedances that are generated with various electrode materials.[16]

Finally, the distribution of the ohmic and polarization impedances in space are quite different. Although the major ohmic impedance at the electrolyte-myocardial tissue interface is widely and essentially uniformly distributed throughout the electrolyte solution and at the solution tissue interface, the activation and concentration impedances are very localized to within a 1.0- to 2.5 μm radius of the electrode in the electrolyte solution.[16] With maturation during chronic lead implantation, a 0.2-mm fibrous tissue layer surrounds the electrode. Thus, while the ohmic overpotential generated at the electrolyte-tissue interface is directly involved in initiating tissue activation, changes in the polarization overpotentials will have no contribution to tissue depolarization. This implies that by maximizing the contribution of the electrolyte-tissue impedance to the total impedance, or conversely, by minimizing the contribution of the activation and concentration impedances to total impedance, increments in total voltage output will be more effectively transmitted to the electrolyte-tissue interface, thereby maximizing the efficiency of energy transfer from the pulse generator to the tissue. This can be accomplished by altering electrode and circuit design in a number of ways.

Polarization impedance varies directly with current density and inversely with electrode surface area, and thus increasing electrode surface area would decrease polarization impedance. Unfortunately, increasing electrode surface area would also increase current threshold and adversely affect the safety margin. However, the net activation and concentration impedance (Z_{ac}) is the sum of Z_{ac} at the cathode and at the anode, and since the passage of stimulating current requires only a single local electrode, the cathode, which has a lower current threshold, can be used as the proximate current-passing electrode, whereas the anode is made the remote electrode. If the surface area of the anode is increased, this would reduce its polarization impedance and thus also reduce the net polarization impedance without affecting the ohmic impedance (which is independent of surface area) or current threshold. Thus this change in circuit and electrode design would improve efficiency of energy transfer to the tissue.[16]

The electrode material affects polarization impedance as well as the ohmic impedance. Selection of the electrode material to give the lowest ratio of polarization impedance to ohmic impedance will minimize the contribution of polarization impedance to total impedance and thereby improve energy transfer to the myocardium.

Two other characteristics that can be altered to reduce the contribution of polarization impedance to total impedance are the pulse duration and pulse amplitude. Ohmic impedance is not time dependent and is therefore unaffected by pulse duration, whereas polarization impedance varies directly with pulse duration. By shortening pulse duration, the ratio of polarization to ohmic impedance will decrease, thereby improving efficiency of energy transfer.[16]

Reduction of pulse duration must be countered by an increase in pulse amplitude by the strength-duration relation, to maintain the current above threshold level. Fortunately, at increased pulse amplitude, the ohmic impedance contributes a greater proportion to total impedance than does polarization impedance, which decreases with increased pulse amplitude.[16] Thus the combination of decreasing pulse width and an increased pulse amplitude reduces the amount of voltage that must be dissipated in overcoming polarization overpotentials and thereby maximizes energy transfer from the pulse generator to the tissue to initiate membrane depolarization. In practice, pacing parameters should be chosen with the shortest pulse width and appropriate (high) pulse amplitude, within the limits of the output voltage capabilities of the power source and considerations of the safety margin.

The measurement of output impedance is not an academic exercise. It has important implications for energy threshold and therefore for safety margins for pacemaker function, as well as for pulse generator longevity.

Threshold energy (E_{th}) is the product of threshold voltage (V_{th}), threshold current (I_{th}), and pulse width (T) ($E_{th} = V_{th} \times I_{th} \times T$). Since threshold voltage, by Ohm's law, is equal to the product of threshold current and threshold impedance ($V_{th} = I_{th} \times Z_{th}$), the expression for threshold energy can be rearranged as the product of threshold current squared times threshold impedance, times pulse width ($E_{th} = I_{th}^2 \times Z_{th} \times T$). Thus threshold energy varies directly with threshold impedance but varies geometrically with threshold current. For a given tissue interface, threshold current varies inversely with threshold impedance, and an increase in threshold impedance results in an associated decrease in threshold current. Since threshold energy is so much more dependent on threshold current than on impedance, the net effect of increasing threshold impedance is to reduce threshold energy.[17]

Threshold energy is the critical factor in determining the safety margin for pacemaker function. The measured voltage threshold has been shown to vary substantially throughout the day, depending on alterations in physiologic conditions.[12] The threshold energy has similarly shown such swings varying ± 50 per cent of its mean value.[18] Threshold energy can show a threefold variation from the minimum to the maximum. Assuming the measured threshold energy at any time may be the minimum, then the maximum energy output of the pulse generator should be three times threshold energy, or $E/E_{th} \geq 3.0$. Since energy can be expressed in terms of voltage and current as $E = V \times I \times T$, the ratio of maximum output voltage and threshold voltage may be given in terms of threshold and output energy:

$$
\begin{aligned}
E_o/E_{th} &= V_o/V_{th} \times I_o/I_{th} \times T/T \\
&= V_o/V_{th} \times \frac{V_o/Z}{V_{th}/Z} \\
&= V_o^2/V_{th}^2
\end{aligned}
$$

For an adequate safety margin, $E_o/E_{th} = V_o^2/V_{th}^2 \geq 3$ or $V_o/V_{th} \geq \sqrt{3} = 1.75$. Since most constant-voltage sources have a maximum voltage output of 5.00 volts, V_{th} should not exceed 5.0/1.75 or 2.90 volts. Since chronic voltage threshold is usually about three times the acute threshold due to the maturation process, acute threshold voltage should not exceed .97 volts.

The implications of output impedance for battery longevity are important. The major factor determining battery drain is the amount of current drawn with each output pulse. The current output of a pulse generator normally exceeds threshold current by a substantial margin. An increase in output impedance would reduce the current output per pulse, and as long as it exceeds threshold, would continue to stimulate the myocardium. This would reduce pulse generator dissipation and lengthen battery life.

Threshold Measurements and Their Clinical Implications

The measurement of threshold parameters for the pacing system is important for determining the minimum current and voltage necessary to achieve successful pacing. From these parameters a number of other important threshold parameters may be derived, specifically charge threshold, energy threshold, and output impedance. The measured and derived threshold values have significant implications for evaluating the integrity of the pacing system and for projecting the feasibility of successful long-term pacing (Table 3–1).

Threshold measurements can be made either with bipolar or unipolar pacing leads. In the latter case, cathodal stimulation threshold is lower[1] and is the preferred modality of unipolar stimulation. In addition, the remote anode in unipolar pacing should have a large surface area (>50 mm^2), since smaller surface areas confer an unnecessarily large output impedance and will therefore artificially increase threshold voltage.

Voltage threshold for the pacing system is the minimum stimulus voltage required to drive the excitatory current at a specified pulse duration. The voltage threshold may possibly be considered the preferred measurement of threshold for constant-voltage pulse generators in the clinical setting,[17] because voltage threshold is relatively independent of electrode surface area[19] and therefore can be compared from lead system to lead system. In addition, the rated maximum voltage output is essentially independent of output impedance, since voltage-limiting impedances are not usually encountered in the clinical setting. Furthermore, measurement of voltage threshold in conjunction with output impedance is helpful in judging the integrity of the lead system. A defective lead system with a fracture will have a normal current threshold but a high output impedance and voltage threshold.[17]

Current threshold for the pacing system is the minimum current in milliamperes necessary to evoke a propagated response. It should be measured in late diastole, with a constant-current source at the time of pacer implantation. Current

Table 3–1. Implantation Problems: Effects on Threshold and Impedance

Problem	Voltage Threshold	Current Threshold	Lead Impedance
Lead displacement	↑	↑	Normal
Lead fracture	↑	Normal	↑
Lead insulation tear	↓	↑	↓↓
Faulty lead connection or faulty generator	Normal	Normal	Normal

threshold primarily reflects myocardial tissue responsiveness and for a given electrode system is linearly and directly related to the actual tissue current threshold.[20] It is very well suited for investigative measurement of excitability characteristics and the effects of pharmacologic or metabolic interventions on excitability.

Charge threshold for the pacing system is the product of the current threshold in milliamperes and the pulse duration in milliseconds and represents the minimum amount of charge in microcoulombs necessary to stimulate an evoked response. Charge threshold may be compared to the total amount of charge stored in the battery, and the maximum battery longevity can be determined.[17] The actual battery longevity can be calculated by determining the output charge per pulse and dividing it into the total battery charge (i.e., total battery charge/charge per pulse = number of pulses).

The integrity of the pacing system can be fully evaluated by measuring threshold voltage and current simultaneously and thus allowing calculation of threshold impedance (see Table 3–1). A normally functioning ventricular pacing system with good electrode contact and a normal lead will have threshold currents of 0.5 to 0.9 ma, threshold voltages of 0.4 to 1.0 volts, and a calculated impedance of 500.0 to 1000.0 ohms.[17]

Poor lead contact has no effect on lead impedance but increases the effective lead surface area (as current traverses blood and reaches tissue, the lines of current have expanded), thereby reducing current density and increasing threshold current and proportionately increasing voltage threshold by interposing the higher impedance of the intervening blood. The lead impedance remains unchanged because the voltage and current thresholds increase proportionately. With a lead fracture, current threshold is unaffected, but lead impedance increases markedly as does voltage threshold. Finally, a break in the lead insulation will markedly reduce lead impedance by introducing a low-impedance shunt pathway from the pacing wire to the blood. Current threshold will remain constant or increase, as a substantial amount of the current necessary for depolarization will be diverted. Threshold voltage will either remain constant (if threshold current rises proportionately to the fall in impedance) or will fall (if current rises minimally). Thus lead impedance is an important guide to the integrity of the pacing system.[17] Current threshold is a good indicator of lead position and electrode contact but gives little information on lead integrity. Voltage threshold is also an indicator of lead position and in some cases is an indicator of lead integrity.

Measurement of lead impedance should best be made at maximum output voltage and current to minimize contribution of polarization effects to the measured impedance.[21] The actual measurement should be made from the simultaneous analogue pulse signal of voltage and current with time.[22] The time during the signal at which the threshold voltage and currents are measured will influence the amplitude of the system impedance, as polarization effects are absent in the initial 90 msec of the pulse, causing a higher threshold current. Finally, system impedance will vary with the time after implantation, since impedance falls during the first 10 days after implant.[23]

Sensing (Input) Circuit

The function of the input circuit is to sense the intrinsic cardiac electrical signal (i.e., the endocardial or epicardial surface electrogram) and thereby inhibit the output circuit from generating a pacer stimulus. Optimum functioning requires that the input circuit be able to discriminate between the P wave or QRS signal and other intracardiac signals (e.g., T wave) and extrinsic signals (e.g., noise, 60-cycle artifact, myopotentials). The intracardiac electrogram is sensed as a potential difference between cathode and anode. In bipolar systems both poles are intracardiac, while in unipolar systems the cathode is intracardiac and the anode is a remote, indifferent electrode. The sensing threshold for the pacing system is the minimum potential difference measured by the input circuit that will inhibit the output circuit.

Sensing threshold is dependent on a complex interaction between specific characteristics of the intrinsic cardiac signal, the impedance of the pacing system, and the sensitivity of the pulse generator's sensing circuit. The factors intrinsic to the input circuit that influence the ability to sense include the matching of the sensing circuit's input impedance to its load impedance. Factors intrinsic to the cardiac signal include the amplitude and configuration of the cardiac electrogram and the slew rate, or frequency spectral content, of the electrogram.[26]

Factors Intrinsic to Input Circuit that Influence Sensing

Appropriate matching of the sensing circuit's input impedance and the load (tissue-electrode interface) impedance has an important effect on the transmission of the intrinsic signal to the input circuit, unattenuated.[17] The equivalent circuit for the input or sensing circuit is shown in Figure 3–14. The total circuit impedance is the sum of the load impedance (Z_{load}—composed of the tissue impedance, polarization impedance at the tissue-electrode interface, and the lead impedance) and the pulse generator input impedance (Z_g). The higher the load impedance, the greater the voltage drop from the EMF generated by the myocardium to the voltage at the pulse generator's sensing circuit. Polarization effects are greater for sensing than pacing, because the R wave has a longer duration than the pacer spike.[28] Thus the load impedance for sensing is greater than for pacing.

As with the output circuit, a number of factors affect the load impedance of the input circuit, including the electrode surface area, the electrode material composition, and the signal duration and amplitude.[17] The load impedance is inversely proportional to lead surface area, so that smaller electrodes, used more commonly because of lower pacing thresholds and less battery drain, have larger sensing impedances. Longer duration intracardiac signals cause increased polarization effects, yielding increased load impedance. Finally, load impedance is inversely proportional to signal frequency, such that low-frequency signals generate higher load impedances.[24] More important than the absolute value of the load impedance in determining sensing capability is the amplitude of the

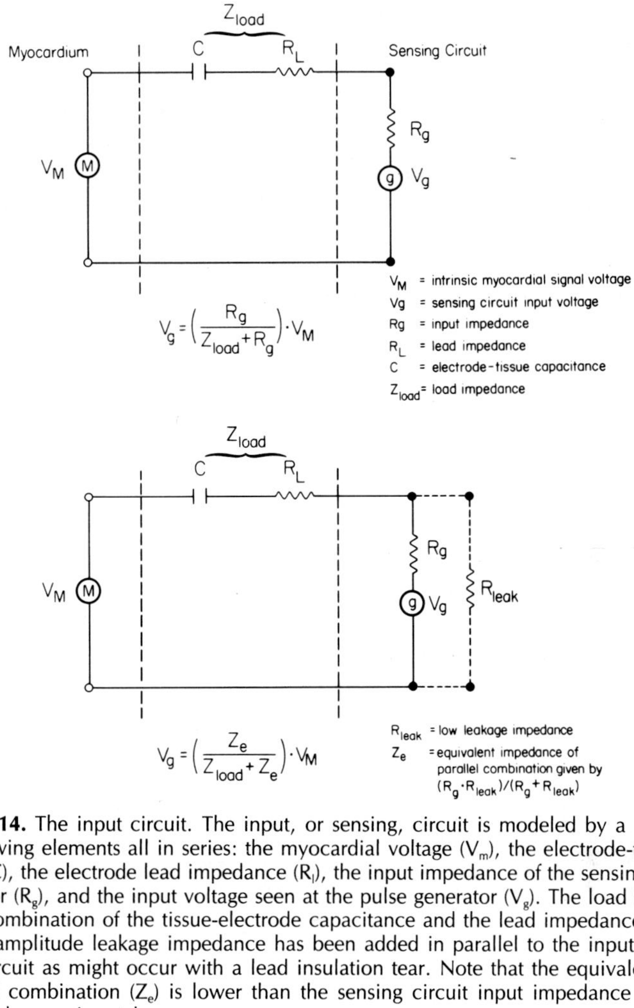

Figure 3–14. The input circuit. The input, or sensing, circuit is modeled by a lumped circuit with the following elements all in series: the myocardial voltage (V_m), the electrode-tissue interface capacitance (C), the electrode lead impedance (R_l), the input impedance of the sensing circuit of the pulse generator (R_g), and the input voltage seen at the pulse generator (V_g). The load impedance (Z_l) is the series combination of the tissue-electrode capacitance and the lead impedance. In the lower panel, a low amplitude leakage impedance has been added in parallel to the input impedance of the sensing circuit as might occur with a lead insulation tear. Note that the equivalent impedance of the parallel combination (Z_e) is lower than the sensing circuit input impedance alone causing potential impedance mismatch.

load impedance relative to the pulse generator input impedance.[24] As shown in Figure 3–14, the load and input impedances function as a voltage divider, such that the percentage of the signal voltage generated by the myocardium (V_m) that is seen by the sensing circuit inside the pulse generator (V_g) in terms of the load impedance (Z_{load}) and the pulse generator impedance (R_g) is given by the relation $V_g = [R_g/(R_g + Z_{load})] \times V_m$. The degree to which the cardiac signal is attenuated when it reaches the sensing circuit of the pulse generator is dependent on the relative amplitudes of the load and pulse generator impedances. If they are similar, the signal will be attenuated by 50 per cent, whereas if the pulse generator input impedance is at least an order of magnitude larger, then the signal will be attenuated only minimally. Most pulse generators are now made with very high input impedances (>40,000 ohms), so that significant signal attentuation at the pulse generator is obviated.

The major cause of impedance mismatch between the electrode-tissue load and the pulse generator is the development of an insulation break causing a leakage impedance that effectively shorts out the input impedance, as illustrated in Figure 3–14. The parallel combination of the input impedance (Z_g) and the low-leakage impedance (Z_{leak}) is an equivalent impedance given by $Z_e = Z_{leak} \times Z_g/(Z_{leak} + Z_g)$, which is much smaller than Z_g alone. Thus the effective input impedance generated by the insulation leak is markedly reduced and may approach the same order of magnitude as the load impedance. This would result in significant signal attenuation of the intrinsic electrogram and loss of sensing.

Another factor that is intrinsic to the input circuit and that affects sensing capability is the filtering characteristic of the input circuit.[25] The equivalent circuit of the pulse generator input circuit, pacer leads, and electrodes and heart muscle is best represented by an RC circuit that functions as a differentiator, as shown in Figure 3–14. The voltage generated by the myocardium (V_m) is altered by the RC circuit, and the resultant voltage (V_g) seen at the pulse generator sensing circuit is given by $V_g = V_m \times \frac{S\,R_g\,C}{(1 + S\,R_g\,C)}$, where R_g is the generator input impedance, C is the capacitance at the tissue-electrode interface, and S is the product of 2π and the signal frequency. If the circuit were a perfect differentiator, all myocardial signals, regardless of frequency, would be attentuated by being differentiated (i.e., output signal proportional to the slope of input signal). But the circuit is an imperfect differentiator because it has a cutoff frequency of $\omega = 1/R_gC$, such that all signals or components of signals having frequencies less than ω are differentiated, whereas all signal components with frequency greater than ω are transmitted to the pulse generator unchanged. Thus the circuit functions as a high-pass filter. The greater ω, the more signal components that are attenuated, whereas the smaller ω, the more signal components transmitted unattenuated to the sensing circuit. The circuit will therefore tend to accentuate higher frequency components of a signal and attenuate the lower frequency components.[25] Those signals composed primarily of low-frequency components will not be sensed.

Factors Intrinsic to Input Cardiac Signal that Influence Sensing

The factors intrinsic to the cardiac signal that influence the ability to sense include the electrogram amplitude, configuration, and slew rate (dV/dt), or frequency spectral content.[26]

It has been reported that intrinsic cardiac electrograms have a limited number of configurations. For unipolar ventricular endocardial electrograms, 58 per cent are biphasic, with the characteristic intrinsicoid deflection and equal R and S waves; 30 per cent are monophasic, with predominant negative deflections; and 12 per cent are monophasic, with predominant positive deflections.[27] Unipolar atrial endocardial electrograms from the coronary sinus almost uniformly have a biphasic configuration (89 per cent), and the remaining 11 per cent have monophasic positive deflection configuration.[27] Bipolar ventricular endocardial or atrial electrograms are the algebraic sum of the unipolar signals seen at each electrode, with a weighting factor due to differences in the time of arrival at the signal at each pole. If the bipolar lead is precisely perpendicular to the spread of the wave front, the two unipolar tip electrograms may cancel, yielding a very low amplitude signal (Fig. 3–15). This can lead to sensing problems that can be corrected by switching from bipolar to unipolar sensing. On the other hand, if the bipolar leads are parallel to the spread of the wave

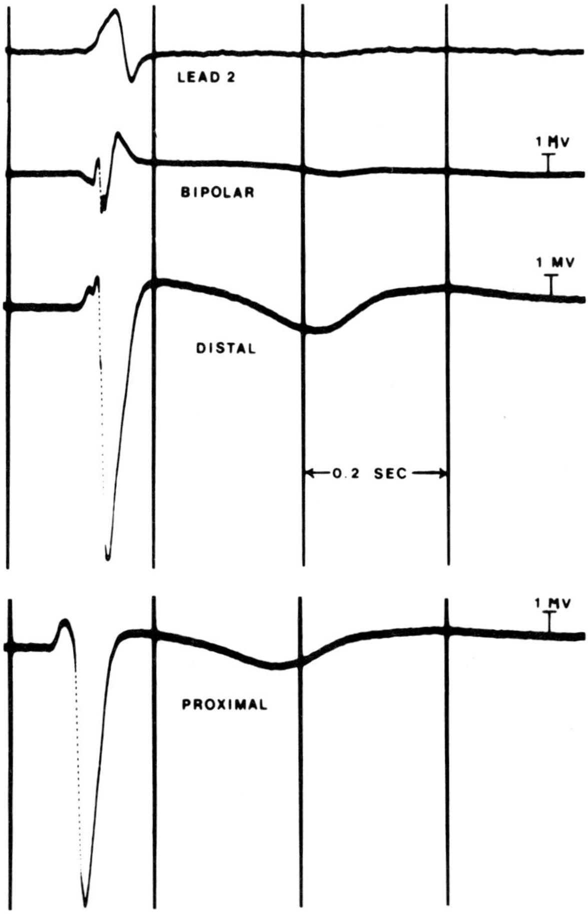

Figure 3–15. The relation between bipolar and unipolar electrograms when the sensing electrode is oriented perpendicular to the axis of the intrinsic signal. Surface ECG lead II and intracardiac electrograms recorded in bipolar fashion between the proximal and distal electrodes, in unipolar fashion from the distal electrode, and then the proximal electrode from an implanted pacer lead are shown from top to bottom. Note that despite the large-amplitude unipolar electrograms recorded, the bipolar electrogram, which is an algebraic summation of the two unipolar electrograms over time, is very low amplitude and unable to be sensed. (Reprinted from Furman et al: Am Heart J 93:794, 1977.)

front, a difference in arrival time at the two leads may actually augment signal amplitude and improve the capability for sensing.

The effect of signal configuration on the ability to sense is demonstrated by comparing the regions of pacer inhibition, based on pulse amplitude and slew rate for artificial pulses of varying configuration applied to a pacer sensing circuit. On a graph of signal slew rate (ordinate) compared with amplitude (abscissa) (Fig. 3–16), the set of coordinates for which the pacer is inhibited is the region of sensing. Note that not only do different signal configurations (e.g., monophasic triangular vs. biphasic triangular) have differing regions of inhibition, but for a given signal configuration, different polarities of the same waveform yield different regions of inhibition.[26]

For appropriate sensing, the intrinsic signal must have an adequate amplitude. Generally the minimum signal amplitude for sensing is between 1.5 to 4.0 mv, but because signal amplitude is reduced after chronic implantation because of fibrous-tissue reaction,[20] the minimum acceptable signal amplitude at acute implantation is 5.0 mv for the R wave and 2.0 mv for the P wave.

In actuality, as shown by the graphs of signal amplitude compared to slew rate, adequate amplitude alone does not determine ability to sense. Rather a combination of signal amplitude and slew rate is necessary to allow sensing. The effect of slew rate in determining the ability of a signal to be sensed is related to the filtering characteristics of the sensing circuit. Although the range of slew rates, or dV/dt, that will be sensed varies among pacers, the minimum dV/dt necessary for sensing at any pulse amplitude is fairly uniform at 0.2 volts/sec. On the other hand, the upper limits of slew rate that can be sensed are

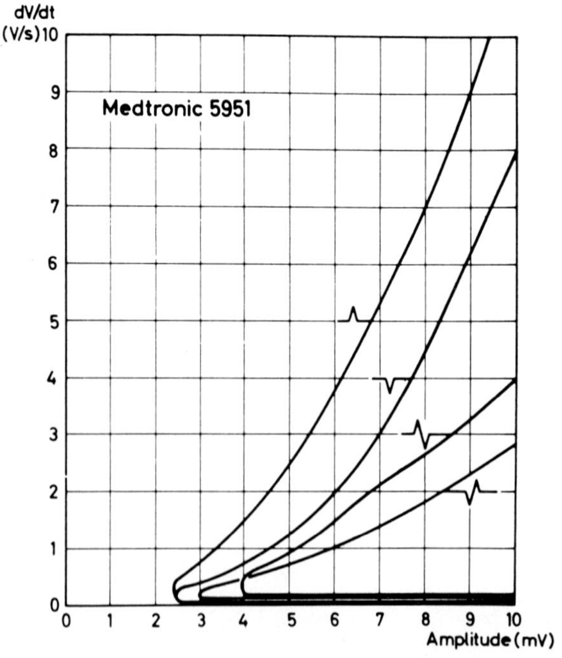

Figure 3–16. Input circuit regions of inhibition. The signal slew rate (in volts per second) is plotted on the ordinate and signal amplitude (in millivolts) is plotted on the abscissa for 5 generated signals with different configurations. The region of sensing circuit inhibition consists of all coordinates contained within the borders of the curve. Note that the requirements of slew rate and amplitude that will inhibit the sensing circuit vary with signal polarity and configuration. (Reprinted from Ohm OJ: PACE 3:318, 1980.)

quite variable and must be correlated with the pulse amplitude. For example, at low signal amplitudes (1.0 to 3.0 mv), maximum dV/dt that can still be sensed may vary from 1.5 to 9.0 volts/sec; whereas at a higher signal amplitude (7.0 to 10.0 mv), maximum dV/dt that still allows sensing may range from 3.0 to 30.0 volts/sec. At acute implantation a typical R-wave slew rate is 3.0 volts/sec, which puts the signal in a good range for sensing. Generally problems arise in the lower signal amplitude domain, when the signal slew rate exceeds the maximum acceptable for sensing in a given pacer input circuit. Since the R-wave signal amplitude decreases during maturation, this type of sensing problem sometimes develops.[28]

The last factors that are intrinsic to the signal and that affect the ability to sense, and more specifically the ability of the sensing circuit to discriminate between different cardiac signals and extraneous signals, are the frequency spectral characteristics of the intracardiac electrogram.[25] That is, the electrogram signal can be broken down via Fourier transform into various component parts with differing energies based on frequencies. The energy profile of a signal in terms of its frequency content is given by the bandwidth—that is, the range of frequencies that contain the bulk of the signal amplitude when signal amplitude is plotted as a function of frequency (Fig. 3–17). The limits of the bandwidth are

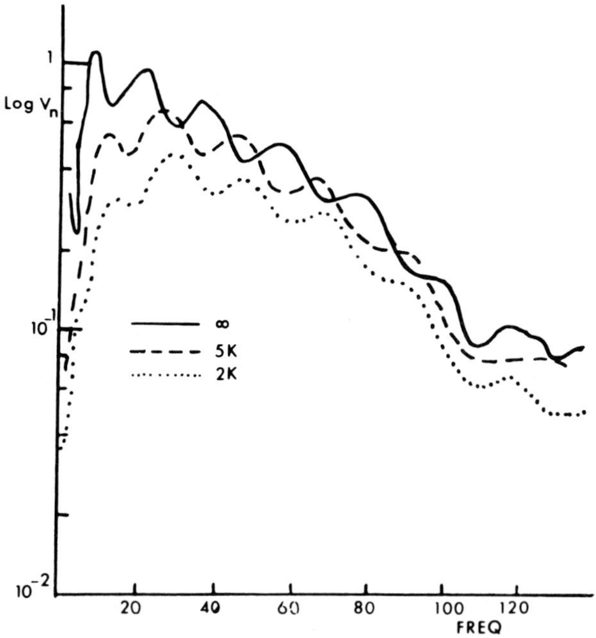

Figure 3–17. Spectral analysis of the endocardial signal in the frequency domain. The intrinsic signal amplitude (in volts) on a log scale on the ordinate is plotted against the signal frequency (in Hertz) on the abscissa. The three different curves are for input circuits with different input impedances (infinite, 5000, and 2000 ohms). Note that as input impedance is reduced, the low frequency components of the signal (0 to 30 Hz) are more attenuated than the high frequency components (30 to 120 Hz). (Reprinted from Barold et al: Prog Cardiovasc Dis 24:1, 1981.)

defined by the frequency at peak amplitude and the frequency at which the amplitude has fallen to a specific percentage of the maximum (either 50 percent or 25 percent). If such a time-varying signal is processed by an RC circuit such as the pulse generator sensing circuit (with the characteristics of a high-pass filter), the configuration of the signal that will be passed as the output will be dependent on the limits of the bandwidth compared with the cutoff frequency of the RC circuit as a filter. If the signal's bandwidth is well below the cutoff frequency, almost all of the signal will be attenuated. If the bandwidth of the signal straddles the cutoff frequency, the higher frequency components of the signal will be transmitted and accentuated, whereas the lower frequency components will be filtered out. Finally, if the bandwidth of the signal exceeds the cutoff frequency, the entire signal will be transmitted unchanged as the output signal.[27]

Manipulating the signal bandwidth relative to the input circuit's cutoff frequency can allow for discrimination between the intrinsic cardiac signal and other, extraneous signals. This can be done by taking advantage of the changes in bandwidth and cutoff frequency induced by changes in input circuit loading conditions and electrode size.

The intrinsic signal's bandwidth varies inversely with the input circuit load impedance.[25] That is, with increasing load impedance, the major amplitude content of the signal is shifted to the lower frequencies and the maximum frequency is reduced, making the bandwidth narrow. Electrode surface area, which alters load impedance, affects the bandwidth of an intrinsic signal in the same way as does the load impedance. Furthermore, the loading characteristics of the sensing circuit alter the cutoff frequency of the high-pass filter characteristic of the sensing circuit. The cutoff frequency is inversely proportional to load impedance, sensing circuit input impedance, and electrode capacitance.[25] Again, because electrode surface area alters both load impedance and capacitance, it has major effects on cutoff frequency. Thus the character of the sensing circuit's output signal is strongly influenced by the loading conditions of the sensing circuit, which modify both the bandwidth of the intrinsic signal and the cutoff frequency of the sensing circuit. Specific alterations in electrode size, load impedance, and electrode capacitance can be used to allow better discrimination between the R wave and other cardiac and extraneous signals.

The normal R wave has a frequency range of 0.5 to 200.0 Hz. The bulk of its energy spectrum is <20.0 Hz, but it does have higher frequency components as great as 80.0 Hz. The sensing circuit will, depending on its cutoff frequency, attenuate the major part of the R-wave signal, i.e. the low-frequency components <20.0 Hz, but accentuate the high-frequency component at about 80.0 Hz. Both the T wave and ventricular premature depolarizations have much lower bandwidths than the R wave, with no significant high-frequency components.[25] By altering the loading impedance and sensing circuit input impedance (i.e., decreasing both) or using smaller surface electrodes, the cutoff frequency of the sensing circuit could be increased. The entire frequency spectrum of both the T wave and VPD would be attenuated because of their lower bandwidths, whereas portions of the R wave will be accentuated and transmitted, thus allowing good discrimination of the R wave.

More recently, the sensing circuit has been designed to function as a bandpass filter—that is, the combination of a high- and a low-pass filter, with upper and lower cutoff frequencies above and below which all energy components of a signal are attenuated. Thus only those components of the signal in the narrow bandwidth of frequencies will be transmitted as the output signal. This can be used to refine the discrimination function of the sensing circuit to filter out extraneous signals (e.g., 60-cycle noise and myopotentials, both of which have mainly high-frequency components around 50 to 70 Hz). By setting the bandpass of the sensing circuit at 10 to 40 Hz, the lower cutoff frequency will cause attenuation of T waves and allow VPDs and the R wave to be transmitted as output signals, whereas the higher cutoff frequency will filter out 60-cycle noise and myopotentials.

Clinical Applications

By applying these engineering concepts, a number of important observations about sensing intrinsic cardiac signals can be better understood. For example, in general bipolar and unipolar recording techniques are equally adequate for sensing intrinsic cardiac signals. Furman and colleagues[27] noted that the bipolar intrinsicoid deflection was smaller than the simultaneously recorded tip unipolar signal in 51 per cent of cases, and only 2 per cent of the bipolar signals were too small to be sensed when the unipolar signal was adequate. In 43 per cent of cases the bipolar intrinsicoid deflection was larger than the tip unipolar, and in 6 per cent the two signals were equal. The major advantage of the bipolar recording technique is the attenuation of far-field signals, which were smaller than corresponding signals in the unipolar recording in 96 per cent of cases. This is attributable to the simultaneous arrival of the noise signal at both poles of the electrode in equal strength and the subtraction out of the signals with the differential recording technique. Thus when myopotential inhibition is a problem for a unipolar pacing system, switching to a bipolar recording system may correct the difficulty. In dealing with atrial pacing, far-field effect from the ventricular electrograms can confuse the sensing circuit. Again, this interference from far-field signals can be almost completely overcome by using bipolar recordings.

The disadvantage of the bipolar system arises when the recording electrodes may be oriented perpendicular to the main vector of the electrical wave front, which can yield a lower amplitude signal with a reduced slew rate. In this case sensing problems may be corrected by switching from a bipolar to a unipolar recording system, which would still yield a reasonable size electrogram signal since there is no differential recording. In addition, the bipolar recording system is more susceptible to changes in the R-wave signal because of cyclical variation in position with coughing and respiration, which can cause transient reduction in R-wave amplitude. Again, this can be corrected by switching to unipolar signal recording.

The role of electrode maturation in the development of late sensing failure can be understood in terms of the adequacy of signal amplitude and slew rate. Maturation of the electrode not only alters pacing threshold but may also alter sensing threshold by increasing the lead impedance, thereby reducing both the slew rate and amplitude of the intrinsic electrogram. If the signal amplitude at the lower end of the frequency spectrum falls despite even a 40 per cent reduction in slew rate, the slew rate often still exceeds the maximum slew rate that at low amplitudes allows sensing (see Figure 3–16). This problem can in part be obviated by using so-called "high-sensitivity" pacers, which are specifically designed to have higher maximum allowable slew rates (>15 to 20 mv/sec) at the lower signal amplitude range (2 to 4 mv). However, these high-sensitivity pacers themselves have the additional problem of showing a susceptibility to myopotential inhibition. Myopotentials are high-frequency (50 to 70 Hz), low-amplitude signals that normally are filtered out by the bandpass characteristics of the sensing circuit. But with high-sensitivity pacers, myopotentials and other forms of high-frequency, low-amplitude noise are sensed and can cause pacer inhibition.[25] In fact, the incidence of this complication approaches 80 per cent with these pacemakers.

All in all, sensing failure in clinical practice is rarely related to transmission of a poor signal to a normally functioning pulse generator sensing circuit (5 percent).[29] In these cases, the causes of an inadequate signal for sensing include: low-amplitude signal at the time of implantation, inadequate slew rate at initial implantation, generally too high a slew rate in association with a low-amplitude signal, and segmentation of the signal (i.e., the signal changes polarity abruptly in multiple steps, yielding many segments, each of which has too small an amplitude to exceed sensing threshold).[29] In these circumstances, repositioning the lead to obtain more adequate intrinsic signals is the best approach. Although exchange for a higher sensitivity pacemaker may be contemplated, this technique is frequently associated with interference problems.

The most common cause of sensing failure is inadequate electrode-surface contact. This results from electrode displacement. The major causes for loss of electrode position include: inadequate anchoring at the time of implant, abnormal tension on the leads where secured in the pocket, myocardial perforation, and Twiddler's syndrome. Finally, loss of sensing can result from defects in the sensing circuitry (e.g., mismatch of load impedance and sensing circuit input impedance, increased lead impedance due to lead fracture, and intrinsic failure of the sensing circuitry).

To maximize the sensing capability of the pacer's input circuit and minimize sensing failure a number of design modifications can be made to enhance R-wave signal transmission and filter out noise and far-field or extraneous signals. As Furman and colleagues[27] indicate, ideally the sensing threshold of the input circuit should be reduced to a level of approximately 2 mv, which would allow for sensing almost all atrial and ventricular electrograms. Second, the frequency response of the input circuit should be adjusted to a narrow bandpass of approximately 10 to 40 Hz, thus passing unattenuated the intrinsic deflection of the R and P wave and filtering out the T wave and any high-frequency noise components. Finally, the sensing circuit input impedance should be adjusted to be at least two orders of magnitude greater than the lead impedance, so that the myocardial signal is not unduly attenuated by the voltage divider effect of the input circuit configuration.

REFERENCES

1. Hoffman BF, and Cranefield PF: Electrophysiology of the Heart. Mt. Kisco, Futura, 1976, pp. 211–256.
2. Jenerick HP, and Gerard RW: Membrane potential and threshold of single muscle fibres. J Cell Comp Physiol 42:79, 1953.
3. Hodgkin AL: The Croonian lecture: Ionic movements and electrical activity in giant nerve fibres. Proc R Soc Lond 148:1, 1958.
4. Hodgkin AL: Evidence for electrical transmission in nerve. J Physiol (Lond) 90:183, 1937.
5. Hodgkin AL: The ionic basis of electrical activity in nerve and muscle. Biol Rev 26:339, 1951.
6. Weidmann S: Effect of current flow on the membrane potential of cardiac muscle. J Physiol (Lond) 115:227, 1951.
7. Weidmann S: The electrical constants of purkinje fibres. J Physiol (Lond) 118:348, 1952.
8. Jack JJB, Noble D, and Tsien RN: Electric Current Flow in Excitable Cells. Oxford, Clarendon Press, 1975.
9. Orias O, Brooks MCC, Suckling EE, et al: Excitability of the mammalian ventricle throughout the cardiac cycle. Am J Physiol 163:272, 1950.
10. Furman S, Parker B, and Escher DJW: Decreasing electrode size and increasing efficiency of cardiac stimulation. J Surg Res 11:105, 1971.
11. Weidmann S: The effect of the cardiac membrane potential on the rapid availability of the sodium-carrying system. J Physiol (Lond) 127:213, 1955.
12. Sowton E, and Barr I: Physiologic changes in threshold. Ann NY Acad Sci 167:679, 1969.
13. Preston TA, Fletcher RD, Lucchesi BR, and Judge RD: Changes in myocardial threshold. Physiologic and pharmacologic factors in patients with implanted pacemakers. Am Heart J 74:235, 1967.
14. Davies JG, and Sowton E: Electrical threshold of the human heart. Brit Heart J 28:231, 1966.
15. Tyers GF, Brownlee RR, Hughes HC Jr, et al: Myocardial stimulation impedance: The effects of electrode, physiologic, and stimulus variables. Ann Thorac Surg 27:63, 1979.
16. Mansfield PB: Myocardial stimulation: The electrochemistry of electrode-tissue coupling. Am J Physiol 212(6):1475, 1967.
17. Barrold SS, Ong LS, and Heinle RA: Stimulation and sensing thresholds for cardiac placing: Electrophysiologic and technical aspects. Prog Cardiovasc Dis 24:1, 1981.
18. Preston TA, Fletcher RD, and Lucchesi BR: Changes in myocardial threshold: Physiologic and pharmacologic factors in patients with implanted pacemakers. Am Heart J 74:235, 1967.
19. Irnich W, Parsonnet V, and Myers GH: Compendium of pacemaker technology. II. Definitions and Glossary. Part I. PACE 2:88, 1977.
20. Tarjan PP: Engineering aspects of implantable cardiac pacemakers. *In* Samet P (ed): Cardiac Pacing. Grune and Stratton, New York, 1973, p. 54.
21. Furman S, Parker B, and Escher DJW: Decreasing electrode size and increasing efficiency of cardiac stimulation. J Surg Res 11:105, 1971.
22. Barold SS, and Winner JA: Techniques and significance of threshold measurements for cardiac pacing. Relationship to output circuit of cardiac pacemakers. Chest 70:760, 1976.

23. Fontaine G, Kevorkian M, and Welti JJ: Comparison between endocardial versus myocardial and unipolar versus bipolar thresholds after long-term pacing. *In* Cardiac Pacing: Proceedings of the 4th International Symposium. VanGorcum, Assen, 1973, p. 304.
24. Amundsen DC: Sensing properties of pacemaker electrodes. Proc Engl Med Bio 17:83, 1975.
25. Myers GH, Kresh YM, and Parsonnet V: Characteristics of intracardiac electrograms. PACE 1:90, 1978.
26. Barold SS: Current problems with demand pacemakers. Eur J Cardiol 1:339, 1974.
27. Furman S, Hurzeler P, and DeCaprio P: Cardiac pacing and pacemakers. III. Sensing the cardiac electrogram. Am Heart J 93:794, 1977.
28. Ohm OJ: Inhibition/filter characteristics and input impedances of QRS-inhibited demand pacemakers determined by in vitro studies. PACE 3:318, 1980.
29. Furman S, Hurzeler P, and DeCaprio V: The ventricular endocardial electrogram and pacemaker sensing. J Thorac Cardiovasc Surg 73:258, 1977.

4

Hemodynamics of Pacing

A-HAMID HAKKI, M.D.,
and ABDULMASSIH S. ISKANDRIAN, M.D.

With the recent giant strides in pacemaker technology and with the large numbers of patients requiring pacemakers, today more than ever it is necessary to understand the changes in cardiac performance induced by pacing. During the past 20 years extensive experimental and clinical work has been carried out to evaluate the metabolic and hemodynamic changes induced by cardiac pacing.[1–38] Assessment of ventricular performance during atrial, ventricular, or atrioventricular (AV) sequential pacing has been performed using invasive hemodynamic measurements and contrast angiography, and more recently, noninvasive echocardiography and radionuclide ventriculography (Table 4–1). The last method is particularly suited for this purpose, since it permits measurement of left ventricular regional function, global function, and volume.

When interpreting the hemodynamic alterations induced by pacing, factors such as patient population, the site of pacing, heart rate during pacing, patient position, and effect of medications should be taken into consideration. Thus hemodynamic changes in patients with coronary artery disease are different from those in normal subjects.[1–2] Also, the hemodynamics of atrial and AV sequential pacing may be different from that of ventricular pacing, especially in patients with coronary heart disease, since a properly timed atrial systole enhances ventricular function,[3–5] particularly in patients with compromised left ventricular function and in patients with impaired diastolic distensibility of the left ventricle.

Atrial pacing results in gradual prolongation of PR interval until Wenckebach AV block appears.[6, 7] In many patients the development of AV block appears to be the limiting factor during pacing.

$M\dot{V}O_2$ is dependent upon left ventricular size, systolic pressure, heart rate, and intropic condition of the ventricle.[8, 9] Pacing results in a decrease in end-diastolic and end-systolic volumes and usually in insignificant change in systemic pressure.[10, 11] Therefore, the overall change in $M\dot{V}O_2$ will depend on relative changes in heart rate, volume, and intropic state. Development of myocardial ischemia in patients with coronary artery disease during pacing is probably the net result of the increase in $M\dot{V}O_2$ (due to tachycardia), which exceeds the decrease in $M\dot{V}O_2$ as a result of decrease in ventricular size.

Table 4–1. Advantages and Disadvantages of Cardiac Pacing

Advantages of Pacing
Permits rapid termination of pacing (ischemia)
Enables measurement of pulmonary artery pressure and cardiac output
Permits measurement of ejection fraction and wall motion abnormalities when combined with radionuclide angiography
Can be particularly suitable for patients with peripheral vascular disease or physical disability
Can be performed during routine diagnostic catheterization
Disadvantages of Pacing
Invasive—requires insertion of catheters

Myocardial ischemia (imbalance between the supply and demand ratio) results in changes in systolic and diastolic function of the left ventricle[39] and is manifested by angina, ST depression, changes in ejection fraction, wall motion abnormalities, elevation in left ventricular end-diastolic pressure, wedge pressure, pulmonary artery pressure, lactate production, and arrhythmias. If it is severe and global, it may result in a decrease in cardiac output and hypotension. Some patients may develop mitral regurgitation due to papillary muscle dysfunction.

It should be noted that normally the left ventricular end-diastolic pressure decreases[10] with pacing because of a decrease in end-diastolic volume; thus if the left ventricular end-diastolic pressure fails to decrease or if it increases, this represents an abnormal response.[2] Some patients with coronary artery disease who respond with a decrease in left ventricular end-diastolic pressure with pacing demonstrate an overshoot phenomenon upon sudden cessation of pacing.[12] This is most likely because of aggravation of myocardial ischemia due to a sudden increase in end-diastolic volume, which raises $M\dot{V}\dot{O}_2$.

Radionuclide ventriculography is an extremely useful method for evaluating cardiac performance during pacing,[13, 14] since it makes assessment of biventricular function possible. Recently several laboratories described and validated methods not only for measuring ejection fraction but also for measuring end-diastolic volume, end-systolic volume, systolic volume, and cardiac output by either first-pass[40, 41] or gated equilibrium radionuclide angiogram.[42] Each method has advantages and disadvantages, and detailed analyses of these methods are beyond the scope of this presentation. The reader may refer to one of many excellent publications about this topic.[40–43]

In this presentation we will summarize some of the work carried out with atrial pacing in normal subjects and in patients with coronary artery disease.

LEFT VENTRICULAR PERFORMANCE IN NORMAL SUBJECTS

Ross and colleagues[15] studied 17 normal subjects with right atrial pacing and demonstrated no change in the cardiac index with the stepwise increase in heart rate between 80 and 121 beats per minute. This indicated a reduction in stroke volume with increases in heart rate. At heart rates of 148, a small reduction in the cardiac index was observed. In addition to the reduction in stroke volume there was a decrease in left ventricular ejection period and in the left ventricular ejection rate. The role of the heart rate in the hemodynamic response to exercise was examined in 7 patients who performed supine exercises while the heart rate was held constant by atrial pacing at rates comparable to those occurring spontaneously during exercise. These patients demonstrated an increase in both cardiac index and stroke volume. Furthermore, isoproterenol infusion in 5 patients resulted in an increase in cardiac index and heart rate but inconsistent alterations in stroke volume. When the heart rate was subsequently held constant by electrical stimulation at a level previously attained during isoproterenol infusion, reinfusion resulted in similar augmentation of the cardiac index—an increase entirely mediated by an increase in stroke volume. These studies indicate that in the absence of augmented metabolic requirements, homeostatic mechanisms maintain the cardiac output relatively constant, despite marked changes in heart rate. When metabolic demands are increased by muscular exercise or catecholamines, however, the cardiac output will increase by an increase in stroke volume, even when alterations in heart rate are prevented.

Samet and colleagues[3] studied 20 subjects without demonstrable heart disease with atrial and ventricular pacing at rates varying between 60 and 140 beats per minute. They demonstrated that the cardiac index during atrial pacing was significantly greater than during ventricular pacing. They concluded that the atrial contribution to ventricular function is significant even in normal subjects. These authors later demonstrated the similarity between the hemodynamics of AV sequential pacing and atrial pacing.[4, 5]

Benchimol and Leggitt[16] studied eight normal subjects using right atrial and right ventricular pacing at heart rates between 80 and 180 beats per minute. They demonstrated that for any given rate of atrial or ventricular pacing there was no significant difference in cardiac index, stroke volume index, mean blood pressure, or systolic ejection time. These results indicated that the contribution of atrial systole to cardiac function was minimal in these normal subjects. These authors then compared right ventricular to left ventricular pacing in three normal subjects at heart rates varying between 80 and 180 beats per minute and found no significant change in cardiac index, stroke volume index, mean blood pressure, stroke work, or ejection time—regardless of the site of pacing.

Linhart and colleagues[2] performed atrial pacing in 10 normal subjects who presented with atypical chest pain and demonstrated decreases in both the left ventricular end-diastolic pressure and stroke volume but no significant change in either the cardiac output or the systemic blood pressure.

Parker and colleagues[17] found no change in myocardial lactate utilization during atrial pacing in two normal subjects. As in previous studies, these patients demonstrated a decrease in the left ventricular end-diastolic pressure and no change in the cardiac index.

Befeler and colleagues[18] studied the effect of posture in 4 normal subjects during atrial and ventricular pacing at heart rates varying from 101 to 120 beats per minute. They concluded that atrial contribution to ventricular performance is important in both supine and upright positions. Parker and colleagues[1] performed right atrial pacing in 21 normal subjects and found no significant change in the cardiac output, whereas the stroke volume decreased as an inverse function of the pacing rate. They demonstrated that left ventricular end-diastolic pressure decreases with increasing heart rate. Their data and those of others emphasize the importance of considering the heart rate when interpreting changes in the left ventricular end-diastolic pressure.

Dwyer[10] studied left ventricular function, pressure-volume relationship, and wall motion using sequential cineventriculography in 3 normal subjects. At mean pacing heart rates of 117 beats per minute there was no change in the cardiac index and systolic blood pressure, a decrease in left ventricular end-diastolic pressure and end-diastolic volume, and no significant change in the ejection fraction.

DeMaria and colleagues[19] measured changes in chamber dimensions by echocardiography in 25 normal subjects during atrial pacing with heart rates varying between 50 and 150 beats per minute. They demonstrated a decrease in the left ventricular end-diastolic dimension and the end-systolic dimension without change in the shortening fraction. In addition, they demonstrated a decrease in left atrial dimension with increased pacing rate, which reached a plateau at rates of equal to or greater than 120 beats per minute.

Recently, Hung and colleagues[20] performed equilibrium gated radionuclide ventriculography in 20 patients who had normal ventricular function but had had surgery for recurrent supraventricular tachycardia. Atrial pacing at rates of 120, 140, and 160 beats per minute was performed in 10 patients. In the other 10 patients, sequential AV pacing was performed and compared with simultaneous ventricular and atrial pacing at rates of 100 and 160 beats per minute. They demonstrated no significant change in the left ventricular ejection fraction with atrial pacing, despite a progressive decrease in the end-diastolic volume. During simultaneous ventricular and atrial pacing at 160 beats per minute, the reduction in the end-diastolic and stroke volumes was greater than with sequential AV pacing, as a result of the loss of atrial transport mechanisms. They concluded that the hemodynamic consequences of supraventricular tachycardia in patients with normal ventricular function were primarily a result of a decrease in the ventricular volume as the heart rate increased and the loss of atrial contribution, rather than a result of any change in left ventricular ejection fraction.

In our laboratory we studied eight normal subjects at rest and during coronary sinus pacing (Table 4–2; Fig. 4–1). We monitored changes in pulmonary artery pressure and cardiac output by a Swan-Ganz thermodilution catheter and measured ejection fraction by first-pass radionuclide ventriculography using a computerized multicrystal camera. The method and its validation have been described previously from our laboratory.[41] With atrial pacing there was no change in pulmonary artery pressure, aortic pressure, or cardiac index. There was no significant change in ejection fraction, despite an increase in heart rate

Table 4–2. Hemodynamic Data at Rest and During Pacing in Normal Subjects

	Control	Pacing	p Value (C vs. P)
HR	72 ± 8	123 ± 11	<0.001
$(\overline{PA})$	16 ± 5	16 ± 6	NS
$(\overline{AO})$	96 ± 7	101 ± 5	NS
CI	3.2 ± 0.6	3.3 ± 0.6	NS
EDVI	79 ± 13	47 ± 8	<0.001
ESVI	35 ± 6	21 ± 5	<0.001
EF	54 ± 3	56 ± 5	NS

Abbreviations: C = control; P = pacing; HR = heart rate (beats/min); $(\overline{PA})$ = mean pulmonary artery pressure (mm Hg); $(\overline{AO})$ = mean aortic pressure (mm Hg); CI = cardiac index (L/min/M^2); EDVI = end-diastolic volume index (ml/M^2); ESVI = end-systolic volume index (ml/M^2); EF = ejection fraction (percent); NS = not significant; EDVI and ESVI are derived from the thermodilution and radionuclide angiographic measurements. (From Iskandrian AS, Hakki AH, Bemis CE, et al.: Am J Cardiol 51:1057, 1983.)

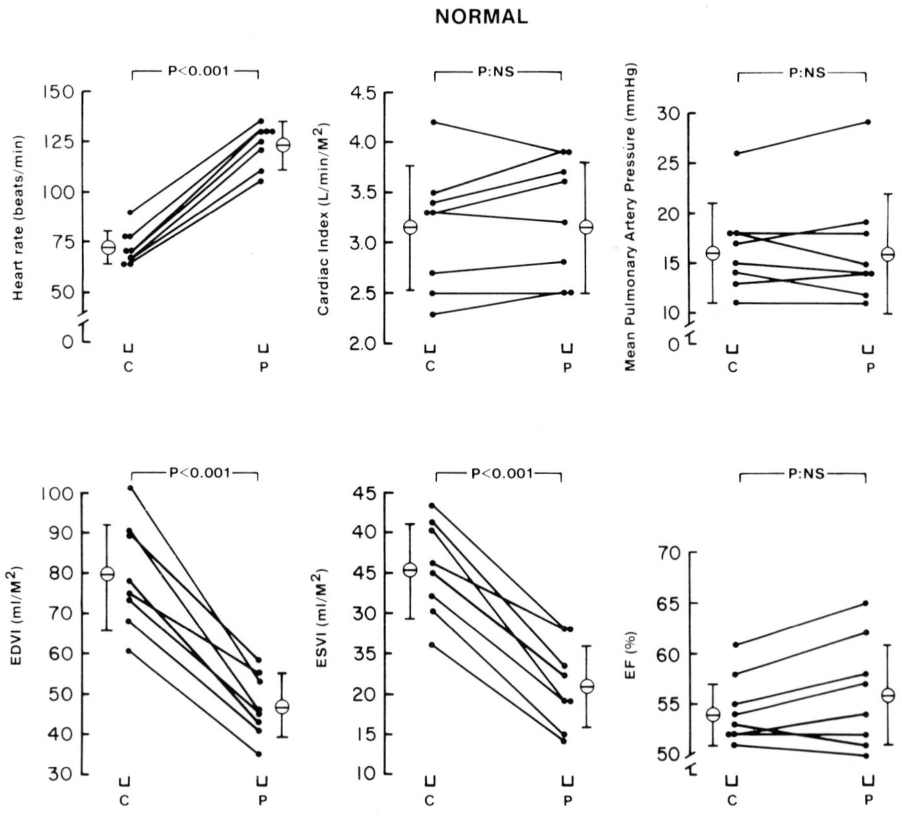

Figure 4–1. Hemodynamic and radionuclide ventriculographic data in normal subjects at rest (C) and during coronary sinus pacing (P).

Table 4–3. Hemodynamic Changes During Exercise in Normal Subjects

	Rest	Exercise	p Value
EF	61 ± 60	73 ± 5.0	<0.001
EDVI	77 ± 13	86 ± 17	NS
ESVI	30 ± 9	24 ± 9	NS
CI	3.8 ± 0.6	9.4 ± 2.0	<0.001
HR	79 ± 11	157 ± 14	<0.001
SBP	130 ± 13	188 ± 24	<0.001
Ex. Load (kpm/min)	—	700 ± 200	—
Ex. Duration	—	9.9 ± 2.8	—

Abbreviations: EF = ejection fraction (%); CI = cardiac index (L/min/M^2); HR = heart rate (beats/min); SBP = systolic blood pressure (mm Hg); Ex. = exercise; NS = not significant; EDVI = end-diastolic volume index (ml/M^2); ESVI = end-systolic volume index (ml/M^2); ESVI and EDVI are derived from radionuclide angiographic measurements.

and a decrease in end-diastolic volume. This is in contrast to the increase in ejection fraction during exercise in normal subjects[41] (Table 4–3). There were significant decreases in end-diastolic volume and end-systolic volume during pacing. Volume measurements in our study were derived using two methods. In the first we used the radionuclide ejection fraction and thermodilution stroke volume, thus avoiding the use of a geometric assumption for measuring volumes. In the second method, the end-diastolic volume was calculated by radionuclide angiography using the area-length method of Dodge and colleagues.[44] The two methods correlated quite well in measuring the end-diastolic and end-systolic volumes. The ratio of aortic systolic pressure to end-systolic volume increased significantly with rapid pacing. This may indicate improvement in contractility. Enhanced inotropic function has previously been reported by other investigators.[19, 21, 22] None of our normal subjects complained of chest pain or developed wall motion abnormalities during pacing.

PATIENTS WITH CORONARY ARTERY DISEASE

Atrial pacing has been used diagnostically in patients with coronary artery disease, particularly in those in whom exercise testing is contraindicated or not feasible (e.g., patients with peripheral vascular disease). Sowton and colleagues[23] introduced the technique of atrial pacing to measure angina threshold in patients with coronary artery disease. They were able to induce angina pectoris in 17 of 22 patients at a mean pacing rate of 117 beats per minute. In patients with pacing-induced angina there was no change in the cardiac output (as determined by dye-dilution technique), but as expected there was a decrease in the stroke volume. There was also a modest increase in the mean aortic pressure and a decrease in stroke work. These authors described a threshold level of pressure

× rate (which reflects myocardial oxygen consumption) above which angina pectoris occurred.

Linhart and colleagues[24] studied 16 patients with coronary artery disease and induced angina pectoris by atrial pacing in 9. The hemodynamic changes were different in patients who developed angina compared with patients in whom neither angina nor ST depression was induced by pacing. Thus in the latter group there was a decrease in the left ventricular end-diastolic pressure, a decrease in the stroke volume, and no significant change in the blood pressure or cardiac output. In the 9 patients with pacing-induced angina there was either an elevation or no change in the left ventricular end-diastolic pressure, inconsistent change in the blood pressure, and a slight increase in the cardiac output in some patients. These authors also demonstrated that ST depression occurred prior to the onset of chest pain. Ischemic chest pain was relieved, and the EKG changes normalized with either elimination of atrial pacing or the administration of sublingual nitroglycerin. In some patients, abnormal hemodynamic responses were elicited even in the absence of angina pectoris.

Parker and colleagues[17] measured myocardial lactate metabolism in 21 patients with coronary artery disease during atrial pacing. Lactate production by the myocardium was demonstrated in 13 of the 17 patients with pacing-induced angina and ST-segment depression. It should be noted that normally the myocardium extracts lactate. In the patients in whom angina was not induced by pacing, the hemodynamic changes were similar to those observed in normal subjects, with a decrease in the left ventricular end-diastolic pressure, which remained normal upon termination of pacing. On the other hand, patients with pacing-induced angina may have an initial decrease in the left ventricular end-diastolic pressure with pacing, but upon cessation of pacing the left ventricular end-diastolic pressure rises abruptly over two to three beats. The increase in end-diastolic pressure upon termination of pacing is thought to reflect myocardial ischemia as a result of a sudden increase in end-diastolic volume resulting in increase in $M\dot{V}\dot{O}_2$. There was no significant change in the cardiac index during atrial pacing in these patients.

Dwyer[10] studied 10 patients with coronary artery disease, 9 of whom had sustained previously documented transmural myocardial infarction. Sequential cineventriculography was performed during atrial pacing. Myocardial ischemia manifested by angina was induced in 7 patients and was characterized by marked ST-segment changes in 3. There was no demonstrable change in cardiac index or systolic blood pressure with pacing. The changes in left ventricular end-diastolic pressure were variable: there was an increase in 4, a decrease in 5, and no change in 1 patient. On the other hand, left ventricular end-diastolic volume decreased in 9 of 10 patients, although the magnitude of reduction was less when compared to normal subjects. Eight of 10 patients had a decrease in ejection fraction with pacing associated with regional wall motion abnormalities.

Pasternac and colleagues[25] performed left ventricular cineangiograms in 10 patients with coronary artery disease during incremental atrial pacing. In 8 patients, left ventricular asynergy occurred during pacing in the distribution of obstructed coronary vessels. The left ventricular end-diastolic volume decreased irrespective of the development of asynergy, but ejection fraction decreased markedly in patients with pacing-induced asynergy. There was no significant change in the left ventricular end-diastolic pressure and cardiac index.

Recently, Stone and colleagues[13] studied ventricular function using contrast and radionuclide angiography in 13 patients with coronary artery disease who developed angina during pacing. There was a decrease in the ejection fraction and wall motion abnormalities during pacing in most of the patients.

Both atrial pacing and exercise testing have been valuable in the evaluation of patients with angina pectoris and provide a wealth of diagnostic and prognostic information. Although these methods of stressing the heart have been used extensively, only a few studies compared the two methods in the same patient population. Thus Bahler and MacLeod[12] determined anginal threshold by atrial pacing in 23 patients with coronary artery disease. Twelve of those patients also performed supine exercises at progressively higher workloads until the onset of angina. The heart rate was higher in pacing-induced angina compared with exercise-induced angina. The cardiac output during exercise was higher than during pacing. The left ventricular end-diastolic pressure during exercise was higher compared with that during pacing; however, assumption of the feet-up position during supine exercise alone produced an increase in left ventricular end-diastolic pressure in 10 of 12 exercising subjects. With exercise, further increase in left ventricular end-diastolic pressure occurred with the development of angina. Similarly, left ventricular stroke work and minute work were higher during exercise than during pacing. These authors demonstrated that pacing rate at the onset of angina had little correlation with the angiographic severity of coronary artery disease. This is in contrast to the good correlation between external workload producing angina pectoris during exercise and the severity of coronary artery disease.

Keleman and colleagues[26] compared the symptomatic and EKG responses to graded maximal exercise treadmill testing and atrial pacing in 49 patients with severe coronary artery disease and in 25 normal subjects. One patient and one normal subject underwent atrial pacing but were not exercised. They demonstrated that occurrence of chest pain during maximal exercise testing or right atrial pacing was an excellent indicator of obstructive coronary artery disease. On the other hand, pacing-induced ischemic ST-segment depression was an unreliable indicator of the presence of arteriographic obstructive coronary disease, with 26 percent false-negative and 60 percent false-positive results.

Slutsky and colleagues[14] evaluated left ventricular function using equilibrium radionuclide angiography during atrial pacing in 12 patients with coronary artery disease and found a significant decrease in ejection fraction and end-diastolic volume with pacing except for those patients who experienced angina during pacing, in whom the volume increased. Several studies have indicated that atrial pacing by maintaining atrial contribution to ventricular filling results in better hemodynamics than does ventricular pacing. On the other hand, the site of ventricular pacing, whether from the right ventricle or the left ventricle, did not appear to be important in the resultant hemodynamic changes.

We obtained hemodynamic data in patients with angina pectoris secondary to coronary artery disease (defined as 70 percent or more diameter narrowing of one or more coronary vessels by coronary arteriography). Tables 4–4 and 4–5 demonstrate the hemodynamic changes with pacing in comparison with changes with exercise in two different groups of patients. Nine patients had one-vessel disease, 6 patients had two-vessel disease, and 5 had three-vessel disease. Angina pectoris or ST-segment depression (or both) developed during pacing in 13 patients (65 percent). There was no significant change in the cardiac index with pacing. There was an increase in the mean pulmonary artery pressure (an indicator of left ventricular filling pressure) and the mean aortic pressure in our patients with coronary artery disease. The left ventricular ejection fraction (measured by first-pass radionuclide ventriculography) decreased with pacing in most patients who had angina or ST-segment depression (Fig. 4–2). In some patients, a slight increase in ejection fraction was seen with submaximal pacing followed by a decrease with maximal pacing (Figs. 4–3 and 4–4).

The end-diastolic volume and end-systolic volume decreased with pacing in patients with coronary artery disease. Similar findings occurred when radionuclide-derived volume measurements were used. The decrease in end-diastolic volume is a continuous one. This is demonstrated in 13 patients who had hemodynamic measurements at two pacing rates (Fig. 4–3). Left ventricular volume changes during pacing in patients with coronary artery disease are similar in direction to changes in normal patients (Fig. 4–5).

THE EFFECT OF ATRIAL PACING ON MYOCARDIAL BLOOD FLOW

The clinical syndrome of angina pectoris has long been attributed to a disparity between the amount of oxygen delivered to the myocardium by the coronary blood supply and the requirements of the cardiac muscle for oxygen. In order to study the adequacy of coronary blood flow in patients with angina pectoris, Schmidt and colleagues[27] used ^{133}Xenon and a multiple-crystal scintillation camera to quantitate myocardial capillary blood flow in different regions of the heart. They performed atrial pacing in 24 patients with coronary artery disease and in 24 patients with minimal or no coronary artery disease. With increments in heart rate and the double product induced by pacing, patients with coronary artery disease had a less-pronounced increase in left ventricular myocardial blood flow and a significantly lesser decline in coronary vascular resistance compared to patients with no coronary arterial obstruction. In other words, there was a lower increment in the mean left ventricular perfusion per increment of the double product in patients with significant coronary artery disease. They suggested that in their patients with coronary artery disease, angina pectoris resulted when obstructive coronary lesions restricted the total or regional myocardial blood flow response to an increased rate of myocardial oxygen consumption.

Table 4–4. Hemodynamic Data at Rest and During Pacing in Patients with Coronary Artery Disease

	CAD (N = 30)			CAD (N = 13)			p Value		
	Control	*Pacing*	*p Value (C vs. P)*	*Control*	*Pacing$_1$*	*Pacing$_2$*	*C vs. P_1*	*C vs. P_2*	*P_1 vs. P_2*
HR	70 ± 12	126 ± 13	<0.001	68 ± 10	99 ± 5	129 ± 9	<0.001	<0.001	<0.001
$\overline{PA}$	17 ± 5	21 ± 8	<0.01	19 ± 4	19 ± 5	25 ± 8	NS	<0.02	<0.05
$\overline{AO}$	102 ± 10	113 ± 14	<0.001	105 ± 8	113 ± 13	118 ± 13	<0.02	<0.01	NS
CI	2.8 ± 0.4	2.9 ± 0.6	NS	2.9 ± 0.4	3.2 ± 0.5	3.0 ± 0.6	<0.01	NS	NS
EDVI	90 ± 28	58 ± 22	<0.001	97 ± 27	72 ± 25	61 ± 25	<0.001	<0.001	<0.05
ESVI	49 ± 21	36 ± 21	<0.001	53 ± 20	40 ± 21	39 ± 24	<0.001	<0.01	NS
EF	48 ± 9	43 ± 11	<0.05	46 ± 7	47 ± 10	43 ± 13	NS	NS	NS

Abbreviations: CAD = coronary artery disease; P_1 = submaximal pacing; P_2 = maximal pacing; CAD (N = 30) column includes the maximal pacing measurements in 20 patients; CAD (N = 13) column includes the 13 patients shown in the center columns. The CAD (N = 30) columns include the remaining 7 patients who had one level of pacing. C = control; P = pacing; HR = heart rate (beats/min); $\overline{PA}$ = mean pulmonary artery pressure (mm Hg); $\overline{AO}$ = mean aortic pressure (mm Hg); CI = cardiac index (L/min/M^2); EF = ejection fraction (percent); EDVI = end-diastolic volume index (ml/M^2); ESVI = end-systolic volume index (ml/M^2); EDVI and ESVI are derived from the thermodilution and radionuclide angiographic measurements.

Table 4–5. Hemodynamic Changes During Exercise in 41 Patients with Coronary Artery Disease

	Rest	Exercise	p Value
EF	45 ± 14	43 ± 12	NS
EDVI	104 ± 43	117 ± 46	<0.05
ESVI	61 ± 42	69 ± 38	<0.05
CI	3.1 ± 1.2	5.9 ± 2.5	<0.001
HR	71 ± 12	128 ± 22	<0.001
	—	500 ± 180	—
	—	7.6 ± 2.8	—

Abbreviations: P = pacing; EF = ejection fraction (percent); CI = cardiac index (L/min/M^2); HR = heart rate (beats/min); EDVI = end-diastolic volume index (ml/M^2); ESVI = end-systolic volume index (ml/M^2); EDVI and ESVI are derived from radionuclide angiographic measurements.

Knoebel and colleagues[28] measured myocardial blood flow using ^{84}rubidium in ten patients with significant three-vessel coronary artery disease and in 6 patients without coronary artery disease. These determinations were measured at rest, with atrial pacing, and with atrial pacing plus nitroglycerin. There was a decrease in myocardial blood flow by 16 percent with pacing alone but an increase by 22 percent from pacing flows with additional sublingual nitroglycerin at the same pacing rate. They attributed their findings to a redistribution of blood flow, in which there is a decreased flow to the endocardium resulting in a

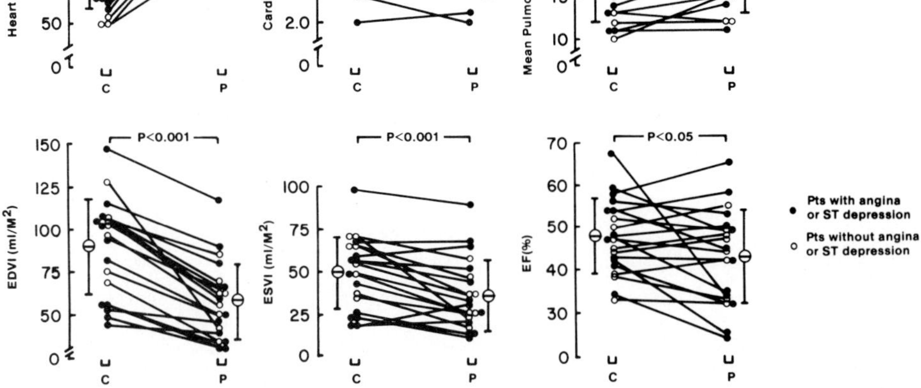

Figure 4–2. Hemodynamic and radionuclide ventriculographic data in patients with coronary artery disease at rest (C) and during coronary sinus pacing (P). Filled circles indicate the occurrence of angina or ST depression during pacing. Open circles indicate the absence of angina or ST depression.

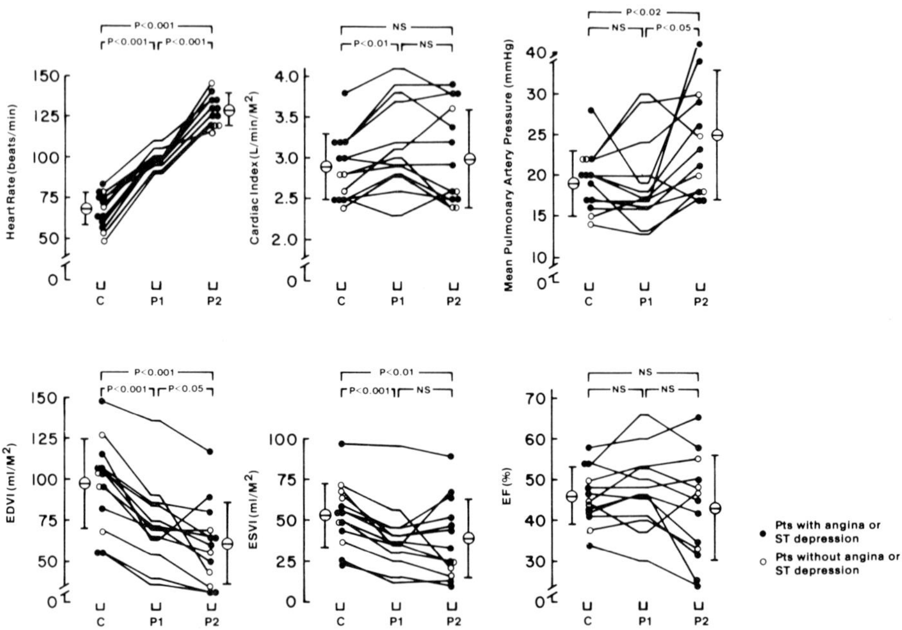

Figure 4–3. Hemodynamic and radionuclide ventriculographic data in patients with coronary artery disease at rest (C) and at submaximal (P) and maximal (P_2) pacing. Filled circles indicate the occurrence of angina or ST depression during pacing. Open circles indicate the absence of angina or ST depression.

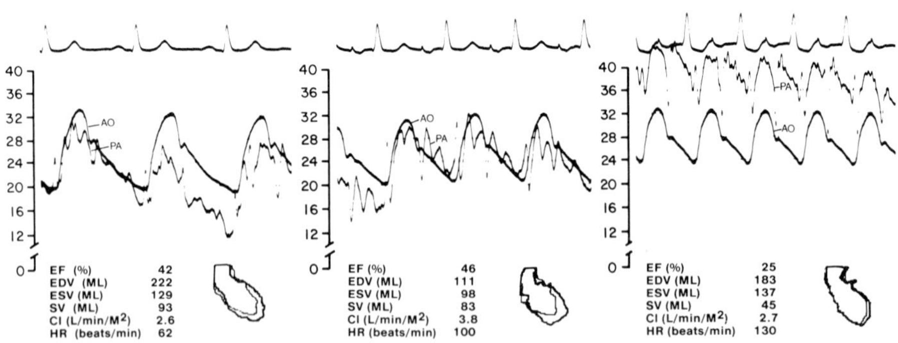

Figure 4–4. A patient with coronary artery disease demonstrating hemodynamic and radionuclide ventriculographic abnormalities at maximum (P_2) but not at submaximal (P_1) pacing. EF, ejection fraction; EDV, end-diastolic volume; ESV, end-systolic volume; SV, stroke volume; CI, cardiac index; HR, heart rate; AO, aortic pressure (mm Hg); PA, pulmonary artery pressure (mm Hg); C, control measurements.

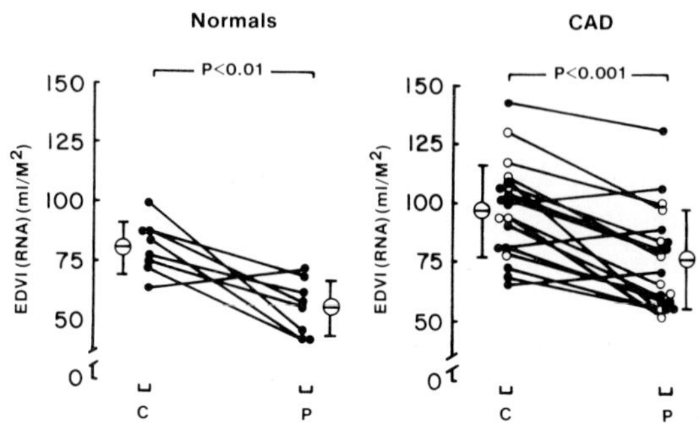

Figure 4–5. Changes in left ventricular end-diastolic volume index (EDVI) by radionuclide angiography (RNA) during coronary sinus pacing in normal subjects (normals) and in patients with coronary artery disease (CAD). C, control measurement; P, pacing.

decreased flow as measured by the uptake of ^{84}rubidium. Nitroglycerin, on the other hand, reduces cardiac work in addition to redistributing blood flow with an increase in the endocardial supply-to-demand ratio.

EXERCISE HEMODYNAMICS WITH FIXED VENTRICULAR RATE

The increased cardiac output observed during exercise is primarily the result of a two- to threefold increase in heart rate. Thus, in patients with complete AV block and in those patients who are dependent on a fixed-rate ventricular pacemaker, the response of the cardiac output to exercise will depend exclusively on changes in the stroke volume. Segel and colleagues[29] performed light supine bicycle exercises in 14 patients with complete AV block (13 with acquired and 1 with congenital heart block) and found an increase in the average cardiac index with widening of the $AV\dot{O}_2$ difference. These responses to exercise were subnormal however. In 2 of the 13 patients with acquired complete AV block the increase in cardiac output was caused by an increase in heart rate (despite a decrease in the stroke volume), whereas in the remaining 11 patients there was an increase in stroke volume (and cardiac output) but either no change or an increase in heart rate of less than 5 beats per minute.

SHORT-TERM AND LONG-TERM EFFECTS OF VENTRICULAR PACING

Of the 100,000 pacemakers implanted yearly worldwide, 86 percent are ventricle inhibited (VVI). The atrial synchronous ventricular pacemaker (VDD) permits an increase in ventricular rate as a response to acceleration of the SA node activity. Short-term studies have shown an increase in exercise capacity after changing from VVI to VDD pacing. In a recent study Kruse and colleagues[30] compared the acute and long-term effects of VVI and VDD pacing in 16 patients. There was an increase in working capacity of 24 percent with VDD pacing compared with VVI pacing. The cardiac output was higher during VDD pacing, particularly during exercise, because of the capability of heart rate increase and despite a substantial compensatory stroke volume increase during VVI pacing. The $A\dot{V}\dot{O}_2$ difference was higher during VVI compared to VDD. During exercise, arterial blood lactate was higher during VVI than during VDD pacing. These studies demonstrate the advantage of VDD over VVI pacing during both short-term and long-term follow-up.

CORONARY SINUS PACING

The coronary sinus provides an alternate method for atrial pacing, particularly in instances in which stability of the pacing electrodes is crucial. Befeler and colleagues[31] found similar hemodynamic response with coronary sinus pacing compared with right atrial pacing. Using both techniques, the cardiac output was consistently higher than that obtained using ventricular pacing.

EXPERIMENTAL STUDIES

Laurent and colleagues[32] studied the effects of heart rate on coronary flow and cardiac oxygen consumption. They measured coronary blood flow and cardiac oxygen consumption during right atrial pacing in 10 open-chest dogs. Sixty observations were made at heart rates between 77 and 310 beats per minute. They showed that coronary flow and cardiac oxygen consumption increased with a rise in heart rate. Heart rate is therefore an important factor in determining myocardial oxygen consumption at each level of cardiac work. An investigation of the intrinsic effects of heart rate on left ventricular performance was performed by Mitchell and colleagues.[33] They studied the effect of increasing heart rate on left ventricular performance in an areflexic dog's right heart bypass preparation. They showed that the left ventricle performed the same amount of stroke work over a wide range of heart rates without an increase in end-diastolic pressure, in spite of the markedly shortened time available for performing this work. This intrinsic adaptive response of the left ventricle was believed to be secondary to an intrinsic increase in contractility without an increase in end-diastolic fiber length, thus the term "homeometric" autoregulation. This is in contrast to the Frank Starling "heterometric" autoregulation, which is brought about by the beat-to-beat variation in end-diastolic fiber length.

The effect of tachycardia on coronary hemodynamics, myocardial metabolism, and coronary efficiency was investigated by Maxwell and colleagues.[34] These authors studied nine intact anesthetized dogs using right atrial pacing. They measured the cardiac output by the Fick principle and the coronary blood flow by the nitrous oxide method. At average heart rates of 193 beats per minute there was no significant change in cardiac output, although the stroke volume decreased significantly. With pacing there was a significant increase in coronary blood flow and a fall in coronary vascular resistance. Coronary flow per beat, however, was unchanged. Arterial and coronary sinus oxygen and carbon dioxide content did not vary, and there was no change in the cardiorespiratory quotient. In the face of tachycardia, the oxygen consumption per beat was unchanged. In summary, these investigators found that in intact anesthetized dogs a close relationship existed between coronary blood flow and heart rate induced by atrial pacing. Pacing resulted in an increase in coronary blood flow, cardiac oxygen consumption, and carbon dioxide production.

In order to elucidate the magnitude of enhancement of the inotropic state of the left ventricle induced by increases in heart rate, Mahler and colleagues[22] inserted left ventricular micromanometers and atrial pacing electrodes in 14 dogs. Endocardial ultrasonic diameter gauges were inserted in 5 animals. During steady-state pacing at rates of 158 beats per minute there was an increase in the left ventricular DP/DT, despite a marked decrease of the left ventricular end-diastolic pressure and diameter. Upon cessation of pacing, the peak DP/DT increased further above control, with an increase in the circumferential fiber shortening. Propranolol had no significant effect on these responses. These investigators concluded that in the conscious animal, the positive inotropic effect of increased frequency of contraction is most apparent after termination of the tachycardia, when the influence of decreased ventricular size on left ventricular performance is obviated.

REFERENCES

1. Parker JO, Khaja F, and Case RB: Analysis of left ventricular function by atrial pacing. Circulation 43:241, 1971.
2. Linhart JW: Myocardial function in coronary artery disease determined by atrial pacing. Circulation 44:203, 1971.
3. Samet P, Castillo C, and Bernstein WH: Hemodynamic consequences of atrial and ventricular pacing in subjects with normal hearts. Am J Cardiol 18:522, 1966.
4. Samet P, Castillo C, and Bernstein WH: Hemodynamic sequelae of atrial, ventricular and sequential atrioventricular pacing in cardiac patients. Am Heart J 72:725, 1966.
5. Samet P, Castillo C, and Bernstein WH: Hemodynamic consequences of sequential atrioventricular pacing in cardiac pacing. Am J Cardiol 21:207, 1968.
6. Lister JW, Stein E, Kosowsky BD, et al: Atrioventricular conduction in man: Effect of rate, exercise, isoproterenol and atropine on the PR interval. Am J Cardiol 16:516, 1965.
7. Massumi RA, Lee D, Ertena G, and Vera Z: Identification of the sites of atrioventricular conduction defects by means of His bundle electrocardiography and atrial pacing. *In* Schlart RC and Hurst JW (eds): Advances in Electrocardiography. New York, Grune and Stratton Inc, 1972, pp. 105–128.

8. Sarnoff SJ, Braunwald E, Welch GH Jr, et al: Hemodynamic determinants of oxygen consumption of the heart with special reference to the tension-time index. Am J Physiol 192:148, 1958.
9. Sonnenblick EH, Ross J Jr, Covell JW, and Braunwald E: Velocity of contraction as determinant of myocardial oxygen consumption. Am J Physiol 209:919, 1956.
10. Dwyer EM: Left ventricular pressure-volume alterations and regional disorders of contraction during myocardial ischemia induced by atrial pacing. Circulation 42:1111, 1970.
11. Slutsky R, Watkins J, Peterson K, and Karliner J: The response of left ventricular function and size to atrial pacing, volume, loading, and afterload stress in patients with coronary artery disease. Circulation 63:864, 1981.
12. Bahler RC, and Macleod CA: Atrial pacing and exercise in the evaluation of patients with angina pectoris. Circulation 43:407, 1971.
13. Stone D, Dymond D, Elliott AT, et al: Use of first-pass radionuclide ventriculography in assessment of wall motion abnormalities induced by incremental atrial pacing with coronary artery disease. Br Heart J 43:369, 1980.
14. Slutsky R, Watkins J, Peterson K, and Karliner J: The response of left ventricular function and size to atrial pacing, volume loading and afterload stress in patients with coronary artery disease. Circulation 63:864, 1981.
15. Ross J Jr, Linhart JW, and Braunwald E: Effects of changing heart rate in man by electrical stimulation of the right atrium. Circulation 32:549, 1965.
16. Benchimol A, and Liggett MS: Cardiac hemodynamics during stimulation of the right atrium, right ventricle, and left ventricle in normal and abnormal hearts. Circulation 33:933, 1966.
17. Parker JO, Chiong MA, West RO, et al: Sequential alterations in myocardial lactate metabolism, ST segments and left ventricular function during angina induced by atrial pacing. Circulation 40:113, 1969.
18. Befeler B, Cohen LS, Hildner FJ, et al: Atrial contribution to ventricular function in the sitting position. Chest 60:240, 1971.
19. DeMaria A, Neuman A, Schubart P, et al: Systematic correlation of cardiac chamber size and ventricular performance determined with echocardiography and alterations in heart rate in normal persons. Am J Cardiol 43:1, 1979.
20. Hung J, Kelly DT, Hutton BF, et al: Influence of heart rate and atrial transport on left ventricular volume and function: Relation to hemodynamic changes produced by supraventricular tachycardia. Am J Cardiol 48:632, 1981.
21. Ricci D, Orlick A, Alderman E, et al: Role of tachycardia as an inotropic stimulus in man. J Clin Invest 63:695, 1979.
22. Mahler F, Yoran C, and Ross J Jr: Inotropic effect of tachycardia and post-stimulation potentiation in the conscious dog. Am J Physiol 227:569, 1974.
23. Sowton E, Balcon R, Cross D, and Krick MH: Measurement of the anginal threshold using atrial pacing: A new technique for the study of angina pectoris. Cardiovasc Res 1:301, 1967.
24. Linhart JW, Hildner FJ, Barold SS, et al: Left heart hemodynamics during angina pectoris induced by atrial pacing. Circulation 40:483, 1969.
25. Pasternac A, Gorlin R, Sonnenblick EH, et al: Abnormalities of ventricular motion induced by atrial pacing in coronary artery disease. Circulation 45:1195, 1972.
26. Kelemen MH, Gillilan RE, Bouchard JR, et al: Diagnosis of obstructive coronary disease by maximal exercise and atrial pacing. Circulation 48:1227, 1973.
27. Schmidt DH, Weiss MB, Casarella WJ, et al: Regional myocardial perfusion during atrial pacing in patients with coronary artery disease. Circulation 53:807, 1976.
28. Knoebel SB, McHenry PL, Bonner AJ, and Phillips JF: Myocardial blood flow in coronary artery disease: Effect of right atrial pacing and nitroglycerin. Circulation 47:690, 1973.
29. Segel N, Hudson WA, Harris P, et al: The circulatory effects of electrically induced changes in ventricular rate at rest and during exercise in complete heart block. J Clin Invest 43:1541, 1964.
30. Kruse I, Arnman K, Conradson TB, and Ryden L: A comparison of the acute and long-term hemodynamic effects of ventricular inhibited and atrial synchronous ventricular inhibited pacing. Circulation 65:846, 1982.
31. Befeler B, Hildner FJ, Javier RP, et al: Cardiovascular dynamics during coronary sinus, right atrial, and right ventricular pacing. Am Heart J 81:372, 1971.
32. Laurent D, Bolene-Williams C, Williams FL, et al: Effects of heart rate on coronary flow and cardiac oxygen consumption. Am J Physiol 185:355, 1956.
33. Mitchell JH, Wallace AG, and Skinner NS Jr: Intrinsic effects of heart rate on left ventricular performance. Am J Physiol 205:41, 1963.

34. Maxwell GM, Castillo CA, White DH Jr, et al: Induced tachycardia: Its effect upon the coronary hemodynamics, myocardial metabolism and cardiac efficiency in the intact dog. J Clin Invest 37:1413, 1958.
35. Leighton RF, Zaron SJ, Robinson JL, et al: Effects of atrial pacing on left ventricular performance in patients with heart disease. Circulation 40:615, 1969.
36. DeSanctis RW: Diagnostic and therapeutic uses of atrial pacing. Circulation 43:748, 1971.
37. Benchimol A, Ellis JG, and Dimond EG: Hemodynamic consequences of atrial and ventricular pacing in patients with normal and abnormal hearts. Am J Med 39:911, 1965.
38. Rowe GG, Stenlund RR, Thomsen JH, et al: Coronary and systemic hemodynamic effects of cardiac pacing in man with complete heart block. Circulation 40:839, 1969.
39. Karliner JS, Peterson KL, and Ross J Jr: Left ventricular myocardial mechanics: systolic and diastolic function. *In* Grossman W (ed): Cardiac Catheterization and Angiography. Philadelphia, Lea and Febiger, 1980, pp. 245–267.
40. Rerych SK, Scholz PM, Newman GE, et al: Cardiac function at rest and during exercise in normals and in patients with coronary heart disease: Evaluation by radionuclide angiocardiography. Ann Surg 303:1404, 1978.
41. Iskandrian AS, Hakki A-H, Kane SA, and Segal BL: Quantitative radionuclide angiography in assessment of hemodynamic changes during upright exercise: Observations in normal subjects, patients with coronary artery disease and patients with aortic regurgitation. Am J Cardiol 48:239, 1981.
42. Strauss HW, Zaret BL, Hurley PJ, et al: A scintiphotographic method for measuring left ventricular ejection fraction in man without cardiac catheterization. Am J Cardiol 28:575, 1971.
43. Papapietro SE, Yester MV, Logic JR, et al: Method for quantitative analysis of regional left ventricular function with first-pass and gated blood pool scintigraphy. Am J Cardiol 47:618, 1981.
44. Dodge HT, Hay RE, and Sandler H: An angiocardiographic method for directly determining left ventricular stroke volume in man. Circ Res 11:739, 1962.

II

CLINICAL APPLICATIONS

5

Indications for Cardiac Pacing

JOSEPH R. CARVER, M.D.

INDICATIONS FOR PACING

It has been 30 years since Zoll introduced temporary cardiac stimulation for the emergency treatment of severe bradycardia and cardiac standstill.[1] Since then technological advances have led to therapeutic success and have generated enthusiasm for expanding the uses of pacemaker implantation beyond its initial use for heart rate support. Applications now include prevention and termination of tachycardia and bradycardia arrythmias and the provision of physiologic atrioventricular (AV) conduction for augmentation of cardiac output. In this review, the current indications for pacemaker implantation will be discussed.

Permanent Pacing

Acquired AV Block

In the infancy of artificial pacemakers, most units were implanted for complete heart block in which there was dissociation of atrial and ventricular activity. This must be distinguished from first-degree AV block, defined by prolonged AV conduction (PR interval greater than 200 msec), and from second-degree AV block (in which there is variable AV conduction either with [type I] or without [type II] progressive increments in AV conduction time). First-degree and type I AV blocks are benign, nonprogressive abnormalities because the site of block is intra-atrial or intranodal in the majority of patients, compared with type II second-degree and complete (third-degree) AV blocks, which are almost always the result of distal block in the His-Purkinje system. The presence of the former findings does not require intervention with a pacemaker, whereas the latter conditions should be paced regardless of whether the block is permanent or transient. Physicians should carefully examine patients with acute, high-degree AV bock, to rule out drug-induced (digitalis, verapamil), ischemia-induced (acute myocardial infarction), and metabolically induced (potassium balance, hypothyroidism) diseases.

Complete heart block was once thought to be secondary to ischemic heart disease in the majority of cases. It has become clear, however, that other diseases, including idiopathic fibrosis of the conduction system (Lev's and Lenegre's diseases), calcification resulting from aging or valvular disease or both, inflammatory myo- and endocarditis, metabolic disease (diabetes mellitus), infectious disease (syphilis, diphtheria), and collagen vascular disease contribute more frequently than other diseases to the development of high-degree AV bock.[2] Regardless of the cause, symptoms of abnormal impulse conduction most often take the form of dysfunction of the central nervous system and result in a decrease in cardiac output and cerebral perfusion. These symptoms range from vague complaints of light-headedness and dizziness to overt syncope (Stokes-Adams), convulsions, or transient ischemic attacks. Pacing with restoration (when AV block is permanent) or continuation (when AV block is intermittent) of an adequate ventricular rate abolishes symptoms when they are temporally related to a slow subsidiary cardiac pacemaker (below the sinoatrial [SA] node), improves hemodynamics, and hopefully prolongs life. Correlation of AV block with symptoms can be accomplished by routine EKG, prolonged Holter monitoring, transtelephonic monitoring with or without memory loops, or in the electrophysiology laboratory.

Symptomatic high-grade AV block is a clear, uncontested indication for pacing, but controversy continues to surround the use of pacing in the asymptomatic patient with intraventricular conduction delay manifested by bifascicular block (left anterior or posterior hemiblock with right bundle branch block) with or without PR interval prolongation—that is, the high-risk patient. While prophylactic pacing[3,4] or careful monitoring [5,6] in this population has been suggested, recent studies caution against implanting pacemakers prophylactically, since the risks of syncope and sudden death are low and, in most patients, heart block can be recognized and successfully treated once it is confirmed.[7] In the symptomatic, high-risk patient in whom type II or complete heart block is not documented with routine study, His bundle EKG and electrophysiologic studies should be performed.

Congenital AV Block

Congenital complete AV block may be isolated or associated with other congenital cardiac lesions.[8] A narrow complexed QRS (less than 100 msec) is usually associated with intranodal block, and in the absence of symptoms (similar to acquired intranodal block) no pacing is required. When associated with symptoms of diminished cardiac output that cannot be attributed to an associated lesion, these symptoms usually improve following pacemaker insertion. When the QRS is wide or the ventricular rate is slow (less than 40 beats per minute), an electrophysiologic study should be performed even in the asymptomatic individual, to determine the site of block (usually His-Purkinje system) and the integrity of "escape" pacemakers (junctional and beyond).

Surprisingly, it has been my experience and that of others[9] that this lesion is not benign and that the quality and duration of life can be improved dramatically with permanent pacing, especially when the normal sequence of AV contraction can be reestablished by dual-chamber physiologic pacing units.

Sick Sinus Syndrome

Replacing complete heart block as the major indication for pacing is the "wastebasket" diagnosis of sick sinus syndrome, in which impulse formation is impaired. It is manifested on EKG by sinus bradycardia, inappropriate sinus rhythm, post-tachycardia atrial or ventricular standstill, sinus arrest, SA block, bradycardia alternating with tachycardia, and atrial fibrillation with either a slow ventricular rate or with long pauses (greater than 3.5 seconds) in the absence of drug therapy. Symptoms similar to those associated with high-degree AV block result from loss of atrial contribution to ventricular filling, decreased diastolic ventricular filling, or the abrupt cessation of an effective cardiac output. When temporally correlated with any of the above rhythm disturbances these symptoms require permanent pacing. Individual discretion must be maintained for patients with vague symptoms that do not reliably coincide with rhythm disturbances and for asymptomatic patients in whom rhythm abnormalities are uncovered. When in doubt, electrophysiologic study can be used to guide the decision of whether or not to pace.

Sick sinus syndrome is commonly thought to occur as a result of aging and is uncommonly diagnosed in the young population. Recently Kay and colleagues[10] reviewed their experience by studying 18 young adults between 20 and 40 years old who, on the basis of long-term ambulatory EKG monitoring, showed evidence of symptomatic SA node dysfunction. They ruled out causes such as surgical damage to the SA node, previous viral illness, and familial predisposition to sick sinus syndrome by history; associated valve disease was ruled out by physical examination. Unlike trained athletes with physiologic bradycardia, all of Kay's patients were symptomatic with syncope, near-syncope, or light-headedness that abated after pacemaker placement. Thus a young age is not a contraindication to the diagnosis or treatment of the sick sinus syndrome.

A variant of the sick sinus syndrome is carotid sinus hypersensitivity manifested by syncope secondary to excessive vagal stimulation. Normally, either carotid sinus pressure or Valsalva's maneuver produces some slowing of the SA node discharge. In patients with an exaggerated response, sinus arrest or transient AV block occurs with loss or near-loss of consciousness. Symptoms are easily ameliorated by permanent pacing.

Tachyarrhythmias

Even as our knowledge of electrophysiology expands and we are guided by new and rational diagnostic methods, permanent pacing for tachycardia is becoming more widely accepted as a significant number of patients continue to be refractory to standard and investigational drugs. Pacing is now an accepted treatment choice for control of bradycardia when drugs for supraventricular tachycardia prevention induce symptomatic bradycardia, for prevention of drug-resistant supraventricular tachycardia, and for tachycardia resulting from brady-arrhythmias.[11] The last occurs because of maximal disparity of refractoriness favoring reentry during slow heart rates (rule of bigeminy).

Similarily, when tachycardia is followed by hemodynamic compromise that makes predicting the effects of various drugs potentially disastrous or when ventricular tachycardia occurs as an escape rhythm, permanent pacing for prevention is a logical therapeutic choice.

In addition, pacing can also be used to terminate an established tachycardia.[12] It has been shown consistently that a critically timed premature stimulus or stimuli can enter a reentrant pathway and interrupt a tachyarrythmia. A pacemaker supplying that stimulus to a predetermined "termination zone" (established in the electrophysiology laboratory) can be activated either manually with a magnet or automatically to terminate either supraventricular or ventricular tachycardia effectively, reliably, and consistently. A variety of pacing modes are presently available.[13]

Physiologic Pacing

A more recent development in pacing is the ability to maintain or reestablish physiologic conduction—that is, the normal AV sequence of contraction to maximize cardiac output using dual-chamber units with pacing or sensing in both chambers. Potential indications for use of these devices are low-output states (congestive heart failure), patients who decompensate with ventricular pacing,[14] and young active patients with normal atrial function who would benefit from the augmentation of cardiac output in proportion to atrial rate, enabling them to achieve a high level of physical activity.[15,16] These systems are more complex and expensive than single-chamber units, and complete hemodynamic and electrophysiologic studies should precede implantation.

Temporary Pacing

In general, indications for temporary pacing include any life-threatening arrhythmia or its precursor. These may be either primary (due to conduction system disease) or secondary to a correctable situation such as acute ischemia, digitalis excess, calcium- or β-blocking drugs, disorders of electrolytes or acid-base system, and thyroid disease. Secondary disorders generally require a brief period of pacing while the associated abnormalities are corrected with medical therapy.

Temporary pacing should precede a permanent unit whenever possible, to provide hemodynamic stability and allow the surgeon to achieve optimal electrode positioning for the permanent unit. This practice provides a brief delay, during which a correctable cause of the indication for pacing can be ruled out. It also permits the selection of those patients who require AV sequential units to provide the atrial contribution to ventricular filling to maintain cardiac output, blood pressure, or both. This added filling of the ventricle may conribute up to 30 percent of the total cardiac output. Those patients who thus decompensate with temporary pacing require either an atrial sequential or an atrial synchronous pacemaker system. We greatly encourage the use of temporary pacing, because in experienced hands it poses virtually no risk of mortality or morbidity but does provide multiple benefits.

Cardiac and Noncardiac Surgery

Another area in which pacing has paralleled technological growth is rate support in the perioperative period of bypass and valvular surgery. At our institution we routinely place temporary epicardial pacing wires at the time of open-heart surgery. This enables us to maintain AV conduction in postoperative patients with temporary suppression of the SA node (junctional rhythm) or AV nodal conduction (AV block) resulting from anesthesia, surgical manipulation, hypothermia, or medication. Similarly, cardiac output is often rate related in this period and can be maximized by atrial or AV sequential pacing at a rate faster than the intrinsic heart rate. Because these events are usually transient and self-limited, permanent pacing is seldom required. On the other hand, after repair of complex congenital lesions the conduction system is often irreversibly damaged, and permanent pacing is often necessary.[17]

We are often consulted regarding prophylactic placement of a temporary pacing wire in noncardiac surgical patients with chronic bifascicular block prior to general anesthesia and surgery. Recently it has become clearly evident that the risk of developing high-degree AV block is not influenced by the stress of surgery or anesthesia, and these chronic EKG abnormalities neither influence surgical morbidity or mortality nor require treatment.[18]

Acute Myocardial Infarction

In the presence of acute myocardial infarction, the following rhythm disturbances require temporary pacing:

1. Acute bifascicular block (left anterior or posterior hemiblock with right bundle branch block), acute left bundle branch block, or alternating bundle block regardless of infarct location.

2. Type II second-degree AV block or third-degree AV block in association with anterior wall myocardial infarction.

3. Symptomatic type II second-degree AV block or complete heart block in association with inferior wall myocardial infarction. Symptoms include hypotension, congestive heart failure, recurrent or persistent angina, or premature ventricular depolarizations.

4. Bradycardia of less than 45 beats per minute in the absence of drug suppression.

No pacing is required with asymptomatic sinus bradycardia, first-degree AV block,[19] or type I second-degree AV block,[20] or in the presence of myocardial infarction with preexisting bifascicular or bundle branch block.[21]

Much controversy surrounds the decision to place a permanent pacing unit in the peri–myocardial infarction period, because discordant studies in the literature either support[22] or refute[23] its benefits. A rational guideline is to pace survivors of high-degree AV block concomitant with acute myocardial infarction when they suffer the new onset of left bundle branch bock or bifascicular block.

Although it is clear that many of the above patients die of power failure or complex ventricular rhythm disturbances, the development of high-degree AV block is an independent predictor of sudden death, and prophylactic pacing eliminates this variable and should affect survival in a positive manner. A word of caution and individual judgment is necessary in recommending permanent pacing for the patient with profound congestive heart failure (Killip class III or IV).

No permanent pacing is required for the patient who develops the above-mentioned intraventricular block but does not proceed to manifest AV block during hospitalization.

CONCLUSIONS

We have presented an overview of indications for permanent and temporary pacing. The state of the science is relatively new, and further technological advances will most certainly continue to broaden those indications to encompass conditions unimaginable today and improve the quality and duration of life in the years to come.

REFERENCES

1. Zoll PM: Resuscitation of the heart in ventricular standstill by external electric stimulation. NEJM 247:768, 1952.
2. Lenegre J: Etiology and pathology of bilateral bundle branch block in relation to complete heart block. Prog Cardiovasc Dis 6:409, 1964.
3. Scheinman MN, Peters RW, Modin G, et al: Prognostic value of intranodal conduction time in patients with chronic bundle branch block. Circulation 53:240, 1977.
4. Vera Z, Mason DT, Fletcher RD, et al: Prolonged His-Q interlude in chronic bifascicular block: Relation to impending complete heart block. Circulation 53:47, 1976.
5. Peters RW, Scheinman MN, Modin G, et al: Prophylactic permanent pacemakers for patients with chronic bundle branch block. Am J Med 66:978, 1979.

6. Surawicz B: Prognosis of patients with chronic bifascicular block. Circulation 60:40, 1979.
7. McAnulty J: Natural history of "high-risk" bundle branch block. NEJM 307:137, 1982.
8. Nakamura FF and Nadas AS: Complete heart block in infants and children. NEJM 270:1261, 1964.
9. Besley DC, McWilliams GJ, Moodie DS, et al: Long-term follow-up of young adults following permanent pacemaker placement for complete heart block. Am Heart J 103:332, 1982.
10. Kay R, Estioko M, and Wiener I: Primary sick sinus syndrome as an indication for chronic pacemaker therapy in young adults: Incidence, clinical features, and long-term evaluation. Am Heart J 103:338, 1982.
11. Fisher JP, Cohen HL, Mehra, R, et al: Cardiac pacing and pacemakers. II. Serial electrophysiologic-pharmacologic testing for control of recurrent tachyarrhythmias. Am Heart J 93:658, 1977.
12. Engel TR: Pacing techniques to guide the therapy of tachycardias. Ann Intern Med 90:266, 1979.
13. Fisher JD, Kim SG, Forman S, et al: Role of implantable pacemakers in control of recurrent ventricular tachycardia. Am J Cardiol 49:194, 1982.
14. Johnson AD, Laiken SL, and Engler RL: Hemodynamic compromise associated with ventriculoatrial conduction following transvenous pacemaker placement. Am J Med 65:75, 1978.
15. Karlof I: Hemodynamic effect of atrial-triggered versus fixed-rate pacing at rest and during exercise in complete heart block. Acta Med Scand 197:195, 1975.
16. Furman S: Therapeutic uses of atrial pacing. Am Heart J 86:835, 1973.
17. Hofshire PF: Postoperative complete heart block in 64 children treated with and without pacing. Am J Cardiol 39:559, 1977.
18. Pastore JD, Yurchak PM, Janis KM, et al: The risk of advanced heart block in surgical patients with right bundle branch block and left-axis deviation. Circulation 57:677, 1978.
19. Lie KI, Wellens HJ, and Schuelenburg RM: Bundle branch block and acute myocardial infarction in the conduction system of the heart: *In* Wellens HJ, Lie KI, Janse MJ, et al (eds): The Conduction System of the Heart: Structure, Function, and Clinical Implications. Philadelphia, Lea and Febiger, 1976, pp. 662–672.
20. Mullins CB: Editorial: Indications for pacing after acute myocardial infarction in patients with fascicular block. J Electrocardiol 8:297, 1975.
21. Gann D, Balachandran PK, El-Sherif N, et al: Prognostic significance of chronic versus acute bundle branch block in acute myocardial infarction. Chest 67:298, 1978.
22. Hindman MC, Wagner GS, Jaro M, et al: The clinical significance of bundle branch block complicating acute myocardial infarction. II. Indications for temporary and permanent pacemaker insertion. Circulation 58:609, 1978.
23. Atkins JM, Leshen SJ, Blomqvist G, et al: Ventricular conduction blocks and sudden death in acute myocardial infarction: Potential indications for pacing. NEJM 288:281, 1973.

6

Temporary Cardiac Pacing: Indications, Techniques, and Management

LEONARD N. HOROWITZ, M.D.

TEMPORARY CARDIAC PACING

The use of electrical stimuli to initiate depolarization and hence contraction of the heart is a commonly used therapeutic modality in both acute and chronic abnormalities of the cardiac rhythm. This chapter discusses the use of temporary pacemaking modalities for the treatment of acute rhythm disorders. Temporary cardiac pacing was made clinically feasible in the early 1950s by Paul Zoll, when he developed external transthoracic pacing.[1] Although this was far from an ideal method, it showed that temporary cardiac pacing for disorders that would otherwise be life-threatening was possible and effective. Since then, substantial advances have been made in the field of temporary pacing. These advances include the development of transvenous electrodes and methods for inserting them in the heart. Subsequent development of external pacing devices has now made temporary pacing a varied and complex subject. The indications for temporary cardiac pacing, the equipment and procedures for temporary pacing, the management of the patient with a temporary cardiac pacemaker, and the complications of temporary pacing will be discussed in this chapter.

INDICATIONS

The primary indications for temporary cardiac pacing are bradyarrhythmias that are either symptomatic or associated with a poor prognosis (Table 6–1). Symptomatic bradyarrhythmias generally produce a significant decrease in cardiac output with resultant decreases in cerebral and cardiac function; dysfunction

Table 6–1. Indications for Temporary Pacing

Emergency Therapy

1. Complete heart block producing symptoms or complicating acute myocardial infarction
2. SA node disease, especially the "tachy-brady" syndrome
3. Symptomatic bradycardia of any cause
   Drug therapy of tachycardias
   Drug overdose
4. Overdrive suppression of tachyarrhythmias
5. Termination of tachyarrhythmias

Prophylactic Therapy

1. Following cardiac surgery
2. During angiographic cardiac catheterization
3. During acute myocardial infarction associated with new right bundle branch block with left- or right-axis deviation of left bundle branch block
4. In patients with Mobitz II AV block
5. Prior to replacement of a failing permanent pacemaker

of other major organ systems may occasionally occur. The major symptoms are disorientation or syncope as a result of cerebral hypoperfusion and angina and congestive heart failure as evidence of cardiac hypoperfusion. In these situations temporary pacing is therapeutic. In other situations temporary cardiac pacing can be instituted as a prophylactic measure, as in patients with Mobitz type II atrioventricular (AV) block or right bundle branch block and left-axis deviation in the setting of acute myocardial infarction. Although these conditions generally do not cause symptoms in and of themselves, they are highly suggestive of a patient at risk of developing high-grade AV block with significant bradycardia, which is frequently symptomatic and life-threatening.

The indication for temporary cardiac pacing for the treatment of symptomatic bradyarrhythmias is usually obvious (Fig. 6–1). The bradycardia may be produced by dysfunction of the sinoatrial (SA) node or the AV conduction system. In patients with sick sinus syndrome, symptomatic sinus bradycardia unresponsive to pharmacologic management may occasionally produce symptoms that are related purely to the low heart rate. More often, in patients with sick sinus syndrome bradyarrhythmias are related to sinus exit block or prolonged pauses following the termination of tachyarrhythmias. In either of these situations the institution of pacemaking can maintain the cardiac rate at an acceptable level and assure adequate cardiac output. The effectiveness of temporary pacing in patients with AV conduction disturbances is similarly obvious when high-grade AV block and slow ventricular escape rhythms are present.

Certain conduction disturbances, although asymptomatic, are likely to progress to symptomatic bradyarrhythmias and, depending upon the clinical context, are indications for the insertion of a temporary pacemaker. The occurrence of second-degree AV block (Mobitz type II), particularly during acute myocardial infarction or following cardiothoracic surgery, is attended by a very high incidence of high-grade AV block and should be managed with a temporary pacemaker.[2] First-degree AV block or second-degree AV block of the Wenckebach or Mobitz type I AV block, on the other hand, rarely proceeds to high-

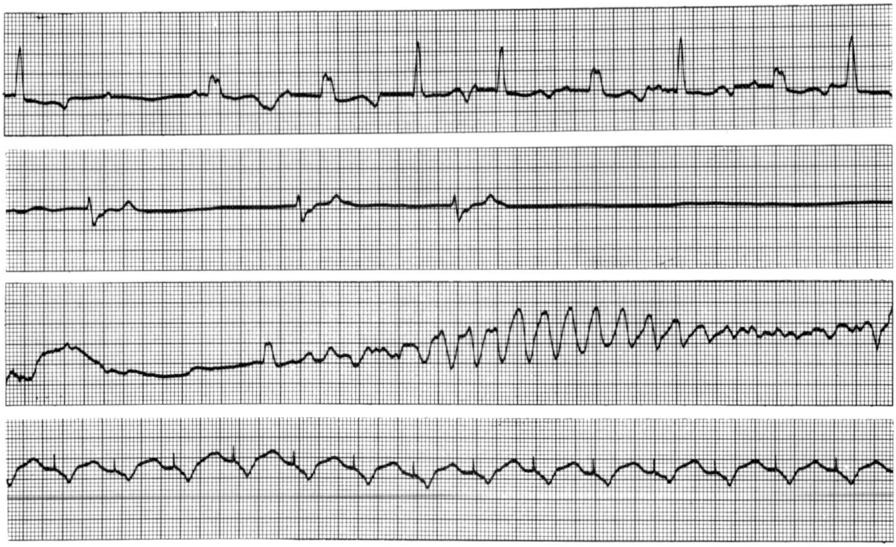

Figure 6–1. Heart block and ventricular tachyarrhythmias in acute myocardial infarction. These EKG rhythm strips were recorded in a patient who had recently suffered an acute myocardial infarction. In the top tracing complete heart block is seen with a wide QRS escape rhythm. Frequent ventricular premature depolarizations are present. Ten minutes later asystole was present. The asystolic interval was terminated in the third strip by the ventricular complex, which induced ventricular fibrillation. In the bottom strip it can be seen that ventricular pacing prevented the bradyarrhythmias as well as the ventricular tachyarrhythmias.

grade block with inadequate ventricular escape rhythm and thus neither are indications for temporary pacing. During the course of acute myocardial infarction the development of right bundle branch block with left anterior hemiblock or left posterior hemiblock (patterns frequently referred to as bifascicular block) is associated with a significant incidence of progression to complete heart block with slow ventricular escape rhythms.[3] Temporary pacing in patients with acute inferior myocardial infarction with AV block or symptomatic bradycardia is more controversial. There are those who prefer the use of atropine to temporary pacing because the bradyarrhythmia is usually readily reversible and frequently does not progress to produce significant symptoms. The insertion of a temporary pacemaker even in this situation is preferable because it is a low-morbidity procedure and provides the physician with complete control of the heart rate, an advantage that is not possible with pharmacologic manipulation. Unexpected and uncontrollable responses to atropine can occur, and in fact, paradoxical worsening of the conduction disturbance may occasionally be seen in these patients.

Temporary pacing is commonly employed prophylactically during cardiac catheterization and following cardiac surgery. Transient bradyarrhythmias are so common in these clinical settings that the immediate availability of pacing is desirable.

Temporary pacing may be required when drugs that produce bradycardia are needed for the treatment of cardiac disease (e.g., angina or arrhythmias). Such is sometimes the case when a β-blocking or calcium-channel-blocking agent is needed for the treatment of coronary artery disease in a patient in whom these agents significantly reduce the heart rate or produce SA node or AV conduction disturbances. Such is also frequently the case in the treatment of patients with the tachycardia-bradycardia syndrome, in which the drug is used to treat the tachycardia.

Temporary cardiac pacing has also been used in the treatment of tachycardias. Pacing can be used for both suppression and termination of tachyarrhythmias. Pacing the heart at rates faster than that of an automatic arrhythmia results in pacemaker capture of the site of abnormal automaticity and overdrives the abnormal rhythm. This is useful when supraventricular pacing can be used to overdrive a ventricular tachyarrhythmia (Fig. 6–2). On occasion, once such overdrive pacing has assumed control of the cardiac rhythm gradual decrease in the pacing rate can be accomplished with continued control of the arrhythmia. In addition, rapid bursts of pacing have been used to terminate reentrant arrhythmias such as atrial flutter and ventricular tachycardia[4,5] (Fig. 6–3). Pacing can interrupt arrhythmias by disrupting the relationship between conduction and refractoriness within the reentrant circuit that produces the arrhythmia, thus causing extinction of the reentrant process. The management of tachyarrhythmias by temporary pacing is indicated for patients in whom pharmacologic management has failed or in whom arrhythmias recur frequently.

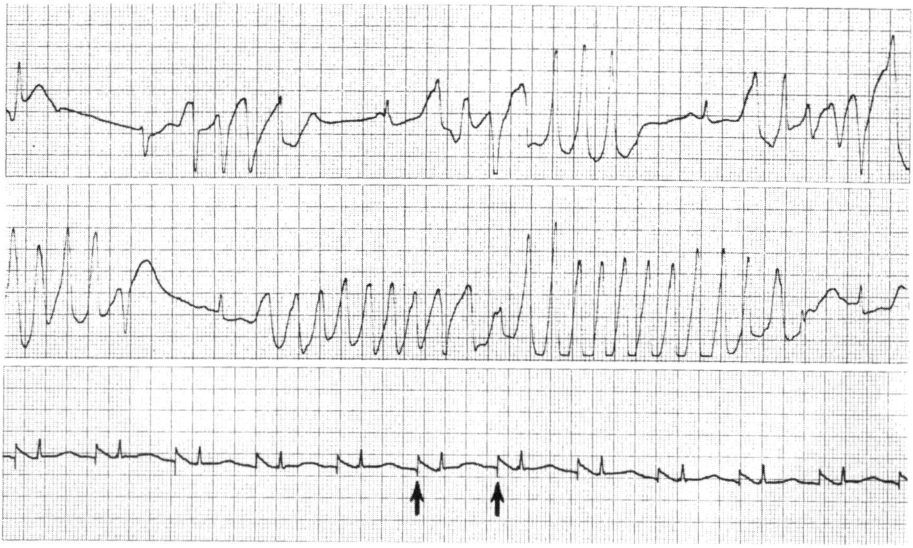

Figure 6–2. Atrial overdrive pacing for prevention of ventricular tachycardia. These EKG tracings were obtained in a patient with marked sinus bradycardia and paroxysmal episodes of torsades de pointes. Note the characteristic varying QRS morphology, which interrupted the extremely slow sinus rhythm. In the bottom tracing atrial pacing indicated by the stimulus artifact producing a P wave (arrows) suppressed the ventricular tachyarrhythmia.

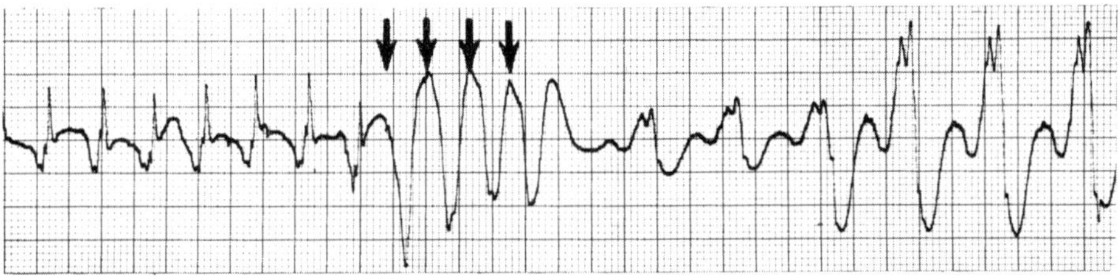

Figure 6–3. Termination of ventricular tachycardia by rapid ventricular pacing. This EKG recording was obtained in a patient who was having frequent episodes of ventricular tachycardia, which required cardioversion. Ventricular tachycardia was present on the left at a rate of 190 per minute. After the seventh complex a four-complex burst of rapid ventricular pacing was introduced and terminated ventricular tachycardia. Sinus tachycardia with bundle branch block was present on the right after termination of the ventricular tachycardia. The change in complex size on the right side of the tracing results from a change in amplitude setting.

The most common type of temporary cardiac pacing is ventricular pacing, in which the temporary electrode is positioned in the ventricle—usually the right ventricle. Temporary atrial pacing is less often used because it is not necessary and because stability of temporary atrial pacemaking electrodes is less reliable than ventricular electrodes. Specific indications in which an atrial pacemaker is necessary or desirable include pacing for termination of atrial arrhythmias and pacing for overdrive suppression of ventricular or atrial arrhythmias. A more common type of temporary pacing that is particularly useful in certain circumstances is AV pacing. In this type of temporary cardiac pacing, both the atria and ventricles are paced. This type of pacing restores normal AV synchrony and improves cardiac performance. AV pacing is indicated in patients with poor left ventricular function.

TECHNIQUES

Equipment

The basic equipment required for temporary cardiac pacing includes the catheter electrodes and the external pacemaker units that initiate and control the pacing stimuli.

The most common type of electrode used for temporary cardiac pacing is a transvenous catheter, which is positioned in the heart via the venous system. A variety of transvenous catheters are available (Figs. 6–4 and 6–5). Catheters are either firm (generally constructed of woven Dacron) or flexible (constructed of extruded plastic). The latter catheters are usually referred to as semifloating. Balloon-tipped and semifloating catheters are primarily designed for flow-assisted placement when fluoroscopic guidance is not available.[6,7] They can be inserted

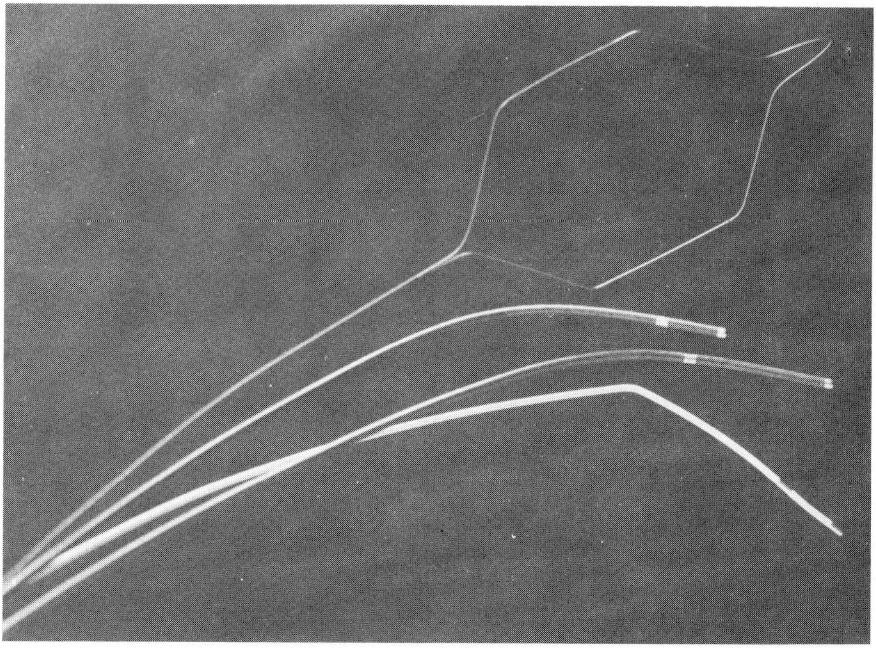

Figure 6–4. Types of transvenous electrode catheters. A variety of electrode catheters are shown in this figure. From bottom to top they include a semifloating preformed catheter, two woven Dacron catheters with wide and close electrode configurations, and a hexagonal atrial electrode loop.

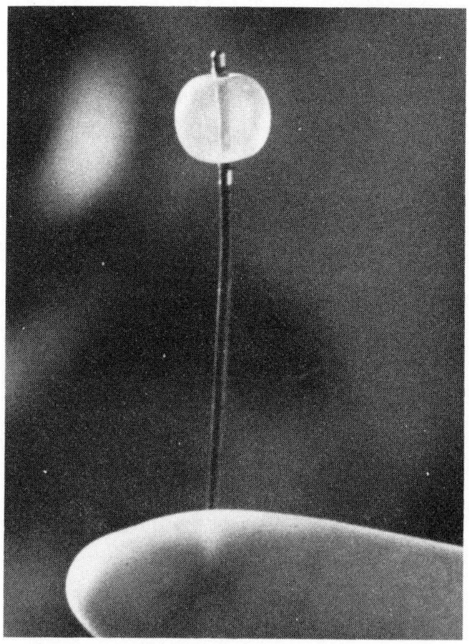

Figure 6–5. Balloon-tipped electrode catheter with the balloon inflated. Note the electrodes on the catheter on either side of the balloon. The size of the balloon can be judged by comparing it with the finger in the photograph.

quickly at the bedside and do not require a radiolucent bed or fluoroscopic equipment; however, electrode stability after initial placement is less reliable than with stiffer catheters. These catheters lack maneuverability, which can prohibit electrode placement in patients with significant structural cardiac alterations such as atrial or ventricular dilatation or tricuspid valve incompetence. Firm catheters, usually woven Dacron, are more easily manipulated but must be inserted with fluoroscopic guidance because they are more likely to perforate vessels or the endocardium when they are inserted without fluoroscopic observation.[8] Woven Dacron catheters maintain their position very well, and because their stiffness decreases when they warm to body temperature, the risk of cardiac perforation after insertion is not a significant problem.

There are a variety of electrode configurations that have been designed to fulfill the specific requirements of temporary cardiac pacing. Temporary pacing can be achieved with either unipolar or bipolar stimulation (see chapter 3). Unipolar catheters have a single electrode, which is used to deliver cathodal stimulation, whereas the anode is located at a distance from the pacing site. Because these are usually more sensitive to external electrical interference, they are not frequently used. Bipolar electrode catheters have two closely positioned (0.1 to 2.0 cm) electrodes. Such electrodes are preferred because bipolar pacing is less susceptible to external interference, and if failure of one electrode occurs, unipolar pacing can be performed through the remaining electrode. Multielectrode catheters are also available for specific indications, primarily AV pacing. Transvenous electrode catheters with two or more pairs of electrodes positioned along the catheter so that they are in contact with the atrial and ventricular endocardium have been designed so that temporary AV pacing is possible with a single-electrode catheter (Fig. 6–6). Furthermore, other design modifications have been made to allow special applications. Electrodes have been incorporated into catheters with a lumen for pressure measurement or drug infusion, and catheters with special shapes and contours have been made to facilitate electrode placement in certain cardiac structures such as the right atrial appendage or coronary sinus.

External pulse generators are typically single-channel, constant-current output sources. Such pulse generators can be used to pace either the atrium or the ventricle. A typical external pacemaker unit allows for control of stimulus output (generally varying from 0 to 20 ma) and stimulus frequency (generally varying from 30 to 150 or 180 per minute). Intrinsic cardiac activity (see chapter 3) is monitored by self-diagnostic circuits that indicate when the pacemaker is sensing and when it is pacing (Fig. 6–7). Another common type of external pulse generator is the AV sequential pacemaker (Fig. 6–8). This unit is a dual-output pacemaker with individual controls for atrial and ventricular stimulus intensity, pacing rate, AV interval, and ventricular sensitivity. Specialized pacemakers have also been developed that can sense atrial activity and pace the ventricle following an AV interval. Pacemakers that can deliver very rapid pacing rates to be used for termination of tachyarrhythmias are also available (Fig. 6–9). Most recently, external pacing using a DDD permanent pacemaker equipped with special connectors for external attachment has become feasible.

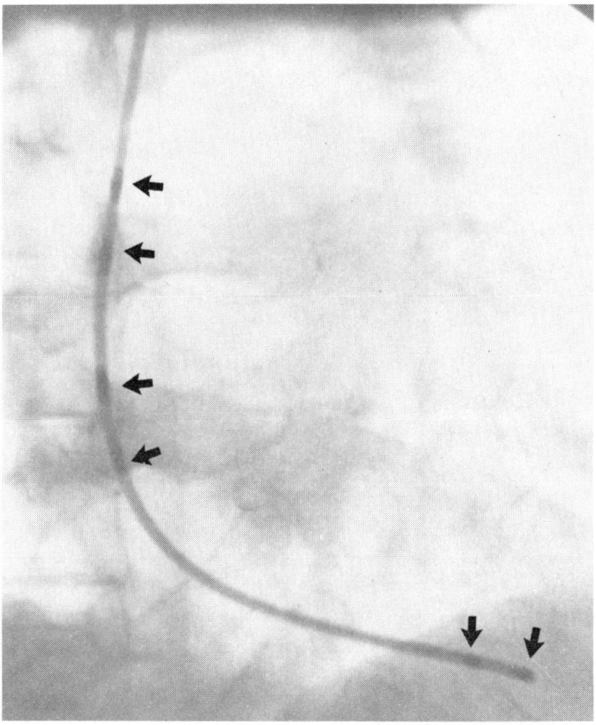

Figure 6–6. Mutipolar electrode catheter for AV pacing. This X-ray shows a hexapolar electrode catheter, which was designed for AV pacing. The electrodes are indicated by the arrows. Two electrodes are located at the distal portion of the catheter for ventricular pacing, and the proximal electrodes are arranged in two pairs for contact with the lateral atrial wall for atrial pacing.

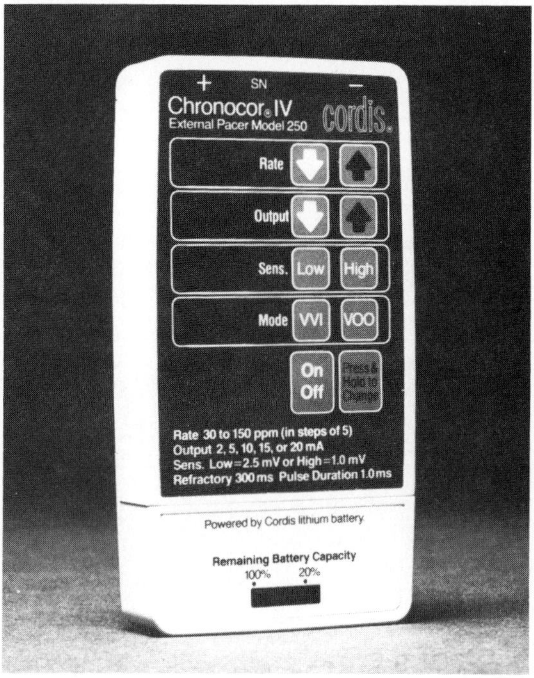

Figure 6–7. External pulse generator. A single-channel external pacemaker is shown. This unit has a lithium battery and has solid state circuitry for selecting rate, output, sensitivity, and pacing mode. The selected settings are shown in a digital display on the face of the unit.

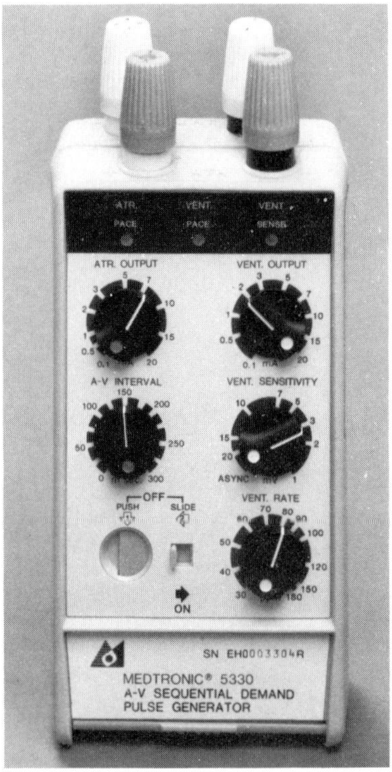

Figure 6–8. External AV pulse generator. This dual-channel output unit is used for AV sequential pacing. Atrial and ventricular outputs are set on the upper dials, and AV interval in milliseconds and ventricular sensitivity in millivolts are set on the middle dials. The ventricular rate is set with the dial at the lower right. There are two sets of connectors on the top of the generator, one each for the atrial and ventricular electrodes.

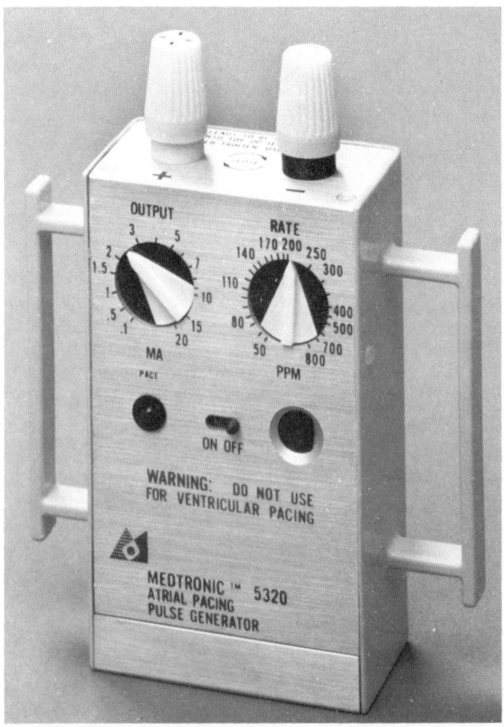

Figure 6–9. External rapid-pacing pulse generator. This pulse generator is designed for pacing at rapid rates without a sensing function. Output is varied as well as pacing rate, which with this unit could be as high as 800 pulses per minute. Particular care must be used with this unit to avoid inadvertently rapidly pacing the ventricle.

Procedure

The insertion of temporary transvenous pacing electrode catheters can be achieved from several sites. Virtually all temporary pacing catheters are positioned in the right heart chambers, and catheters are advanced to these positions through the systemic veins. Venous access can be achieved through the subclavian vein, internal or external jugular veins, brachial veins, or the femoral veins.

The subclavian vein is the favored site of access by many physicians.[9] It is easy to introduce a catheter percutaneously through this vein, and proximity to the heart facilitates catheter placement. The catheter position is usually stable because the catheter can be secured to the chest wall. The use of the subclavian vein for a temporary pacing catheter, however, may preclude the vein's later use for the insertion of a permanent pacemaker. It is also important to remember that the use of a subclavian approach carries the risk of pneumothorax from inadvertent puncture of the apical pleura or hemothorax caused by puncture of the innominate or subclavian arteries. This approach is particularly hazardous in patients with lung disease.

The internal jugular vein also provides direct venous access to the right heart.[10] Once the catheter is positioned its movement is minimal—although neck movement can produce some catheter motion. The risk of carotid arterial puncture during insertion exists and must be considered when using this site. The use of the external jugular vein does not carry this risk of carotid artery injury; however, venous valves and a tortuous course may make catheter manipulation more difficult through this site. Although cutdown on either the subclavian or jugular veins can be performed for the insertion of a temporary pacemaker, the percutaneous approach is by far preferable. Cutdown in these areas requires considerable surgical skill and is generally not recommended.

The brachial vein provides ready access to the systemic venous system for catheter placement.[11] The brachial vein can frequently be cannulated percutaneously, but when cutdown is necessary, the risk of damaging associated structures such as the brachial artery is small. Use of the brachial vein avoids disturbing the subclavian vein, which can later be used for permanent pacemaker implantation. Arm movement, however, can produce significant catheter movement and may lead to catheter dislodgement or perforation. The passage of the catheter from the arm to the subclavian vein in some patients may be difficult. Selection of a medial vein in some patients may be difficult. Selection of a medial vein in the antecubital fossa can facilitate a more direct pathway to the central venous circulation. Venous thrombosis is more common using the brachial vein approach.

The femoral vein, although easily cannulated, is less frequently used for insertion of temporary pacing catheters.[12] Catheter maneuverability is very important using the femoral vein approach, and it is almost mandatory that a stiffer, woven Dacron catheter be used. This requires the use of fluoroscopy equipment in the pacemaker insertion. In addition, mobility of the patient is severely restricted, since the patient cannot sit or move out of bed with a catheter inserted in the femoral vein. There are increased risks of thromboembolic complications with the catheter in this position in immobilized patients. Furthermore, the proximity to the perineum increases the risk of infection.

In extremely emergent situations the transthoracic approach of electrode placement can be used.[13,14] Although there is some disagreement regarding the efficacy of transthoracic pacing, it is probably justifiable during resuscitation efforts when time and facilities are not available for transvenous approaches. The transthoracic needle, which contains a pacemaker wire, is inserted 1 to 2 cm beneath the xiphoid process. The needle is advanced into the right ventricle by directing it superiorly, leftward, and slightly posteriorly. When blood flow is obtained through the needle, the electrode wire is advanced through the needle and the needle is removed. The pacing wire is secured to the skin, and pacing can be performed by placing another wire or needle under the skin as an indifferent electrode. The entire procedure can be completed in less than a minute and is ideal in those situations in which cardiopulmonary resuscitation cannot be interrupted. There is a considerable risk of complications, including perforation or laceration of coronary arteries or cardiac chambers, pneumothorax, hemothorax, or pericardial tamponade; however, in a lifesaving attempt this approach is justified. As soon as it is feasible a transvenous electrode catheter should be inserted, since transthoracic wires inserted in this manner are frequently unstable.

Temporary myocardial pacing electrodes are routinely affixed to the atrium and ventricle following cardiac surgery.[15] These plastic-insulated 0 or 00 wires are inserted in the myocardium and brought through the skin. They are easily dislodged and have unstable thresholds but are useful for several days after surgery.

The ideal catheter position for ventricular pacing is the right ventricular apex. The electrode catheter tip becomes wedged in the trabeculae of the right ventricular apex, and movement is minimized. The sweep of the catheter when inserted from either the femoral vein or veins leading to the superior vena cava provides pressure on the electrode tip, keeping it in position. Electrode placement either on the free wall or in the right ventricular outflow tract is less desirable because the catheter can be moved by the blood flow toward the pulmonary artery. Excessive pressure on the electrode tip must be avoided because the catheter can either perforate the right ventricular wall into the pericardial sac or cross the interventricular septum into the left ventricle.

Atrial pacing can be achieved in a number of ways. An electrode catheter can be positioned in the coronary sinus, through which the left atrium can be paced. Catheterization of the coronary sinus usually requires insertion of the catheter in the jugular, subclavian, or brachial veins. Occasionally an electrode catheter can be manipulated into the coronary sinus from the femoral vein. A coronary sinus position is generally stable when the catheter can be manipulated deep into the coronary sinus. Although uncommon, coronary sinus perforation is a possibility, and patient movement should be minimized. If the catheter migrates further distally into the coronary sinus, left ventricular pacing can sometimes occur. Other atrial pacing positions include the right atrial appendage, which may be very difficult to achieve with standard electrode catheters.

Recently, a preformed J-shaped catheter has been developed for transvenous temporary right atrial pacing.[16] A more common type of electrode catheter that can be used for atrial pacing is a catheter that is designed to be positioned in the right ventricular apex with additional electrodes positioned 10 to 20 cm proximal to the electrode tip. These electrodes will lie along the lateral right atrial wall and will be capable of producing atrial sensing and pacing. Another recent development for atrial pacing is the atrial hexagonal loop electrode.[17] This electrode is positioned in the right atrium in a carrier catheter and then is opened. It expands and contacts the atrial wall in several positions. Dislodgement has been a minimal problem with this electrode, and secure electrode contact is common. The thrombogenicity of this electrode system, however, has been questioned.

The insertion and placement of a temporary electrode catheter should be performed with adequate technical and professional support. Emergency equipment including a defibrillator should be readily available. It is ideal to have fluoroscopy and continuous EKG monitoring available for this procedure. When fluoroscopy is not available, a flow-directed or balloon-tipped catheter should be used. The insertion site must be surgically prepared using the standard aseptic technique. The inserting physician and assistants should wear sterile gowns, as is standard for any surgical procedure. The patient should be draped widely to allow comfortable movement about the insertion site and placement of sterile supplies. Both subcutaneous and deep local anesthesia should be administered. We prefer the use of bupivacaine (0.25 percent) because of its long-acting properties.

The preferred approach is the percutaneous Seldinger technique.[11] Using this technique a needle is inserted into the vein, and once free blood flow has been obtained a flexible guide wire is inserted through the needle, which is then removed. A puncture wound is made with a scalpel blade at the insertion site, and blunt dissection using a hemostat creates a pathway for the introducer. A tapered vessel dilator is then introduced over the guide wire and inserted into the vessel. The introducer is moved over the vessel dilator and positioned in the vein. The guide wire and vessel dilator are then removed. Although a number of introducers are available, we prefer the type with a gasket seal that prevents back-bleeding. Many of these introducers have a side-port infusion assembly that allows the introducer to be used for intravenous fluid or drug administration. The catheter is inserted through the introducer into the venous system and is then advanced to a position within the heart (Fig. 6–10).

In those patients in whom venous access is difficult a surgical cutdown is necessary. When this is the case we prefer the brachial vein approach because cutdown in this area can be performed with minimal risk. When using this technique it is best to introduce the catheter through the skin using a small puncture or introducer entry approximately 0.5 cm distal to the site of the cutdown. This allows the cutdown to be closed without having the catheter exiting through it.

Ideally, electrode catheters are advanced to and positioned in the heart under fluoroscopic guidance. This allows precise catheter movement and posi-

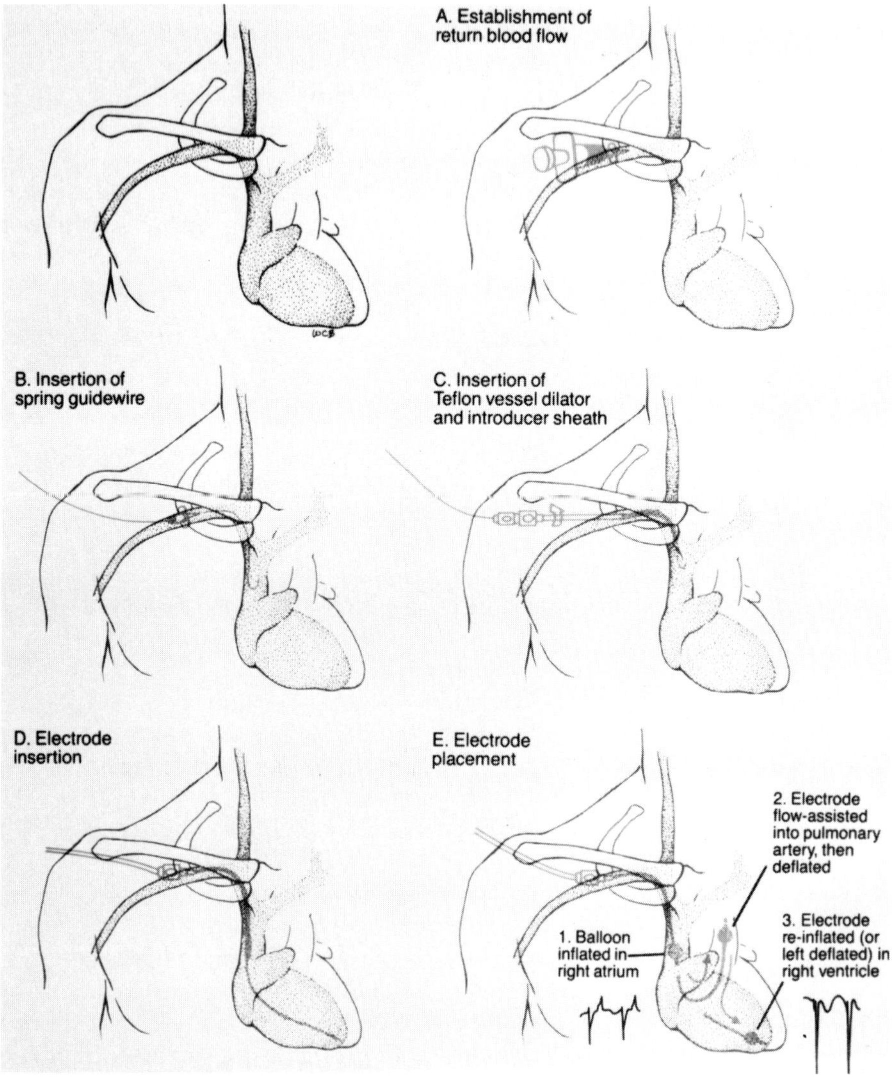

Figure 6–10. Schematic view of pacemaker insertion using the subclavian approach. The venous system and right heart are shown in stippling. Pacemaker insertion begins with insertion of a needle into the subclavian vein using the infraclavicular approach and establishing free blood flow *(A)*. The guide wire is inserted through the needle and the needle removed from the vessel *(B)*. The vessel dilator and introducer sheath are advanced over the wire into the vein *(C)*. The electrode catheter is introduced through the introducer and positioned in the heart (*D* and *E*).

tioning in the cardiac chamber. Positioning the electrode catheter within the right atrial appendage or the coronary sinus requires fluoroscopic monitoring. The positioning of a catheter for AV pacing with electrodes in the atrium and ventricle also usually requires fluoroscopic monitoring.

Although it is ideal to position catheters in the right ventricular apex under fluoroscopic control, this is not absolutely necessary. In those situations in which fluoroscopy is not available, EKG monitoring during catheter insertion is used.

In this technique the patient is attached to a standard EKG recorder, and the distal electrode of the electrode catheter is connected to the chest lead. The recorder is set to record a unipolar V lead, and the position of the catheter can thus be monitored (Fig. 6–11). As the electrode catheter approaches the heart,

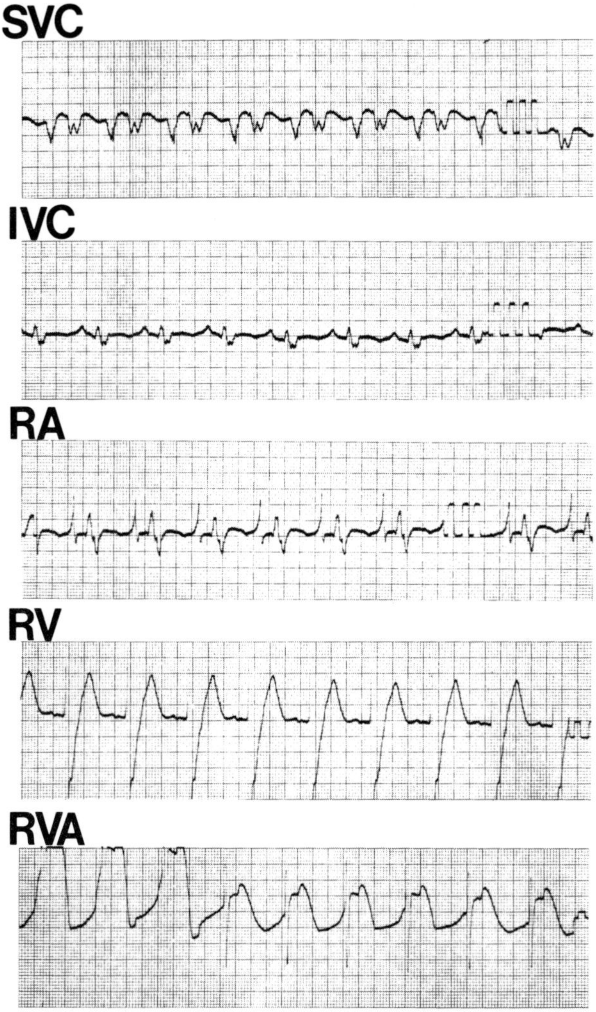

Figure 6–11. EKG monitoring of electrode catheter positioning within the heart. EKG recordings obtained by attaching the chest (V) lead to the distal pole of the electrode catheter as it is advanced through the venous system to the right ventricular apex are shown. Entering the right atrium from the superior vena cava (SVC) in the top tracing or the inferior vena cava (IVC) as shown in the second tracing produced nearly equal atrial and ventricular deflections, which are small. When the catheter is in the superior vena cava the atrial deflection is negative and in the inferior vena cava it is positive. In the right atrium the catheter recorded nearly equal deflections from both atrium and ventricle. The deflections were more rapid and discrete than they were in either vena cava. Advancing the catheter into the right ventricle produced a much larger deflection, and a very small atrial electrogram is recorded. When the catheter was against the RV wall, ST-segment elevation and a very large electrogram were seen. Note the differences in amplitude of the signals as indicated by the standard 1-mv calibration signal, which is shown on the right side of each tracing.

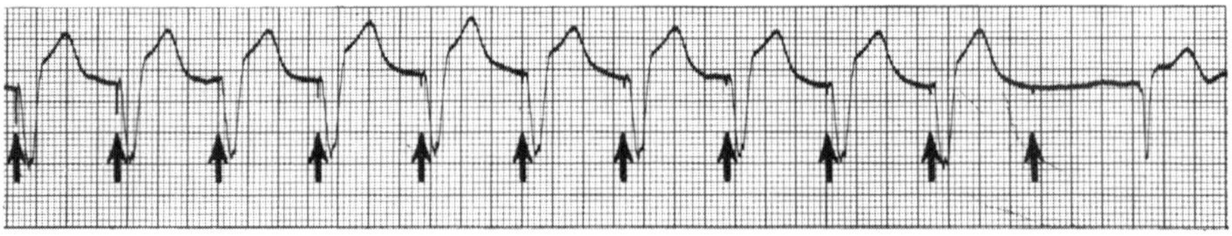

Figure 6–12. EKG recording of threshold testing. Ventricular pacing was present, and the arrows indicate the stimulus artifact that preceded each paced complex. Starting with the complexes on the left, the threshold was continuously decreased, which produced a reduction in the size of the stimulus artifact. Finally, when the stimulus output was 0.5 ma the pacing of the ventricle ceased and capture was lost (last arrow on the right).

atrial and ventricular electrograms are recorded. As the catheter enters the right ventricle the atrial electrogram diminishes in size and the right ventricular electrogram increases markedly. When the right ventricular wall is contacted by the electrode, the electrogram shows very large amplitude and ST-segment elevation.

Immediately after obtaining the desired anatomic position the pacemaker threshold should be determined. The threshold is determined by attaching the pacemaker electrodes to the external pulse generator. The distal electrode should be attached to the cathodal (negative) output and the more proximal electrode to the anode. The pacemaker should be set at a rate at least 10 beats per minute faster than the patient's intrinsic rate and the output of the pacemaker set at maximum. After appropriate pacing is ascertained by EKG monitoring, the output of the pacemaker is gradually decreased until the stimuli fail to produce capture (see chapter 3) (Fig. 6–12). The current setting at which pacing fails to occur is called the pacing threshold. The pacemaker should then be set at an output of 3 to 10 times this threshold. Pacing thresholds may vary with patient movement, drugs, and other physiologic alterations, and considerable margin in pacing output should be provided for these changes. When the pacemaker is used in the demand mode, it is important to ascertain that adequate sensing of the endocardial electrogram is present. This can be ascertained in two ways. The electrogram recorded through the catheter can be recorded on a standard EKG recorder, and using the calibration signal the size of the electrogram can be measured. Most external pacing devices allow the sensitivity to be set based on this measurement. It is important to remember that such sensitivity must be set at a number lower than the measurement of the recorded electrogram. Another method used to check the sensitivity is to set the pacemaker at a rate 10 beats per minute slower than the patient's intrinsic rate. The sensitivity is set at the most sensitive (e.g., the lowest amplitude setting), and gradually sensitivity is decreased (turning to higher numbers). When the pacemaker fails to sense and begins pacing competitively with the patient's intrinsic rhythm, one has determined a level of sensitivity. The sensitivity should then be set at a more sensitive level.

The insertion of dual-chamber temporary pacing systems presents several special problems. It is important to achieve a catheter position that will provide good atrial and ventricular pacing thresholds and the correct ventricular sensing.

This may require several catheter repositionings until the optimal position is achieved. Since most currently available AV pacing external units do not allow atrial sensing but merely atrial pacing and then subsequent ventricular pacing, it is usually necessary to pace the atrium at a rate faster than the intrinsic sinus rate of the patient to produce atrial capture and subsequent restoration of AV synchrony. This may be disadvantageous when the sinus rate is rapid, as may occur in patients with high-grade ventricular block.

Insertion site care after temporary pacemaker insertion is very important. The electrode catheter should be secured to the skin with sutures. In addition, antibiotic ointment should be placed at the insertion site. Although there are several acceptable means for covering the site, we prefer a clear adhesive surgical dressing. This dressing allows the insertion site to be inspected easily. If the electrode catheter is coiled around the insertion site, the clear adhesive surgical dressing will prevent inadvertent dislodgement of the electrode catheter. The external pulse generator should be securely attached to the patient or, if an extending cable is used, to the patient's bed. The controls of the external pacing device should be covered so that they are not inadvertently moved, but they should be able to be easily checked and changed at the bedside. Covering the pacemaker with a plastic shield is ideal for both purposes.

It is very important to remember that the patient now has an electrically conductive pathway from the outside of the body to the heart. Electrical hazards now become critical. It is ideal for patients with temporary electrode catheters to be placed on a nonelectric bed so that the possibility of leakage current is minimized. If this is not possible, the electric bed should be disconnected from power except when movement of the bed is required. The safety of all electrical devices in contact with the patient with the temporary transvenous catheter is of utmost importance.

After pacemaker insertion, the patient should have a portable chest x-ray to document electrode position and, if the subclavian approach is used, to exclude the possibility of a pneumothorax. A 12-lead EKG should be obtained with the pacemaker pacing so that the QRS morphology produced by pacing at the selected site is documented and is available for subsequent review. Continuous EKG monitoring is desirable in patients with temporary pacemakers.

MANAGEMENT

Appropriate daily management of the electrode catheter will maximize the length of time it can be safely left in position and decrease the potential of complications and malfunction. The insertion sites should be inspected daily for inflammation and evidence of infection. The course of the catheter when it is positioned through the brachial vein should be palpated to identify incipient phlebitis. The cardiac examination should include careful auscultation over the precordium. Pacemaker perforation can produce a pericardial friction rub or clicking sounds caused by intercostal muscle contractions. The discovery of a pericardial friction rub may indicate a catheter perforation. The pacing threshold and sensitivity should be checked at least daily. Modest changes in these parameters are common; marked changes in threshold (particularly progressive increases in threshold) may indicate catheter movement. Such changes may require repositioning. Chest x-rays should be obtained daily to ascertain catheter position. A 12-lead EKG during ventricular pacing should be obtained to ascertain that the QRS morphology and axis during pacing are the same as they were following insertion. Changes may indicate catheter movement or perforation. It is also important to assess the need for continued pacing. Since the electrode catheter presents risks of infection, thromboembolism, and perforation, it should not be kept in place longer than is necessary.

Complications

Complications associated with temporary pacing result from the insertion of the electrode or the continued presence of the electrode in the vascular system. The complications of insertion have been discussed previously. The complications caused by temporary cardiac pacing include cardiac perforation, mechanical stimulation of the heart, infection, and thromboembolic events.[18] In addition, external pulse generators can be mishandled and incorrectly used.

Perforation of the endocardium is not uncommon during temporary transvenous pacing, but rarely is it catastrophic except when pacing is lost (Fig. 6–13). Atrial (or coronary sinus) perforation carries a greater risk than does ventricular perforation, and for that reason the multielectrode catheter is preferable to the coronary sinus catheter. Perforation of the ventricular endocardium should be suspected when pacing threshold increases or pacing ceases suddenly, the patient develops shoulder or pericardial pain, or diaphragmatic or intercostal muscle stimulation occurs. The findings of a new pericardial friction rub and extracardiac clicks further support the diagnosis of perforation.

The diagnosis of ventricular perforation can be confirmed by recording intracardiac electrograms from the electrodes (Fig. 6–14). The normal unipolar right ventricular endocardial electrogram is a predominantly negative deflection with ST-segment elevation. Recording a small electrogram without ST-segment elevation suggests perforation, and withdrawal of the catheter several centimeters will confirm repositioning in the ventricular cavity. Pacemaker withdrawal does not usually produce hemopericardium, because the site of perforation is sealed by the contraction of the ventricular myocardium and the inflammatory process evoked by the trauma. Occasionally, significant bleeding and hemodynamic collapse does occur.

Mechanical stimulation of the ventricle can be suspected when ventricular premature depolarizations (VPDs) occur more frequently or appear after pacemaker insertion, particularly if the QRS of the ectopic complex resembles that of the paced QRS. If marked ventricular ectopy (frequent VPDs or runs) occurs

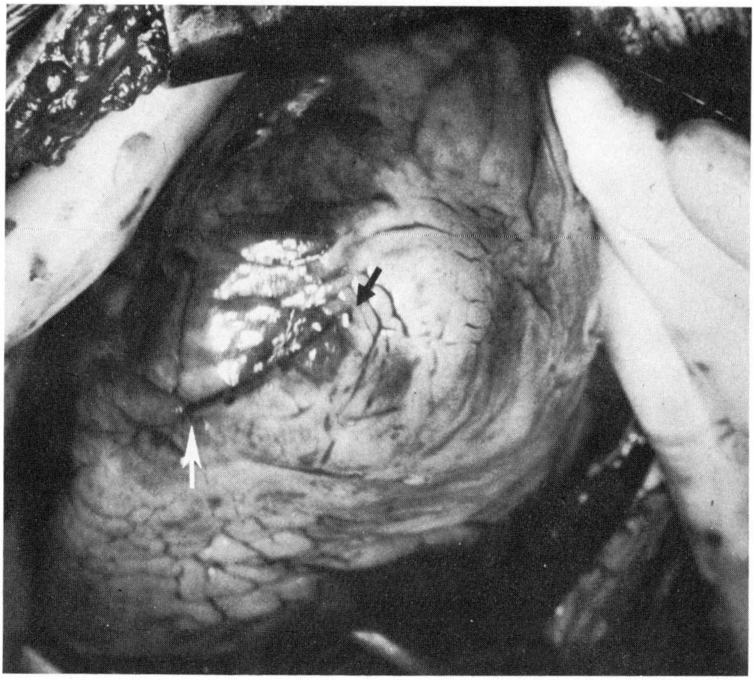

Figure 6–13. Catheter perforation. This photograph was obtained in the operating room in a patient in whom a temporary electrode catheter was inserted prior to cardiac surgery. The catheter perforated the inferior surface of the right ventricle (white arrow), and the catheter protrudes for 3 cm. The tip is indicated by the black arrow. There was no blood in the pericardium, and the perforation was completely asymptomatic, although pacing function was lost.

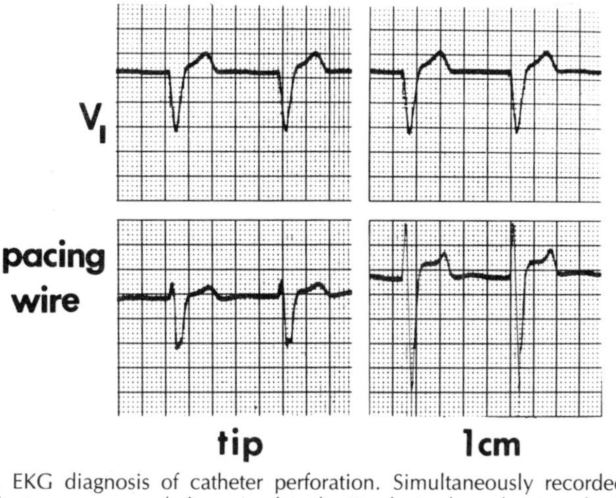

Figure 6–14. EKG diagnosis of catheter perforation. Simultaneously recorded V1 EKGs are shown with the electrograms recorded proximal to the tip electrode and a ring electrode 1 cm from the tip of the pacing catheter. Note that the tip electrode recorded a small electrogram with no ST-segment elevation, indicating that it is not immediately adjacent to the endocardium, whereas the electrode 1 cm proximal to the tip recorded the larger electrogram with ST-segment elevation indicating its proximity to the endocardium. Withdrawal of the catheter using EKG monitoring can document return to correct positioning.

or VPDs fail to respond to drug therapy, catheter repositioning should be attempted to eliminate the possibility that the ectopy is catheter related.

Infection is rarely a major complication when the catheter is inserted under sterile conditions and appropriate care is taken after insertion. If infection is suspected, antibiotics (topical or systemic as appropriate) and catheter removal are indicated.

Venous thrombosis and subsequent embolism occasionally occur following insertion of a transvenous pacing catheter. The vascular trauma and immobility of the patient combine to increase the risk of thrombosis, particularly when the femoral vein is used. Prophylactic low-dose heparinization is useful, but if a high risk of thromboembolism is present, full systemic heparinization should be considered. Routine treatment of complicating thromboembolic events should accompany removal of the catheter.

Troubleshooting Malfunctions

The frequent evaluation of temporary pacemaker function as discussed previously should identify many malfunctions early and allow for appropriate corrective action. The most common malfunctions are failure to capture (non-pacing or noncapture) and failure to sense.

Nonpacing or increasing pacing threshold can result from electrode displacement, generator failure, or electrode catheter disruption. If the pacing threshold progressively increases or pacing capture fails at the highest current output, electrode position should be checked by chest x-ray and function of the pacing generator and its battery should be evaluated. The connection of the catheter to the generator should also be checked. Electrode catheter perforation, a type of dislodgement, can be evaluated as discussed above. Disruption of the electrode catheter is uncommon but can be suspected by the absence or variation of pacemaker stimuli (spikes) on the surface EKG. Immediate evaluation of the exposed catheter and its connections to the pacemaker should be performed. Recording unipolar electrograms from each electrode is useful in diagnosing electrode disruption. Inability to record an electrogram or recording an intermittent signal indicates a physical disruption in the catheter. Until a definitive solution can be achieved, the output of the pulse generator should be increased; if necessary, unipolar pacing can be instituted by using one of the electrodes of a bipolar pair.

Failure to sense or inappropriate sensing is less critical than failure to capture. Failure to sense is caused by pacing generator malfunction, an inadequate endocardial electrogram, or incorrect setting of the generator's sensitivity. Sensitivity can be evaluated (see page 100) and adjusted accordingly. If generator malfunction is suspected, another generator should be connected. Recording of the endocardial electrogram can assure that the signal is of appropriate amplitude. Catheter repositioning may be needed to obtain an electrogram of sufficient amplitude.

Inappropriate sensing (causing the pacemaker to inhibit when it should pace) can be caused by extraneous electrical activity such as leakage current or electrosurgical unit discharge or catheter placement in a location that records atrial activity, such as the right ventricular outflow tract. The T wave or ST segment can sometimes be of sufficient amplitude that the sensing circuit is activated by these signals. Recording the endocardial electrogram can identify signals that may be causing the inappropriate sensing. Either adjusting the generator sensitivity to a lower level or repositioning the catheter should alleviate these problems.

REFERENCES

1. Zoll PA: Resuscitation of the heart in ventricular standstill by external electrical stimulation. NEJM 247:768, 1952.
2. Bigger JT: Mechanisms and diagnosis of arrhythmias. *In* Braunwald E (ed): Heart Disease. Philadelphia, W. B. Saunders Co., 1981, p. 630.
3. Hindman MC, Wagner GS, JaRo M, et al: The clinical significance of bundle branch for temporary and permanent pacemaker insertion. Circulation 58:689, 1978.
4. Wirtzfeld A, Schmidt G, Klein G, and Worzewski W: External electrical stimulation in the management of acute tachyarrhythmias. Pace 4:679, 1981.
5. Barold SS: Therapeutic use of cardiac pacing in tachyarrhythmias. *In* Narula OS (ed): His Bundle Electrocardiography and Clinical Electrophysiology. Philadelphia, F. A. Davis, 1975, p. 407.
6. Schnitzler RN, Caracta AR, and Damato AN: "Floating" catheter for temporary transvenous ventricular pacing. Am J Cardiol 31:351, 1973.
7. Meister SG, Banka VS, and Helfant RH: Transfemoral pacing with balloon-tipped catheters. JAMA 225:712, 1973.
8. Bilitch M, and Berens SC: Insertion techniques and electrode placement. *In* Temporary Transvenous Cardiac Pacing: A Clinical Update. Pro Clinica, 1981, pp. 14–19.
9. Rosenberg AS, Grossman JI, Escher DJW, and Furman S: Bedside transvenous cardiac pacing. Am Heart J 77:697, 1969.
10. Rao G, and Zikria EA: Technique of insertion of pacing electrode through the internal jugular vein. J Cardiovasc Surg 14:294, 1973.
11. Killip T, and Kimball JT: Percutaneous techniques for introducing flexible electrodes for intracardiac pacing. Ann NY Acad Sci 167:597, 1969.
12. Weinstein J, Gnoj J, Mazzarra JT, et al: Temporary transvenous pacing via the percutaneous femoral vein approach. A prospective study of 100 cases. Am Heart J 85:695, 1973.
13. Roberts R: Emergency transthoracic pacemaker—review. Ann Emerg Med 10:600, 1981.
14. Gessman LJ, Wertheimer JH, Davison J, et al: A new device and method for rapid emergency pacing: Clinical use in 10 patients. Pace 5:929, 1982.
15. Weirich WL, Goh VL, and Lillehei CW: The treatment of complete heart block by the combined use of a myocardial electrode and an artificial pacemaker. Surg Forum 8:360, 1957.
16. Littleford PO, and Pepine CJ: A new temporary atrial pacing catheter inserted percutaneously into the subclavian vein without fluoroscopy: A preliminary report. Pace 4:458, 1981.
17. Berens SC, Kohn A, MacAlpin RN, and Lenz MW: New stable temporary atrial pacing loop. Am J Cardiol 34:325, 1974.
18. Lumia FJ and Rios JC: Temporary transvenous pacemaker therapy: An analysis of complications. Chest 64:604, 1973.

7

Permanent Cardiac Pacing: Surgical Technique

A. HADI HAKKI, M.D., F.R.C.S.

Team spirit and collaboration must exist between the surgeon and the cardiologist in making decisions regarding the whole spectrum of pacing. These decisions include the indications for pacing, the mode and type of pacemaker units to be implanted, and the technical aspects of the procedure used and its related potential complications. If all of these considerations are thoroughly discussed by the surgeon and the cardiologist, we can best benefit our patients and reach a situation called "ideal cardiac pacing."

In our institution and in many others across the country, epimyocardial implants are applied, when indicated, in two instances: in patients who are undergoing open-heart surgery or in those rare instances when transvenous pacing is for some reason precluded. The vast majority of pacing procedures used around the world employ the intravenous route.

THE TRANSVENOUS APPROACH

Almost all of the permanent pacemaker implants in our institution are performed transvenously. This is a simple and practical technique, and although it is not free from complications, it carries a significantly lower morbidity and, in some cases, even lower mortality compared with the transthoracic approach.[1] An operating room or a similar sterile room, EKG monitoring, fluoroscopy, and a standby defibrillator are required for all endomyocardial implants.

Except for women beyond the age of 75 years, the sites of pacemaker electrode insertion, in order of preference, are:

1. The subclavian vein
2. The cephalic vein
3. The right jugular vein (external or internal)
4. The left jugular vein (external or internal)

Because we have noticed a higher incidence of pneumothorax following subclavian vein puncture techniques in women beyond the age of 75 years, cephalic vein cutdown would be the first choice for such patients; subclavian vein puncture would be the second choice. We prefer the left side for insertion because most people are right-handed, and for people who are active in sports that side is less subject to trauma. Other reasons include the ease of placement of the pacemaker electrode into the right ventricle with minimal lead manipulation and prevention of a fatal caval hemorrhage that may be associated with right subclavian puncture.[2]

Patients undergoing pacemaker insertion are placed in the supine position with the head turned opposite to the side of the operative field, and a foam wedge is placed under the legs to facilitate the procedure and to prevent air embolism. Preoperative sedation and antibiotics are given routinely to all patients. The antibiotics are discontinued 24 hours after the operation. If shaving is required in the upper chest and lower neck regions, this can be carried out at the time the patient is placed on the operating room table, in order to minimize the incidence of wound infections.[3] If the patient has a temporary pacemaker, the site of insertion of the electrode is exposed in readiness for removal under fluoroscopy toward the end of the permanent implant insertion. Local anesthesia in the form of 1 percent lidocaine or bupivicaine (Marcaine) is used for all patients, usually without an anesthetist standby. In endomyocardial implant, the pacemaker lead is routinely passed under fluoroscopy to the pulmonary artery first, and then it is pulled back to lie in a suitable position in the right ventricle. Correct catheter placement at or near the right ventricular apex, together with good pacing parameter readings, constitutes the hallmark of successful pacemaker insertion. With the advent of active-fixation pacing electrodes like the screw-in transvenous electrode, the site of placement in the right ventricle may be compromised. Ideally, the pacing electrode should describe a gentle curve in the right atrium, with a smooth curve around the battery to prevent perforation of the myocardium, kinking, and fracture of the pacing catheter. Once the pacemaker lead is well positioned, with good pacing parameter readings, it is then tested for stability by asking the patient to cough and to breathe vigorously.

For all patients undergoing pacing implants, postoperative telemetry for EKG monitoring is carried out for at least 48 hours. Chest x-rays, including postero-anterior and lateral projections, are also obtained within 24 hours following pacemaker insertion, along with a 12-lead EKG strip.

With all endomyocardial implants, an infraclavicular incision just below the midclavicular point on the anterior chest wall is made and extended laterally toward the deltopectoral groove. The incision is carried out further laterally, to intersect the deltopectoral groove in cases of cephalic vein cutdown, whereas it may stop just short of the deltopectoral groove in cases of subclavian vein puncture. With the introduction of new, smaller pacemaker batteries, the length of the skin incision may be as little as 2 inches. Sharp dissection is carried down through the subcutaneous tissue and fascia until the pectoral muscle is exposed. A pocket that will accommodate the pacemaker battery is developed by lifting the subcutaneous tissue and fascia off the pectoral muscle in an inferomedial direction using primarily sharp dissection. In some rare instances (mainly in very thin, elderly patients) the pacemaker pocket may be developed posterior to the pectoral muscle—that is, against the chest wall and in an inferomedial position to the skin incision.

The Subclavian Vein Puncture

Once the pacemaker pocket is made, a subclavian puncture is performed similar to the one described by Wilson.[4] Although this technique can be applied to the majority of our patients, some modification of the technique may be applicable. For example, the needle may require insertion more medial to the midclavicular point, depending upon the chest wall configuration in relation to the clavicle, the anterior chest wall, and the first rib.[5] An 18-gauge needle attached to a 5-ml syringe is inserted beneath the middle point of the clavicle in a horizontal plane, with its tip aimed at the posterior aspect of the suprasternal notch. As the needle is being introduced, gentle suction is applied by the syringe plunger until venous blood is aspirated. The syringe is disconnected from the needle, and a J wire is introduced. Any resistance to the introduction of the J wire calls for readjustment by removing the J wire, reconnecting the needle to the syringe, and aspirating while moving the needle back and forth for a few millimeters until a free flow of blood is obtained. If no blood can be aspirated, the needle and the syringe should be removed and another subclavian puncture attempted. Once the J wire is passed into the venous system, the 18-gauge needle is removed and a dilator with its sheath is introduced, guided by the J wire.

Next, the J wire is removed, followed by the dilator, at which time the patient is asked to hold his breath to minimize the risk of air embolism. The pacemaker lead can then be inserted into the venous system via the sheath, as it is pulled out of the subclavian vein and removed by splitting it open while maintaining traction on each side of its proximal end. After the pacemaker lead is positioned in the right ventricle and checked for stability and parameters, it is secured in place to the pectoral muscle with two 2–0 Tevdek sutures. The lead is then connected to the pacemaker battery and placed in the previously made pocket. After adequate hemostasis, the wound is closed in layers (Fig. 7–1).

The Cephalic Vein Cutdown

The cephalic vein lies in the deltopectoral groove, which may be deep and somewhat difficult to find in obese patients or may be too small for insertion of a pacemaker lead. A useful guide for finding the cephalic vein is to feel for the coracoid process of the scapula and dissect in the area of the deltopectoral groove region. When the vein is exposed, it is isolated with 2–0 Tevdek sutures, one proximally and one distally. The distal suture is tied, and a transverse

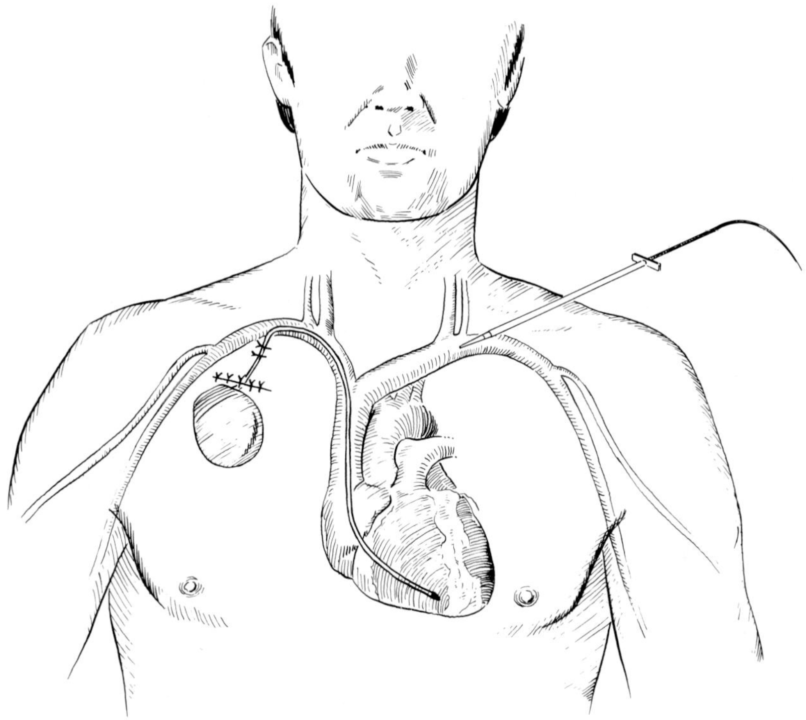

Figure 7–1. A schematic figure showing the introduction of a dilator and sheath over a J wire into the left subclavian vein. After removal of the dilator and the J wire, a pacing electrode can be inserted through the sheath to lie in a suitable position in the right ventricular apex. The lead is secured with nonabsorbable sutures before connecting it to the pacemaker battery.

cutdown is performed in the vein and between the two sutures. Then the pacing electrode is inserted directly into the vein. When successful insertion in the right ventricle is achieved, the previously inserted sutures of 2–0 Tevdek are tied down around the pacemaker lead. Lead fixation to the underlying muscle may be attained by using additional sutures. The lead is then connected to the pacemaker battery and placed in the previously made pocket at the inferomedial aspect of the skin incision (Fig. 7–2).

The External Jugular Cutdown

Although this route can be used with a good rate of success in most patients, the pacemaker lead has to cross over the clavicle to connect to the pulse generator in the infraclavicular area. In some individuals the external jugular vein has a variable course to the superior vena cava, and the introduction of the electrode occasionally proves difficult. Since we instituted the subclavian vein puncture technique in 1980, we have not had to resort to the use of any veins in the neck region for pacemaker lead insertion. The external jugular vein is exposed by making a transverse neck incision about an inch above the clavicle.

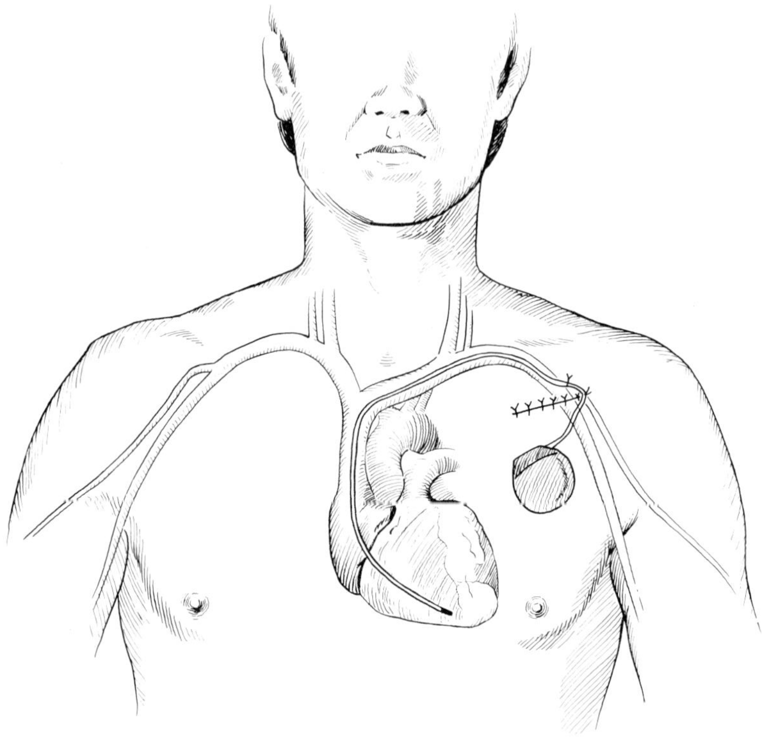

Figure 7–2. The pacing electrode is inserted via the cephalic vein cutdown technique. Note the skin incision going further laterally.

The cutdown technique is similar to the cephalic vein cutdown. After fixing the electrode in the neck region, a tunnel is made subcutaneously to cross over the clavicle, and the electrode is passed through the tunnel to the infraclavicular area to be connected to the pacemaker battery, which is placed in a previously made pocket in that area. Then both the neck and the infraclavicular incisions are closed in layers (Fig. 7–3).

The Internal Jugular Vein Puncture

Although ligation of the internal jugular vein by the usual cutdown technique has been performed, it is not as safe as generally considered.[6] The same equipment that is used for the subclavian vein puncture is used for the internal jugular vein puncture, and the technique is similar to that described by Jernigan.[7] A neck incision is made about an inch above the clavicle and just lateral to the sternocleidomastoid muscle. At this level, the internal jugular vein lies slightly lateral to the midportion of the muscle and is somewhat fixed to the deep surface by fascial attachments. The 18-gauge needle, attached to a 5-ml syringe, is driven by a sharp jab at the outer border of the sternocleidomastoid muscle and

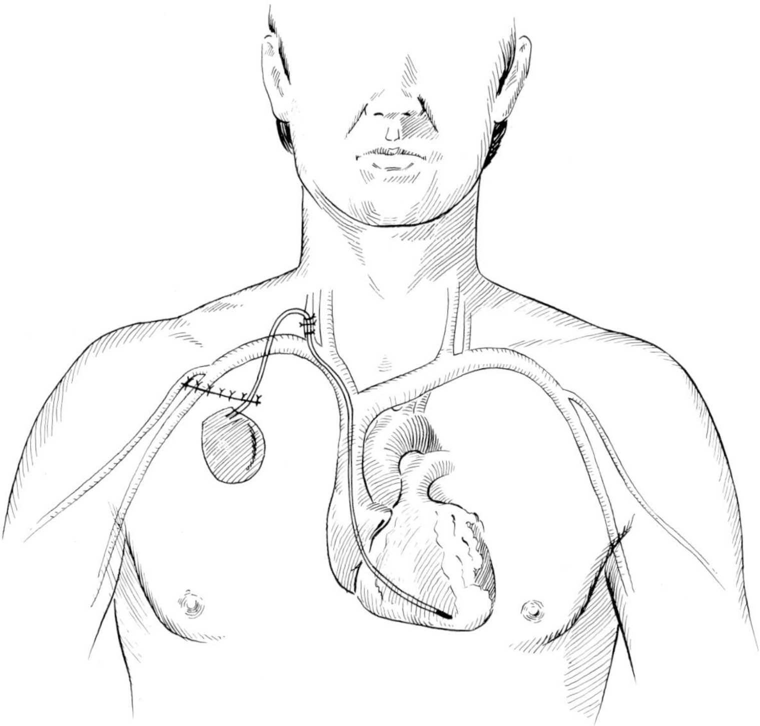

Figure 7–3. A right external jugular vein cutdown technique is noted that would require a neck incision in addition to the infraclavicular incision. As in the internal jugular venipuncture, the pacing electrode has to pass over the clavicle before it can be connected to the pacemaker battery.

directed toward the suprasternal notch. Precautions are taken to avoid puncturing the carotid artery by identifying it anatomically with finger palpation prior to the venipuncture procedure. Once the pacemaker electrode is in place, it is fixed to the fascia in the neck region with two sutures of 2–0 Tevdek material. Then the lead is tunneled subcutaneously to cross over the clavicle and is connected to the pacemaker battery in the infraclavicular area. Finally, both incisions are closed in layers. The older technique exposed the internal jugular vein and passed the pacemaker lead through a purse-string suture applied to the vein. The advent of the subclavian vein puncture technique has eliminated the need for puncture of the neck veins in more than 500 consecutive transvenous implants.

Atrial Pacing

A major limitation of pure atrial pacing is the unpredictable appearance of an AV conduction block; therefore it is usually performed as a part of a dual-chamber pacing procedure. When indicated, it can be performed by either the transvenous endocardial,[8] the transvenous coronary sinus,[9] the transthoracic,[10,11] or the mediastinal-retrocardial approach.[12]

Transvenous Endocardial Pacing

Although much remains to be accomplished in terms of providing stability in transvenous atrial pacing and sensing, there has been a substantial improvement in both surgical techniques and electrode designs. As in the case of ventricular pacing, positioning the atrial lead in the right atrium and obtaining good parameter readings, plus attaining good lead stability during both deep inspiration and expiration, are the hallmarks of successful pacing.

In most of our atrial implants, we use a screw-in J lead. This lead was designed to follow the natural curve that starts from the superior vena cava and extends through the right atrium and into the right atrial appendage. The right atrial appendage, which is the most trabeculated portion of the right atrium, lies in the anterosuperior part of the right atrium. Although destruction of the right atrial appendage by a previous open-heart operation is a known limitation to this type of pacing, we have successfully used it without any complications in many patients.

The screw-in J lead is straightened by fully inserting the stylet. It is then passed transvenously, and once it lies in the right atrium it is maneuvered anteriorly; as the lead is pulled back, a portion of the stylet is also pulled back to establish the curve on the lead. Several attempts may be required to achieve satisfactory positioning in the appendage. The screw is advanced into the atrial tissue by merely rotating the end of the lead clockwise and observing it under fluoroscopy. When in the appendage, the lead tip can be seen under fluoroscopy to move from side to side in synchrony with the heartbeat. This effect is seen when the patient's underlying rhythm is sinus rhythm and obviously is not present with atrial arrythmias or quiescence.

Checking the stability of an atrial appendage implant can be performed by rotating the electrode manually from right to left. This will cause distortion in the loop, but the lead tip should remain in position if it is stable.[13] To prevent early dislodgement, tension in the lead should be maintained so that it is not too tight or too slack. The tension should be adjusted to the type of lead used and the anatomic variation in the right atrial appendage.

The screw-in lead may also be positioned in the lateral wall of the right atrium or in the interatrial septum away from the tricuspid valve and coronary sinus to prevent their potential damage. As in the case of right atrial appendage implants, several attempts may be required before successful fixation of the pacing electrode. A loop must be applied to the stylet in order to successfully guide the pacemaker screw-in lead to these second choice positions. Once good parameter readings are obtained, the screw is advanced into the designated area. Repeat electrical measurements may now show higher current and voltage readings than when the lead was just in contact with the endomyocardium. This situation should improve spontaneously within minutes and is regarded as a temporary change that is probably related to the local trauma caused by the screw. If the electrical parameters do not improve after several minutes, the lead should be repositioned. Finally, the lead is adjusted so that it is neither too tight nor too slack. Another choice of atrial lead includes the tined J lead, which can be positioned in the atrial appendage in a similar manner to that of a screw-in J lead.

Transvenous Coronary Sinus Pacing

The potential hazards of coronary sinus pacing are related to thrombosis or perforation of the vein[9] and early and frequent lead dislodgement.[14] Due to these and other disadvantages encountered (e.g., intermittent capture and sensing and, sometimes, left ventricular pacing), we do not recommend its use for routine permanent atrial pacing.

For easier insertion of the electrode into the coronary sinus, a left-sided venipuncture is preferable. A curve in the stylet will facilitate the insertion of the pacemaker lead into the coronary sinus. Initially, the pacemaker lead has to be advanced for some distance into the coronary sinus vein, and its position in the AV groove is confirmed under fluoroscopy before it is pulled back to its proper position in the proximal portion of the sinus. Further confirmation that the lead is in the coronary sinus is the presence of a left ventricular pacing pattern if the lead is connected to pacing. During the entire maneuvering in the coronary sinus vein, extreme care should be exercised to guard against perforation of this thin-walled vessel. Using a bipolar pacemaker lead for coronary sinus implant may assist the ability to pace proximally or distally. Since the electrode will lie freely in the coronary sinus, it is allowed to describe a smooth curve in the right atrium to aid in passive insertion of the lead and to decrease the incidence of lead dislodgement.

Some of the factors that may influence the success of this technique include the expertise of the surgeon in positioning the electrode into the proximal portion of the sinus; the size of the orifice, which may be small or distorted secondary to severe heart failure; and the pacemaker lead design, which may give better stability and fixation for this type of pacing.

Another approach is the mediastinal-retrocardial technique, which did not gain any popularity—probably because of the complications associated with transmediastinoscopic placement of the lead and the questionable reliability of pacing using this method.

Atrioventricular Pacing

With the introduction of DDD pacemaker batteries, the trend is to insert them whenever indicated, because they are the most effective physiologic units invented to take over the pacing action of the heart. The contribution of the

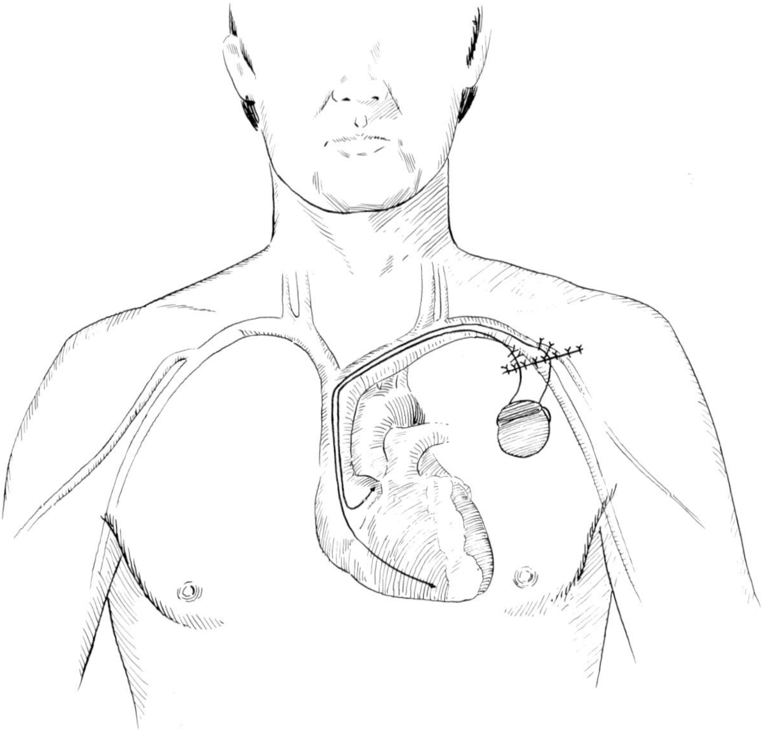

Figure 7–4. Dual chamber pacing with an atrial J lead passed through the subclavian vein and a ventricular lead passed through the cephalic vein. Both leads are secured with nonabsorbable sutures before connecting them to the pacemaker battery. Normally, both leads are inserted through the subclavian vein puncture, and this sketch is for demonstration purposes.

atrial kick to cardiac output is significant in patients with normal and impaired myocardial function.[15–17] Although ventricular pacing is the most commonly used procedure, we are seeing more patients with such units requiring conversion to dual-chamber pacing when the atrial systole contribution to cardiac output is significant.

The technique for dual-chamber pacing requires insertion of a single ventricular pacing electrode and a single atrial pacing electrode with connection of the two electrodes to the atrioventricular sequential battery that is buried in a pocket previously made in the infraclavicular region (Fig. 7–4). Although in some instances we were able to insert both electrodes through a fairly large-sized cephalic vein, our first choice is the subclavian vein puncture technique, except in women beyond the age of 75 years.

As the subclavian vein is punctured, the J wire is left in position as the introducer is removed. Then the ventricular lead is passed alongside the J wire, and the sheath is removed. Next, a second introducer and sheath are inserted into the subclavian vein, guided by the leftover J wire. Then the J wire and the introducer are removed, the atrial pacing electrode is inserted, and the sheath is removed. A purse-string suture is applied around the area of insertion into the subclavian vein and held snug with a hemostat to prevent excessive loss of blood while the pacemaker leads are being manipulated into their final positions. The ventricular lead is positioned first into the right ventricle. In order to allow further lead stability, the stylet is left in the ventricular lead while the atrial lead is being positioned in the right atrium. Once the atrial lead is properly positioned, the stylet is removed from both leads and the tension is then adjusted before transfixing them with sutures to the underlying muscle at the site of venous insertion. Finally, both pacing electrodes are connected to the battery and placed in a previously made pocket inferomedial to the skin incision.

THE TRANSTHORACIC APPROACH

In the U.S.A., the first successful method of long-term cardiac pacing in which both the pacemaker generator and electrode were implanted was performed via a thoracotomy.[18,19] The pacing electrodes were placed directly on the myocardium using a posterolateral thoracotomy. Presently, there are three different incisions used for epimyocardial implants: the anterolateral thoracotomy, the transxiphoid approach, and the transmediastinal approach. The screw-in and the tined transvenous pacing electrodes are currently used for atrial pacing. Both careful technique in inserting the screw-in electrode and correct choice of the area for electrode placement are vital for achieving successful pacing. Areas suitable for pacing on both atria are the appendage or its vicinity, where the wall is slightly thickened. Although the thickest area of myocardium and thus most suitable site for right ventricular pacing is the diaphragmatic surface of the right ventricle close to the apex of the heart, the anterior part of the right ventricle may also be successfully used in many cases, especially if it is thick enough. The spot on the left ventricle most appropriate for epimyocardial implants is the area between the left anterior descending artery anteriorly and the first marginal branch of the left circumflex coronary artery posteriorly. All transthoracic approaches require general anesthesia, but they do not require fluoroscopy.

The Anterolateral Thoracotomy Approach

This was described by Hunter[20] as a procedure in which a limited anterior thoracotomy is performed and entry into the chest is gained through the fifth intercostal space (Fig. 7–5). As the pleura is incised, the left lung is retracted laterally and the pericardium is opened an inch anterior to the left phrenic nerve, with both sides being marsupialized to each side of the chest retractor using nonabsorbable suture material.

The ventricular screw-in lead is twisted 2½ times clockwise with the help of the lead holder until the flange rests on the surface of the ventricle. If the

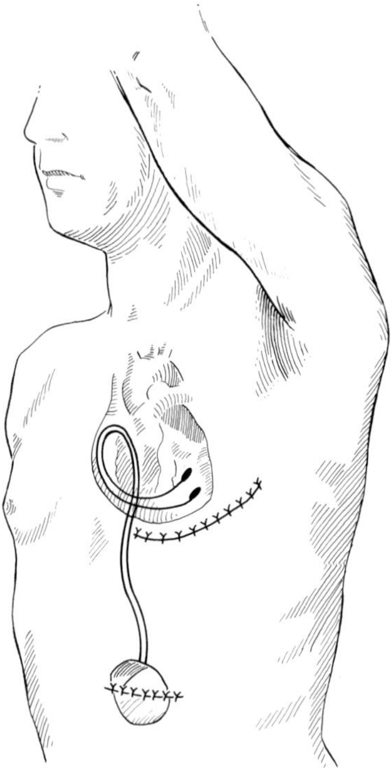

Figure 7–5. A left fifth intercostal space thoracotomy approach is shown. Two epicardial leads are implanted on the left ventricle and connected to a bipolar pacemaker battery. Left atrial pacing can be easily accomplished using this approach. The electrodes should cross over the closed pericardium and ribs diagonally and not acutely in order to prevent lead fracture.

electrical threshold measurements are not satisfactory, removal of the lead can be performed by using the lead holder as a handle to reverse the implantation process. This is accomplished by turning the lead 2½ times counterclockwise. Then the process of lead insertion is repeated at another site of the myocardium. As in endomyocardial screw-in lead insertions, a few minutes should be allowed for repeat electrical pacing measurement before deciding to use this spot or choose another area on the myocardium. Ventricular implants should be about an inch away from the left phrenic nerve at the end of the procedure, when the pericardium is closed; otherwise, hiccups synchronous with cardiac pacing may occur.[21,22] If atrial implants are required for pacing, then the appendage of the left atrium may be the spot of choice. If a screw-in lead is used, the same technique is used as with the ventricular implants. With the screw-in lead, the insertion of the electrode should be perpendicular to the area to be paced. Care should be taken not to use the lead holder as a pushing tool; otherwise, damage to viable myocardium may occur. Also, the electrode may penetrate too deeply and enter the cardiac chamber, causing exit block phenomenon.

A new technique for atrial pacing using a permanent transvenous lead was described by Gordon,[11] and we have successfully used it in four patients with no aftereffects. The lead is inserted into the atrium through a previously inserted purse-string suture, with a guiding suture tied to the tip of the lead and exiting at the area where the atrial appendage is to be paced.

When the pacing thresholds are tested and found to be satisfactory, the pericardium is closed with interrupted sutures. A second incision in the left epigastrium is performed, and a pocket is made for the pacemaker battery to lie between the rectus muscle and its anterior sheath. Both pacing electrodes extending from the closed pericardium and the closed intercostal space should cross over the pericardium and ribs diagonally rather than acutely to prevent lead fracture. A subcutaneous tunnel is made for passage of the leads from the chest area to the left epigastrium to be connected to the pacemaker battery, which is implanted in the previously made pocket. Both incisions are closed in layers, and a chest tube is inserted into the left pleural cavity for drainage and is removed in approximately 24 hours.

The Transxiphoid Approach

This is our first choice for transthoracic approach if only ventricular pacing is required. When atrioventricular pacing is required, then our first choice is the left anterior thoracotomy route. Our technique is the same as described by other surgeons (Fig. 7–6).[23–25]

A longitudinal incision is made over the xiphoid and extending into the lower sternum. The xiphoid process is removed, and the pericardium is exposed, avoiding entry to the pleura. After incising the pericardium, the diaphragmatic surface of the right ventricle is chosen as the spot for insertion of the epimyocardial leads. If for some reason that area is inaccessible because of adhesions, the anterior wall of the right ventricle can be chosen as the site for epimyocardial implant, and further exposure can be gained by chipping off part of the lower sternum using a rongeur. When the electrical measurements of the lead are found to be satisfactory, the lead is then connected to the pacemaker battery and placed in a pocket between the rectus muscle and its anterior sheath. A drain is inserted in the pericardium and removed in approximately 24 hours.

The Transmediastinal Approach

This can be performed through either median sternotomy[26] or a parasternal approach.[27, 28] The former is used in the course of open-heart operations and has the advantage of applying the pacing leads to either atria or ventricles. The parasternal approach limits exposure to the anterior wall of the right ventricle, and like the transxiphoid approach, atrial leads cannot be inserted if indicated because of the technical inaccessibility of the atrium.

With median sternotomy, the insertion of the epimyocardial leads and the

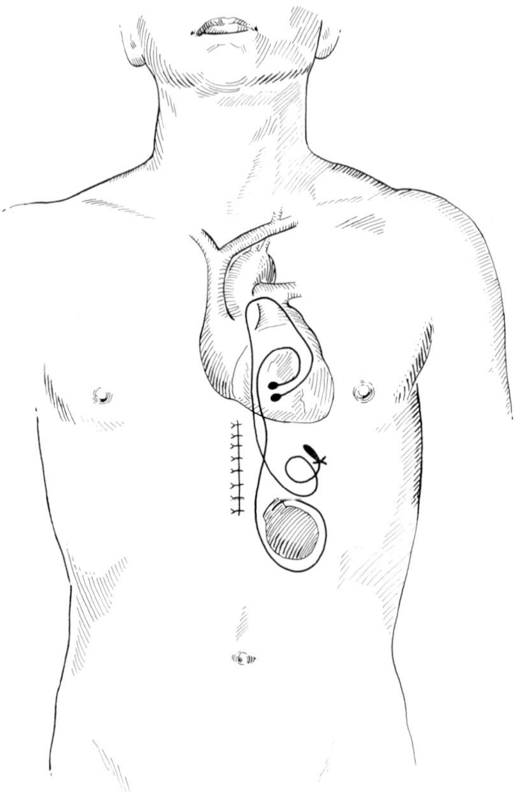

Figure 7–6. Transxiphoid approach showing two right ventricular epimyocardial leads with one of them attached to a unipolar pacemaker battery. The course of the electrodes straight downward as they leave the chest area to be connected to the pacemaker battery makes them far less liable to fracture than is the case with the anterior thoracotomy approach.

pacemaker battery is similar to that of the anterior thoracotomy. However, the pacemaker lead does not cross over the ribs; instead, it follows a straight downward course and is connected to the generator in the same fashion as in the transxiphoid approach.

In the parasternal approach, the cartilage of the left fifth rib is removed, and without entering the pleura the pericardium is exposed and lead insertion lies in the anterior part of the right ventricle. However, the extrapleural method does not neccesarily avoid the same pulmonary complications that can occur with the anterior thoracotomy approach. Also, the incidence of cardiac arrhythmias and pericarditis is significant with this technique.[29]

REFERENCES

1. Siddons H, and Sowton E: Cardiac Pacemakers. Springfield, Charles C Thomas, 1967.
2. Van der Salm TS, Haffajee CI, and Okike ON: Transvenous insertion of double sets of permanent electrodes through a single introducer: Clinical application. Ann Thorac Surg 32:307, 1981.
3. Hunt TK, and Dunphy JE: Fundamentals of Wound Management. New York, Appleton-Century-Crofts, 1979.
4. Wilson JN, Grow JB, Demong CV, et al: Central venous pressure in optimal blood volume maintenance. Arch Surg 85:563, 1962.
5. Romanes GJ: Cunningham's Textbook of Anatomy. Oxford, Oxford University Press, 1981.
6. Griepp RB, Daily PO, Shumway NG: Subclavian-axillary vein thrombosis following implantation of a pacemaker catheter in the internal jugular vein. J Thorac Cardiovasc Surg 60:889, 1970.
7. Jernigan WR, Gardner WC, Mahr MM, and Milburn JL: Use of internal jugular vein for placement of central venous catheter. Surg Gynecol Obstet 130:520, 1970.
8. Rodewald GG, Harms H, and Scheppokat KD: Intravenös-intrakardiale Applikation von vorhofgesteuerten elektrischen Schrittmachern. Z Kreislaufforschung 53:860, 1964.
9. Moss AJ, Rivers RJ, and Cooper M: Long-term perivenous atrial pacing from the proximal portion of the coronary vein. JAMA 209:543, 1969.
10. Nathan DA, Center S, Wu CY, and Keller W: An implantable synchronous pacemaker for the long-term correction of complete heart block. Am J Cardiol 11:362, 1963.
11. Gordon R, Bodell BR, Pearson WT, and Sacks SH: Permanent atrial electrode placement. Ann Thorac Surg 33:86, 1982.
12. Carlens G, Johansson L, Karlof J, and Thornander H: New method for atrial-triggered pacemaker treatment without thoracotomy. J Thorac Cardiovasc Surg 50:229, 1965.
13. Samet P, and El-Sherif N: Cardiac Pacing. New York, Grune and Stratton, 1980.
14. Chung EK: Artificial Cardiac Pacing. Baltimore, The Williams and Wilkins Co., 1978.
15. Samet P, Castillo C, and Bernstein WH: Hemodynamic consequences of atrial and ventricular pacing in subjects with normal hearts. Am J Cardiol 18:522, 1966.
16. Brockman SK: Dynamic function of atrial contraction in regulation of cardiac performance. Am J Physiol 204:597, 1963.
17. Kosowsky BD, Sherlag BJ, and Damato AN: Reevaluation of the atrial contribution to ventricular function. Am J Cardiol 21:518, 1968.
18. Chardack WM, Gage AA, and Greatbach W: A transistorized, self-contained, implantable pacemaker for the long-term correction of complete heart block. Surgery 48:643, 1960.
19. Kantrowitz A, Cohen R., Raillard et al: The treatment of complete heart block with an implanted controllable pacemaker. Surg Gynecol Obstet 115:415, 1962.
20. Hunter SW, Bolduc L, Long V, and Quattlebaum FW: A new myocardial pacemaker lead (sutureless). Chest 63:430, 1973.
21. Sprinkle JD, Takard T, and Scott SM: Phrenic nerve stimulation as a complication of the implantable cardiac pacemaker. Circulation 28:114, 1963.
22. Peleska B, and Buda J: Stimulation of the phrenic nerve as a complication of implanted pacemaker: Management without thoracotomy. J Cardiovasc Surg 6:477, 1965.
23. Carpentier A: Technique d'implantation de pace-maker par une voie d'abord abdominale sous-xyphoidienne. Presse Med 76:75, 1968.
24. Steward S: Placement of sutureless epicardial pacemaker lead by the subxiphoid approach. Ann Thorac Surg 18:308, 1973.
25. Buffle P: Ventricular pacing with epigastric transdiaphragmatic electrodes: Long-term follow-up and comparison with other implantation methods. J Thorac Cardiovasc Surg 72:226, 1976.
26. Guilmet D, Piwnica A, and Pedeferri G: Implantation d'un Stimulateur Cardiaque interne par sternotomie médiane ventricle. Ann Chir Thorac Cardiov 3:443, 1964.
27. Mobin-Uddin K, Smith PG, Lombardo C, and Judge JR: Local anesthesia for insertion of epicardial electrodes. J Thorac Cardiovasc Surg 55:112, 1968.
28. Dixon SH, Penyman RA, Morris JJ, and Young WG: Transmediastinal permanent ventricular pacing. Ann Thorac Surg 14:206, 1972.
29. Brenner AS, Wagner GS, Anderson ST, et al: Transvenous, transmediastinal, and transthoracic ventricular pacing. A comparison after complete two-year follow up. Circulation 49:407, 1974.

8

Cardiac Pacing in Children

JEFFREY M. DUNN, M.D.,
and ASHOK V. MEHTA, M.D.

Although much of the pediatric pacemaker theory and application is derived from experience with adults, it would be unfortunate to ignore the uniqueness of the pediatric population. We will endeavor in this chapter to cover the breadth of pediatric pacing but with weighted consideration of pacemaker application unique to the pediatric population. There seems to be a general pessimistic attitude toward a child's needing a pacemaker. Indeed, this is unfortunate, for recent experience dictates an aggressive and optimistic approach. Pediatric pacing need not be approached with any more trepidation than adult pacing.

TEMPORARY CARDIAC PACING

Indications

Temporary pacing is indicated for arrhythmias that are expected to be short-lived secondary to cardiac infections and drugs,[1] as well as following cardiac surgery,[2,3] as an adjunct to cardiopulmonary resuscitation, in preparation for permanent pacing,[4] and in the catheterization laboratory during pharmacologic and electrophysiologic studies.

Methods

Transvenous Approach

Temporary transvenous endocardial leads are useful in emergency situations in which the arrhythmia to be treated is expected to be self-resolving during electrophysiologic studies and in preparation for placement of a permanent system. We prefer to place temporary wires under fluoroscopic control. However, in emergency situations a balloon electrode catheter may be "blindly" floated. The technique need be no different in children than in adults. Venous cutdown or percutaneous modified Seldinger's technique[5] can be employed. The vein of entry may be antecubital, axillary, femoral, proximal saphenous, internal jugular, or subclavian.

Transthoracic Approach

This pacing mode is reserved for emergency resuscitation when transvenous placement of a temporary wire is contraindicated because of (1) lack of time and (2) difficulty in placing a transvenous lead during resuscitation and when forward flow is minimal, thus negating the efficacy of ballooned floating transvenous systems.

Transthoracic endocardial kits are commercially available. A spinal needle is placed percutaneously below the xiphoid and directed toward the left shoulder into the right ventricle. Position is assured by free blood return. An electrode catheter is then passed through the needle into the ventricular chamber. With removal of the syringe needle, the electrode is secured in the ventricular chamber by its preformed angular tip. Transthoracic pacing should be replaced by transvenous pacing as soon as practical.

Esophageal Approach

Several investigators have reported use of unipolar and bipolar esophageal leads to stimulate the atria and ventricles. Compared with transvenous and epicardial wire pacing techniques,[6–8] esophageal pacing provides a somewhat noninvasive, safe, and rapid bedside method for pacing the atria without fluoroscopy, sedation, cardiac catheterization, or sterile precautions. We have used this technique frequently for diagnosis and management of arrhythmias in children. As suggested by Gallagher and colleagues,[6] a permanent bipolar transvenous wire with electrodes spaced 2.9 cm apart is passed through the nose into the esophagus. The electrode is secured where the greatest unipolar EKG is exhibited. We routinely record the unipolar electrogram from the esophageal leads before pacing, thus limiting the chance of inadvertently pacing the ventricle. Most children tolerate this procedure with only minimal initial discomfort.

Epicardial Approach

Perhaps the most frequent application of temporary pacing is after open-heart surgery for congenital and acquired defects.[9,10] We place temporary epicardial wires prophylactically in virtually all patients at the completion of each open-heart procedure. Their usefulness has been repeatedly proved to us, not only for emergency pacing but also for diagnosis of arrhythmias.

We routinely place two atrial and two ventricular temporary wires. This allows for atrial, ventricular, and sequential pacing modes and provides as well for a backup should one of the leads become dislodged or develop exit block, problems that are frequent with temporary leads. In addition, the atrial leads allow atrial EKG recording for evaluation of supraventricular arrhythmias.

Atrial Wire Placement. Two centimeters of bared electrode are fixated to the right atrial surface with one or two superficial 6–0 Dacron sutures (Fig. 8–1). The two wires are placed about 3 cm apart, on the appendage and body of the right atrium, respectively. The ends are brought out through the skin and fixated.

Ventricular Wire Placement. The ventricular wires are placed in the right ventricular epicardium, clear of obvious coronary arteries. The swedged needle lead is passed through 5 to 10 mm of myocardium at a depth of about 2 mm. Myocardial bleeding is controlled with gentle pressure. The wire is secured with a small Silastic pledget. A small loop of wire is left in the mediastinum, and the distal ends are brought out through the skin. By convention, atrial wires are brought out of the skin to the right of the midline, whereas ventricular wires are brought out to the left.

When not in use, all wires are electrically isolated in latex finger cots or wrapped in gauze. The wires are routinely removed by gentle traction on or about the seventh postoperative day, when they are no longer needed. We have experience of only one complication of removal. In that case, hemopericardium followed removal of an epicardial wire in an anticoagulated patient following double valve replacement. If undue tension is required to remove the wire, the wire can be prepped with povidone-iodine (Betadine) and alcohol and cut at the skin level while the wire is gently tensioned. The end will then permanently retract below the skin. We have experienced no complications with wires left in this manner.

Transcutaneous Approach

Transcutaneous pacing is an important adjunct in pacemaker therapy. It is used to temporarily suppress a ventricular demand pacemaker during electrophysiologic studies, while evaluating intrinsic cardiac rhythm during pacemaker follow-up, and during open-heart surgery when a "cardiopleged" quiet heart is desired.[11] Pacemaker standstill is achieved by placing two surface electrode pads over the left anterior shoulder and pacing these leads with a temporary external generator. If the patient's permanent pacemaker is bipolar, two additional surface electrode pads should be placed over the posterior chest wall and connected to a second temporary pacemaker generator. By increasing the rate of the external temporary pacemaker to just above that of the implanted permanent unit, the permanent unit can be inhibited.

PERMANENT CARDIAC PACING

Indications

During the past 11 years we have implanted pacemakers in 27 pediatric patients at St. Christopher's Hospital for Children (Table 8–1). The single most common indication for permanent pacing in the pediatric age group is symptomatic bradycardia regardless of cause. The indications are summarized below:

1. Third-degree atrioventricular (AV) block (congenital; acquired, nonsurgical, chronic; acquired postsurgical)
2. Progressive second-degree AV block with symptomatic bradycardia
3. Sick sinus syndrome and sinus bradycardia
4. Hypersensitive carotid sinus syndrome
5. Refractory tachyarrhythmias

Methods

Transvenous Approach

We have rarely used permanent transvenous pacing in children, although there are reports advocating this mode. The obvious advantage is in avoiding the morbidity and mortality of mediastinal and transthoracic approaches. The most obvious disadvantages are (1) difficult access in small veins, (2) intracardiac manipulation in the presence of associated cardiac anomalies and intracardiac repairs (such as an intra-atrial baffle), (3) lead dislodgement secondary to growth and increasing distance between the venous fixation site and endocardial contact site, and (4) the risk of systemic embolization in patients with congenital intracardiac shunts.

In older children, the techniques for transvenous pacemaker placement are identical to those in their adult counterparts, reviewed in other sections of this book.

Table 8–1. Indications for Pacemaker Implantation at St. Christopher's Hospital for Children from 1971 to 1982

Indication	Number of Patients
1. Congenital third-degree AV block with no heart disease	3
2. Congenital third-degree AV block with structural heart disease	3
3. Acquired surgical third-degree AV block	7
4. Acquired progressive second-degree AV block and third-degree AV block	6
5. Sick sinus syndrome	4
6. Hypersensitive carotid sinus syndrome	4
Total	27

Epicardial Approach

Epicardial pacing is the most common method utilized for permanent pacing in children. It affords localization of atrial as well as right and left ventricular leads and provides for positive electrode placement without the risk of lead dislodgement as the patient grows.

It is a general impression—although not well documented—that exit block occurs more frequently in children than in adults,[12] especially following open-heart surgery. It is not known whether this is true for transvenous leads as well.

In general, we prefer lead placement via a subxiphoid approach or a limited anterior thoracotomy. Since atrial and ventricular sensing and pacing (DDD mode) offer superior hemodynamics, both right atrial and ventricular leads are placed (Fig. 8–1). This can be accomplished with reasonable exposure through a subxiphoid incision, a right thoracotomy, or a median sternotomy. We generally place two atrial and two ventricular epicardial leads. A small "threshold" probe is employed to locate the most advantageous location before permanent lead implantation.

Because of the inherent thin ventricular walls in children, modification of lead placement from standard adult technique becomes imperative. A lead that perforates the endocardium into the lumen will not only bleed acutely but is more likely to develop exit block with fibrosis around the lead. Thus when

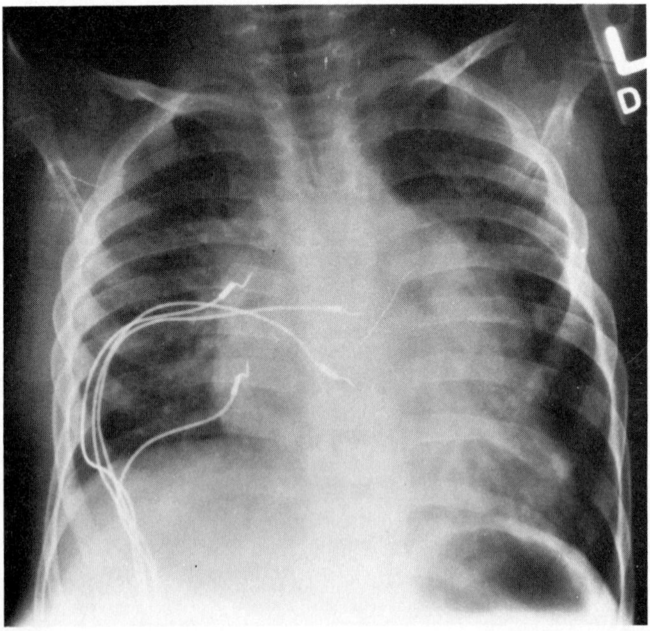

Figure 8–1. Two-year-old child with sick sinus syndrome and syptomatic sinus bradycardia with nodal release. Underlying disease is "upstairs-downstairs" ventricles with levotransposition, ventricular septal defect, and straddling tricuspid valve, after palliative Mustard repair with pulmonary artery banding. Two atrial and two ventricular leads (Medtronic #4951–35).

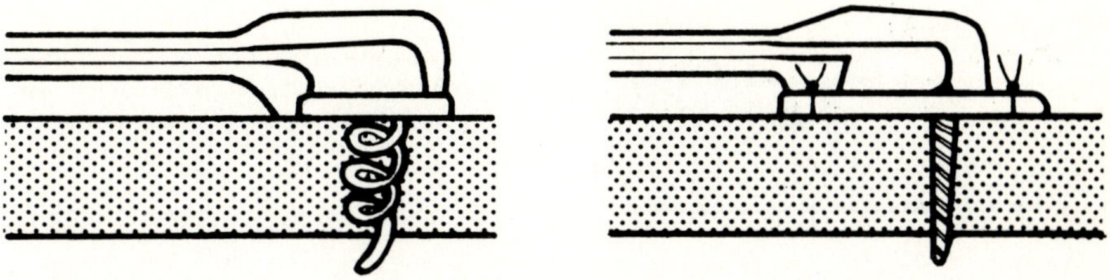

Figure 8–2. Screw-in and post-type leads, which are too deep for the thin pediatric ventricle. Endocardial perforation may produce acute bleeding and ultimately exit block secondary to fibrosis.

bleeding occurs, the leads are removed and replaced. Certain leads are intrinsically too deep for infants and small children and should be avoided. These include "screw-in" leads (Fig. 8–2). Other "post"-type leads such as the Medtronic #6913 and #5815 leads can be modified by bending the post backward so that the electrode protrusion is shallow. We have found this very acceptable in even the smallest infants (Fig. 8–3).

We have found that two lead designs are especially suited for use in infants and small children. The Telectronic lead #030–140 consists of a suture-like extension of the insulated lead. It can be placed at any depth, much like a temporary lead (Fig. 8–4). Recently a shallow "harpoon hook"-type lead (Medtronic #4951–35) has been introduced (Fig. 8–5). It is shallow, is easy to implant, and seems to offer excellent threshold levels, at least for the short follow-up it has afforded.

Permanent placement of the pacing unit continues to be problematic because of the discrepancy between patient and pacer size. Subcutaneous pouches, although easy to make, run the risk of acute erosion secondary to tension and chronic erosion secondary to mechanical trauma in the active child.

Other locations of pacer placement suggested for children include (1) intrathoracic, (2) intra-abdominal, (3) extraperitoneal, and (4) subrectus muscle sites. We prefer placement just deep to the rectus muscle, superficial to the transversalis fascia.[13]

Intrathoracic placement may cause pulmonary compression and atelectasis and necessitates a thoracotomy for battery change. Intra-abdominal placement runs the risk of internal bowel herniation and strangulation, even when attempts at extraperitonealization are made. Extraperitoneal placement above the iliac crest after reflection of the peritoneum can accommodate a pacemaker in a child of any size. One patient in our series, however, has vague abdominal pain when

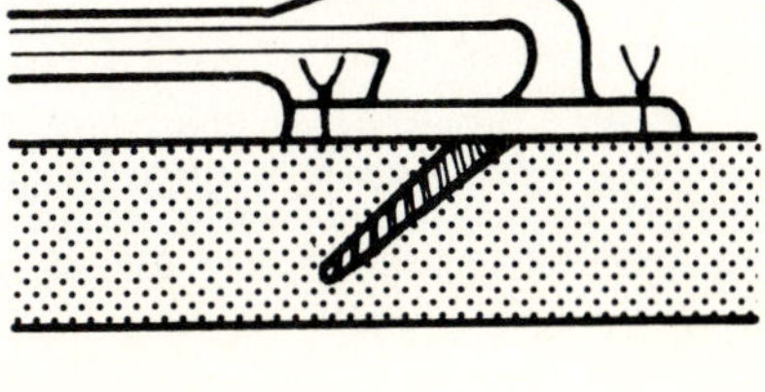

Figure 8–3. A post-type epicardial lead can be bent back on itself with gentle pressure to avoid endocardial perforation.

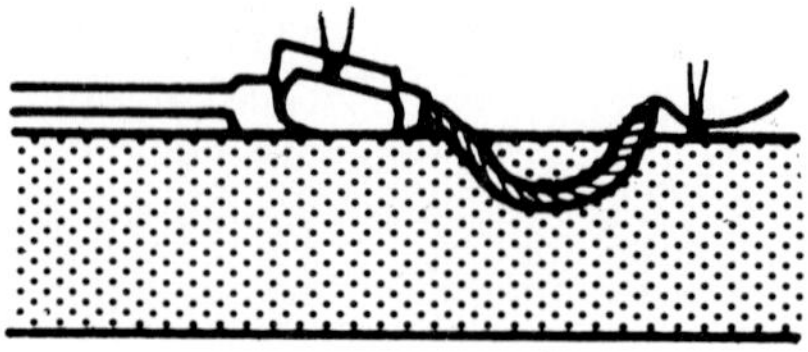

Figure 8–4. Telectronic permanent epicardial lead (#030–140), sutures in place much like a temporary lead. It can be placed to any depth in the myocardium.

she has a full bladder. A cystogram demonstrates indentation of her bladder by the battery pack and 90 degree rotation of the battery pack when her bladder is emptied (Fig. 8–6).

The subrectus muscle position has been uniformly successful in our hands, even in a 3-day-old, 2.5-kg infant with congenital heart block (Fig. 8–7). Through a subxiphoid incision, the anterior rectus sheath is incised longitudinally near the midline. The rectus muscle is reflected off the posterior rectus sheath. This is a relatively avascular dissection except for a few perforating vessels, which are meticulously controlled. After the pacemaker is placed, the rectus sheath is closed without drains.

SURGICAL AV BLOCK

AV block may occur following open-heart surgery for congenital defects,[2, 3, 12, 14, 15] when conduction pathways are surgically violated. Specific congenital lesions (e.g., levotransposition of the great vessels) predispose to spontaneous AV block, especially during stress. Postoperative drug manipulation may also induce AV block.

Surgically, the AV conduction pathway can be encountered in several locations. The AV node and proximal bundle of His are located in the right atrium roughly in the area inscribed by a triangle consisting of the coronary sinus ostium, the tricuspid annulus, and the tendon of Tadoro.[16] This area is surgically vulnerable in repair or replacement of the tricuspid valve, closure of primum atrial septal defects, correction of endocardial cushion defects, and atrial baffle procedures for repair of transposition of the great arteries.[16]

The bundle of His courses from the AV node to the central fibrous body and onto the junction of the muscular and membranous ventricular septum. Immediately the left ventricular bundle branch appears on the left ventricular surface at the junction of the muscular septum and membranous septum. The

Figure 8–5. Medtronic harpoon lead (#4951–35) enters the myocardium only a few millimeters, thus avoiding ventricular perforation. It may be used either as an atrial or ventricular epicardial lead.

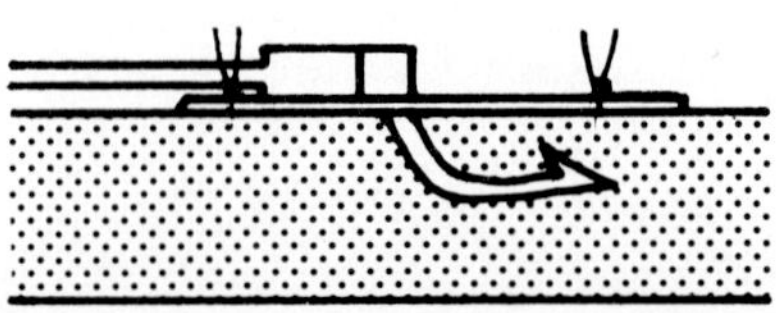

continuation of the bundle of His becomes the right bundle branch and continues toward the papillary muscle of the conus and eventually traverses the septoparietal band and extends into the parietal wall.

When membranous ventricular septal defects occur, the His bundle courses on the edge of the defect in its posterior and inferior portion before diving into the septum. It is here that closure of a ventricular septal defect runs the risk of producing complete heart block.[16] Endocardial mapping of the beating heart can be helpful in localizing the conduction system, especially when it is expected to be aberrant. These techniques, however, are cumbersome, time consuming, and frequently unrewarding. One can generally avoid complete heart block more easily in a quiet, relaxed heart following cardioplegia by relying on knowledge of the conduction pathways for the particular cardiac defect at hand.

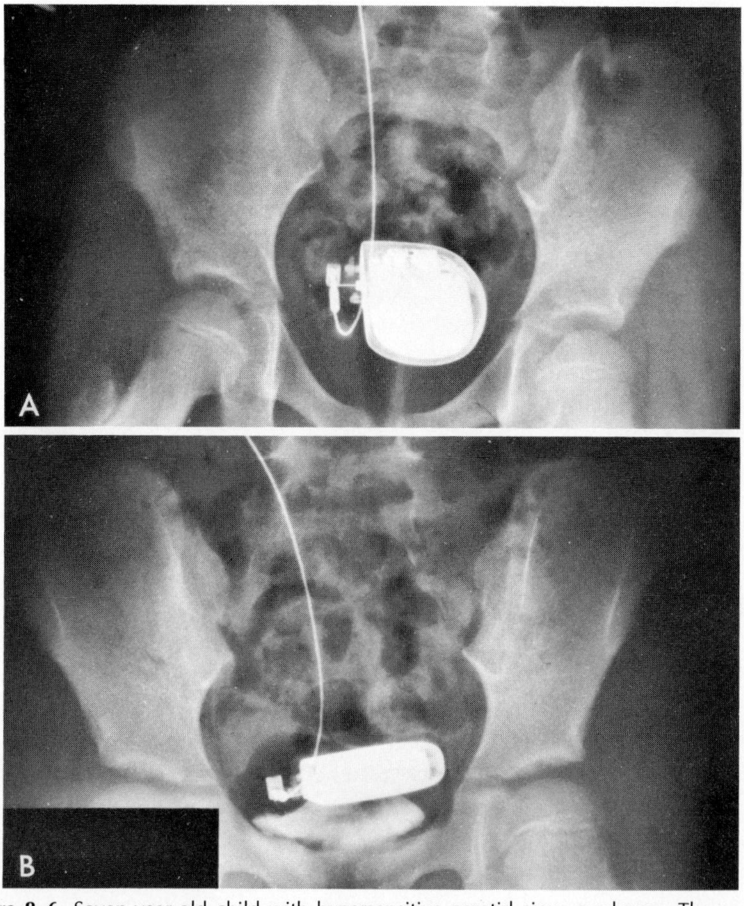

Figure 8–6. Seven-year-old child with hypersensitive carotid sinus syndrome. The pacemaker unit was located in the pre-peritoneal space. Patient complained of chronic low abdominal pain. *A*, Position of pacemaker with bladder full. *B*, Position of pacemaker with bladder empty (barium in rectum). Note the movement of the pacemaker by bladder distension.

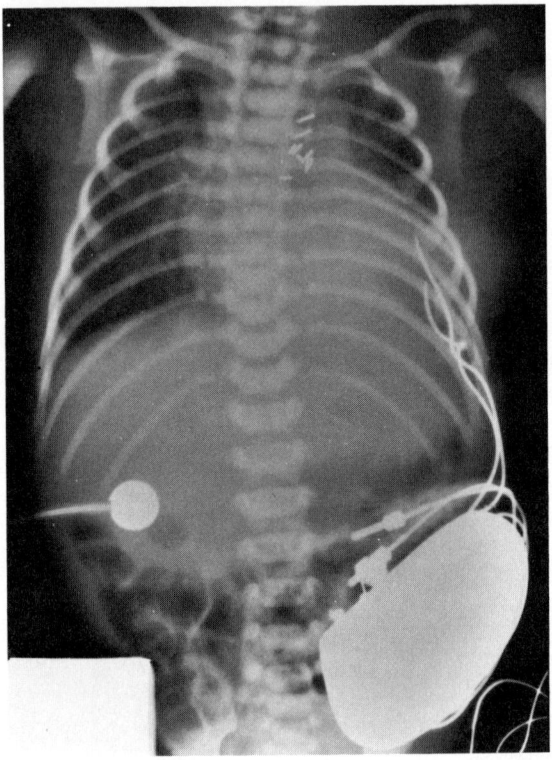

Figure 8–7. Two-day-old child with congenital third-degree AV block and complex congenital heart disease (double-outlet right ventricle, single atrium, total anomalous pulmonary venous drainage, patent ductus arteriosus, and hemiazygos continuation of an interrupted inferior vena cava). Pacemaker unit (Medtronic Spectrax) is placed in the subrectus position. The ventricular leads are Telectronic #030–140.

Right bundle branch block can be produced by most right ventriculotomies and by sutures at the inferolateral aspect of most ventricular septal defects adjacent to the moderator band, an area that is unavoidable if the defect is to be completely closed. These bundle branch block patterns, when isolated, are probably of little or no clinical significance.

The return of a sinus conduction mechanism at the completion of surgery offers no assurance that temporary complete AV block may not occur in the first 24 to 48 hours after surgery. Thus prophylactic temporary epicardial wires are always placed. In our experience, temporary complete AV block may occur anytime in the first few postoperative days. In the majority of cases, the block resolves spontaneously within the first week but may remain for up to 3 or 4 weeks.[15] Beyond 4 weeks resolution of the AV block is extremely unlikely, and we routinely would convert to a permanent implanted epicardial system.

Electrophysiologic studies may be of great help in evaluating the need for permanent pacing. We routinely convert to permanent pacing if the block is intra- or infrahisian.[14] For block above the level of the bundle of His we utilize more conservative indications for pacing, as reviewed below in the section on congenital third-degree AV block.

CONGENITAL HEART BLOCK

Congenital heart block is identified soon after birth but may also be diagnosed during the third trimester of pregnancy by the presence of a fetal heart rate less than 100 beats per minute, which is confirmed by 2-dimensional and M-mode echocardiography. As many as one-half of these infants will also have severe and complex congenital heart disease.[17] Severely affected infants are at risk of fetal wastage and cardiac decompensation upon delivery and separation from the supportive maternal circulation. This can be predicted during the antenatal period by the documentation of decreased fetal tone and movement, echocardiographic evidence of complex cardiac anomalies, or echocardiographic evidence of fetal hydrops, including increased amniotic fluid, ascites, decreased head-to-abdomen ratio (secondary to ascites), pericardial effusion, increased liver size, and increased scalp thickness.

There is much debate regarding the management of hydropic fetus associated with congenital heart block. Early delivery affords the ability to treat the AV block but must be weighed against the risk of delivering an immature infant, especially in the 30- to 35-week gestation period. Transuterine pacing has not been attempted. Certainly the fetus with congenital heart block should be delivered at an institution with perinatal and neonatal services as well as pediatric cardiology and pediatric cardiothoracic surgical facilities.

We routinely use temporary transvenous pacing for any such infant born with congenital heart block and congestive heart failure. These infants usually improve dramatically with the combination of ventricular pacing and medical therapy. Placement of the temporary wire should be accompanied by cardiac catheterization in the infant with structural cardiac anomalies.

In this setting, the temporary pacing system should be replaced by a permanent system without delay. Here medical judgment is important. The combination of temporary pacing and medical therapy will make the patient a better surgical candidate after several days, as congestive heart failure resolves. However, temporary wires can perforate the infant's small and thin-walled right or left ventricle more easily than an adult's. We thus follow the policy of placing a permanent epicardial system as soon as the child is moderately stable and is a reasonable anesthetic risk.

The decision for pacing in the infant without severe cardiac failure is more difficult. A ventricular rate of less than 50 beats per minute represents an absolute indication for pacing.[18] In addition, any symptoms related to cardiac function, such as poor feeding, failure to thrive, heart failure, syncope, and seizures must be considered as relative indications for permanent pacing.[17, 18]

ACQUIRED, CHRONIC, NONSURGICAL THIRD-DEGREE AV BLOCK

Acquired nonsurgical third-degree AV block has been reported with myocarditis, endocarditis, tumor, sclerosis of the cardiac skeleton (Lenegre's disease),[19] rubella, infections, progressive external ophthalmoplegia,[20] rheumatic carditis, Chagas' disease, sarcoidosis, and structural heart lesions (e.g., levotransposition of great arteries),[17] endocardial cushion defects,[17, 21–23] and polysplenia syndrome.[23] We and others have seen progressive second-degree AV block result in third-degree AV block with and without structural heart lesions.[22] Whether the natural history of these patients differs significantly from those with congenital third-degree AV block is unknown. However, the indications for permanent pacing are the same as for congenital third-degree AV block.

PROGRESSIVE SECOND-DEGREE AV BLOCK

Second-degree AV block, either Mobitz type I or II, is an uncommon disease entity in the pediatric age group.[22, 24] In adults, Mobitz type II second-degree AV block is commonly associated with disease of the distal conducting system. We have followed 19 patients with Mobitz type I second-degree AV block. Three of these patients developed third-degree AV block and four developed symptomatic bradycardia with a high degree of AV block (2:1 or 3:1) necessitating permanent pacing.[22] Again, the indication for permanent pacing depends on the symptoms and heart rate as mentioned in the section above on congenital third-degree AV block.

SICK SINUS SYNDROME

Sinus node dysfunction characterized by inappropriate sinus bradycardia, sinus arrest, or sinoatrial (SA) exit block has been reported in children with and without structural heart disease.[25–27] Sick sinus syndrome is commonly recognized as a slow rate alternating with supraventricular tachycardia or atrial flutter (bradycardia-tachycardia syndrome). Sick sinus syndrome is commonly seen in children after Mustard procedure for dextro-transposition of the great arteries, surgical atrial septectomy, and repair of atrial septal defects.[26–28] Permanent pacing in bradycardia-tachycardia syndrome protects against symptomatic bradycardia, and pacing may eliminate supraventricular tachycardia, negating the need for pharmacologic agents to suppress the tachyarrhythmias.[26–28]

HYPERSENSITIVE CAROTID SINUS SYNDROME

At our center we have implanted permanent pacemakers in four children with hypersensitive carotid sinus syndrome. Some of these children have been reported in the literature as having sick sinus syndrome. This syndrome has been seen more commonly in adults than in children. We routinely perform electrophysiologic studies in children suspected of having hypersensitive carotid sinus syndrome to rule out associated SA node or AV node dysfunctions. The diagnosis is usually made from surface EKG or 24-hour Holter recording with long sinus pauses (greater than 2.5 sec) at rest or with vagal stimulation such as unilateral carotid massage.[29] Permanent pacing is the treatment of choice rather than long-term vagolytic agents.[29, 30] Patients with hypersensitive carotid sinus syndrome who demonstrate a significant vasopressor response should be managed by sequential AV pacing.[30]

REFRACTORY TACHYARRHYTHMIAS

With the advent of intracardiac electrophysiologic study, the mechanisms of tachyarrhythmias have been well defined and are well understood. With the advance of more sophisticated and reliable pacemaker technology, the indications for permanent pacing have been increased in the management of tachyarrhythmias. The most common indication for permanent pacing in children with refractory supraventricular tachycardia is the prevention and treatment of bradycardia secondary to pharmacotherapy. This is especially valuable when surgical ablation may not be feasible (e.g., atrial flutter and AV nodal reentry). Resistant cases of ectopic junctional tachycardia may necessitate ablation of the AV node and placement of a permanent pacemaker to assure an adequate ventricular rate. Similarly, ablation of a septal accessory conduction pathway may damage the normal AV conduction mechanisms, necessitating permanent pacing.

In resistant reentrant supraventricular tachycardias, overdrive pacing by radio-frequency transmitter or special antitachycardia pacing (burst pacing) can be therapeutic.[30] Similarly an asynchronous underdrive atrial pacemaker may be useful in selected cases of reentrant supraventricular tachycardia.[31] Scanning pacemakers are a recent adjunct to the management of tachycardias with relatively low rates.[31] With these pacemakers, a single-paced stimulus is emitted after each third QRS complex at a predetermined interval. This is helpful in any reentrant tachycardia in which single or double extrastimuli have been demonstrated by electrophysiologic studies to terminate the tachycardia. Dual-demand pacing is also available to control bradycardias and tachycardias. The future promises the availability of automatic implantable defibrillating and cardioverting units.

REFERENCES

1. Fisch C, and Knoebel SB: Recognition and therapy of digitalis toxicity. Prog Cardiovasc Dis 13:71, 1970.

2. Fryda RJ, Kaplan S, and Helmsworth JA: Postoperative complete heart block in children. Br Heart J 33:456, 1971.
3. Anderson PAW, Rogers MC, Canent RV, et al: Reversible complete heart block following cardiac surgery. Circulation 36:514, 1971.
4. Scott DL: Cardiac pacemakers as an anesthetic problem. Anesthesia 25:87, 1970.
5. Seldinger SI: Catheter replacement of needle in percutaneous arteriography: New technique. Acta Radiol 39:368, 1953.
6. Gallagher JJ, Smith WM, Kerr CR, et al: Esophageal pacing: A diagnostic and therapeutic tool. Circulation 65:336, 1982.
7. Burac B, and Furman S: Transesophageal cardiac pacing. Am J Cardiol 23:469, 1969.
8. Montoyo JV, Angel J, Valle V, and Gansi C: Cardioversion of tachycardia by transesophageal atrial pacing. Am J Cardiol 32:85, 1973.
9. Yabek SM, Aki BF, Berman W, et al: Use of atrial epicardial electrodes to diagnose and treat postoperative arrhythmias in children. Am J Cardiol 46:285, 1980.
10. Waldo AL, MacLean WAH, Cooper TB, et al: Use of temporarily placed epicardial atrial wire electrodes for the diagnosis and treatment of cardiac arrhythmias following open-heart surgery. J Thorac Cardiovasc Surg 76:500, 1978.
11. Hakki HI, Goel IP, and Mundth ED: Pacemaker inhibition in cardiac surgery. Ann Thorac Surg 33:295, 1982.
12. Rowe RD: Permanent cardiac pacing in infants and children. Pace 1:439, 1978.
13. Amato JJ, and Payne DD: Intramuscular abdominal implantation of permanent pacemakers in infants and children. Ann Thorac Surg 25:243, 1978.
14. Driscoll DJ, Gillette PC, Hallman GL, et al: Management of surgical complete atrio-ventricular block in children. Am J Cardiol 43:1175, 1979.
15. Murphy DA, Tynan M, Graham GR, and Bonham-Carter RE: Prognosis of complete atrio-ventricular dissociation in children after open-heart surgery. Lancet 1:750, 1970.
16. Hudson REB: Surgical pathology of the conducting system of the heart. Br Heart J 29:646, 1967.
17. Carter JB, Blieden LC, and Edwards JE: Congenital heart block. Arch Pathol 97:51, 1974.
18. Karpawich PP, Gillette PC, Garson A Jr, et al: Congenital complete atrio-ventricular block: Clinical and electrophysiologic predictors of need for pacemaker insertion. Am J Cardiol 48:1098, 1981.
19. Dianzumba SB, Singer DH, and Megers S: Lenegre's disease in youth. Am Heart J 94:479, 1977.
20. Morriss JH, Eugster GS, and Nora JJ: His bundle recordings in progressive external ophthalmoplegia. J Pediatr 81:1167, 1972.
21. Mehta AV, O'Riordan AC, Sanchez GR, and Black IFS: Acquired non-surgical complete atrio-ventricular block in a child with endocardial cushion defect. Clinical Cardiol 5:603, 1982.
22. Mehta AV, Sanchez GR, Balian A, et al: Natural history of 2° A-V block in children (abstract). Proc. to American Academy of Pediatrics, Cardiology Section, New York, October 22, 1982.
23. Garcia OL, Mehta AV, Pickoff AS, et al: Left isomerism and complete atrioventricular block: A report of six cases. Am J Cardiol 48:1103, 1981.
24. Young D, Eisenberg R, Fish B, and Fisher JD: Wenckebach atrio-ventricular block (Mobitz type I) in children and adolescents. Am J Cardiol 40:393, 1977.
25. Yabek SM, Dillon T, Berman W Jr, and Niland CJ: Symptomatic sinus node dysfunction in children without structural heart disease. Pediatrics 69:590, 1982.
26. Yabek SM, and Jarmakani JM: Sinus node dysfunction in children, adolescents, and young adults. Pediatrics 61:593, 1978.
27. Gillett PC: Recent advances in mechanisms, evaluation, and pacemaker treatment of chronic bradydysrhythmias in children. Am Heart J 102(5):920, 1981.
28. Fleming WH, Sarafian LB, Kuglar JD, et al: Changing indications for pacemakers in children. Ann Thorac Surg 31:329, 1981.
29. Peretz DI, Gevein AN, and Miyagishima RT: Permanent demand pacing for hypersensitive carotid sinus syndrome. Can Med Assoc J 108:1131, 1973.
30. Morley CA, Perrins EJ, Grant P, et al: Carotid sinus syncope treated by pacing; analysis of persistent symptoms and role of atrio-ventricular sequential pacing. Br Heart J 47:411, 1982.
31. Wellens HJJ, Bar FW, Gorgels AP, and Muncharaz JF: Electrical management of arrhythmias with emphasis on the tachycardias Am J Cardiol 41:1025, 1978.
32. Spurrell RAJ, Nathan AW, Bexton RS, et al: Implantable automatic scanning pacemaker for termination of supraventricular tachycardia. Am J Cardiol 49:753, 1982.

9

Cardiac Pacing Following Open-Heart Surgery

IOANNIS P. PANIDIS, M.D.,
and MORRIS N. KOTLER, M.D.

INTRODUCTION

Significant rhythm and conduction disturbances often occur after open-heart surgery, during recovery from cardioplegic arrest.[1–3] The severity of rhythm abnormalities and the time required for the heart to return to normal sinus rhythm appear to be related to the amount of cardioplegic solution used and the duration of aortic cross-clamping.[4] Temporary epicardial wires, inserted at the time of thoracotomy and removed before the patient's discharge, are almost routinely used after open-heart surgery for the effective control of postoperative tachyarrhythmias and the maintenance of an adequate heart rate during bradyarrhythmias.[4,5] Ventricular pacing has been used to enhance cardiac output early after heart surgery, when myocardial function and ventricular compliance are often decreased.[1,6] However, improvement in cardiac output and hemodynamic state is more effectively accomplished postoperatively in critically ill patients by atrial or atrioventricular (AV) sequential temporary pacing.[7,8] The modes, indications (Table 9–1), and complications of temporary epicardial pacing after open-heart surgery will be reviewed in this chapter.

MODES AND TECHNIQUES OF TEMPORARY PACING AFTER OPEN-HEART SURGERY

The exact incidence of rhythm and conduction abnormalities after coronary bypass surgery or valve replacement and the percentage of patients who will require temporary pacing are not known. Morin and colleagues[4] reported that 24 of 100 patients who underwent open-heart surgery required the use of pacing

Table 9–1. Indications for Cardiac Pacing After Open-Heart Surgery

Bradyarrhythmias
Sinus node abnormalities (sinus arrest, sinus bradycardia, slow nodal rhythm)
Second- or third-degree AV block
Tachyarrhythmias
Atrial (atrial flutter, supraventricular tachycardia)
Ventricular (ventricular tachycardia)
Hemodynamic Improvement
Rate augmentation by ventricular pacing
Increase in cardiac output by atrial or AV sequential pacing

for various brady- or tachyarrhythmias. An additional number of patients may need pacing for hemodynamic reasons. Since pacing requirements in patients who have had open-heart surgery are unpredictable, epicardial wires are routinely inserted at surgery.[4] Many centers still use a ventricular-inhibited demand (VVI) temporary pacemaker by implanting pacing wires on the right or left ventricular epicardium. More recently atrial-inhibited (AAI) or AV sequential (DVI) pacing has been used after open-heart surgery.[4,7,8] The DVI pacing is a bipolar, ventricular-inhibited pacing system, which sequentially paces the right atrium and ventricle on demand. The atrium is paced, and if intact AV conduction is present, ventricular pacing is inhibited. In the presence of coexisting AV conduction abnormalities the ventricle is sequentially paced at a preselected AV interval.[9] Two wire electrodes are placed on the right atrial surface and two on the right ventricular epicardial surface at the time of operation. The atrial electrodes are implanted on the right atrium adjacent to the AV groove, approximately 2.5 cm apart. The ventricular electrodes are placed on the right ventricular outflow tract.[8] The atrial wires are exited from the right subcostal area and the ventricular wires from the left subcostal area. The wires usually are gently withdrawn on the fifth postoperative day or before the patient's hospital discharge. Recent advances in the technique of insertion and lead design of epicardial electrodes have minimized the problems of dislodgement, inconsistent electrical performance, and tissue trauma.[10–12]

BRADYARRHYTHMIAS AFTER OPEN-HEART SURGERY

Atrioventricular Block

Postoperative AV block in adults is usually associated with replacement of either the aortic valve or, less frequently, the mitral valve;[3] it may also occur as a complication after septal myotomy-myectomy for hypertrophic cardiomyopathy. The appearance of Mobitz type II second-degree block or complete AV block after cardiac surgery is an absolute indication for temporary pacing (Fig.

9–1).[3,13,14] Patients with Mobitz type I second-degree AV block may not require temporary pacing unless the ventricular rate is slow. Advanced AV block after surgery requires pacing with a temporary device for 2 to 3 weeks postoperatively, before a decision is made to implant a permanent pacemaker. The indications for implantation of a permanent pacemaker in patients with AV block associated with perioperative myocardial infarction after coronary bypass surgery are identical to those for patients with acute myocardial infarction.[15] Bundle branch block following coronary artery bypass surgery, however, does not indicate myocardial necrosis and usually resolves in the early postoperative period.[16] Patients with preoperative right bundle branch block and left anterior fascicular block with or without a prolonged PR interval may rarely progress to complete AV block intraoperatively.[17]

Despite improved surgical techniques, high-grade AV block in children and young adults occurs following surgery for correction of complex congenital cardiac defects.[18–20] Postoperative complete AV block more commonly occurs in children undergoing open-heart surgery for ventricular septal defect, tetralogy of Fallot, transposition of great vessels, and Ebstein's anomaly and carries a poor long-term prognosis;[14,18] delayed onset of heart block may occur several years after surgery.[9,21] Permanent pacing has been recommended for all children with complete heart block that persists for 4 to 6 weeks after intracardiac repair.[18] A high rate of complications is associated with permanent pacing in children.[18,20]

Sinus Node Dysfunction

After cardioplegic cardiac arrest, normal sinus rhythm returns gradually, and there is often a period of atrial quiescence. Thus periods of sinus arrest,

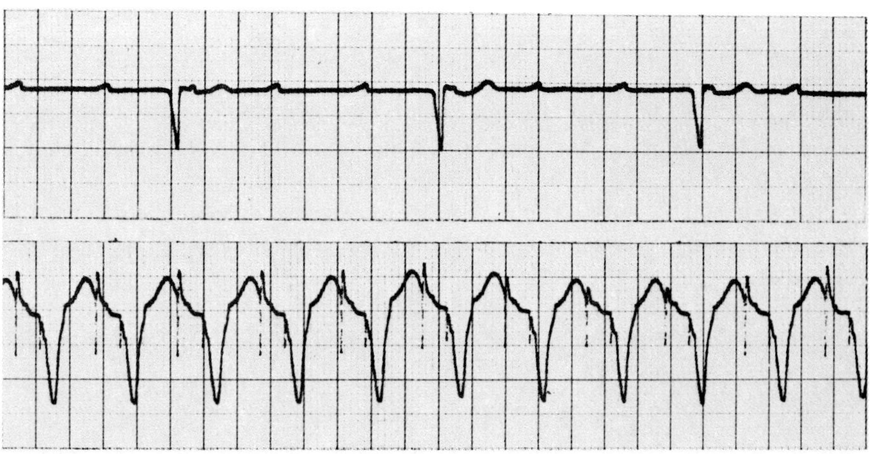

Figure 9–1. Continuous EKG monitoring showing complete heart block after cardiac surgery (upper panel). AV sequential temporary pacing (DVI) is instituted at a rate above patient's atrial rate (lower panel).

sinus bradycardia, and slow junctional or nodal rhythm are not uncommon after open-heart surgery in adults.[4] In children sick sinus syndrome is less frequent after heart surgery, but it may be observed in patients undergoing extensive atrial reconstructive surgery for transposition of great vessels or atrial septal defect.[22,23] A permanent pacemaker is indicated in these children if symptoms occur, the escape rate is inadequate, and dysrhythmia persists for more than a few weeks.[23]

TACHYARRHYTHMIAS AFTER OPEN-HEART SURGERY

Supraventricular and less frequently ventricular tachycardias occur frequently after heart surgery and are caused by hypoxia, increased intramyocardial tension, altered membrane permeability, and disturbed cellular electrolyte balance.[24,25] These tachyarrhythmias can effectively be terminated by temporary cardiac pacing.[26] Forms of pacing stimulation include single stimuli, pairs or triplets of stimuli, and trains or bursts of pacing, which may be applied to either the atria or the ventricles.[27,28] Although most ventricular and supraventricular tachyarrythmias after cardiac surgery are usually managed by pharmacologic agents, refractory cases leading to rapid hemodynamic deterioration are occasionally encountered and respond to pacing therapy.[29] Temporary pacing can also be used for the prevention of certain tachycardias, whereas the atrial electrode may be useful for recording EKGs for the diagnosis of arrhythmias such as atrial flutter and atrial tachycardia.

Supraventricular Tachyarrhythmias

In paroxysmal supraventricular tachycardia due to AV nodal reentry, electrical conversion by pacing is rarely used therapeutically despite its effectiveness. With pacing overdrive suppression, the supraventricular tachycardia is captured by pacing at 10 to 20 beats above the rate of the tachycardia. Atrial pacing and rarely ventricular pacing are employed. Once the arrhythmia is terminated the pacing rate is reduced (Fig. 9–2).[29–31] Interruption of the reentry circuit can also be accomplished by atrial stimulation at a rate less than the atrial rate, AV sequential pacing, or single extrastimuli, especially when the tachycardia is not

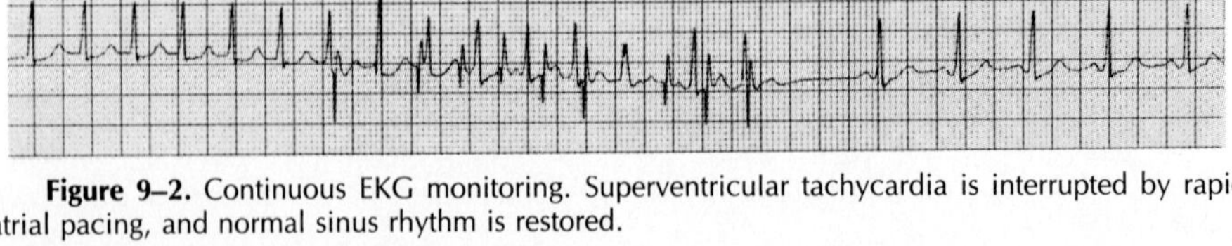

Figure 9–2. Continuous EKG monitoring. Superventricular tachycardia is interrupted by rapid atrial pacing, and normal sinus rhythm is restored.

rapid (less than 180 beats per minute).[32,33] Prevention of the recurrence of tachycardia has been achieved by continuous pacing at a rate of 80 to 160 beats per minute.[31,34]

Direct cardiac stimulation by rapid atrial pacing is an effective therapeutic approach to patients with atrial flutter after heart surgery, when digitalis has not provided adequate control of ventricular rate.[35,36] Rapid atrial pacing at rates of 10 to 25 percent above the flutter frequency (up to 600 beats per minute) is usually successful in converting type I or classic atrial flutter (rate 240 to 338 beats per minute) to sinus rhythm or atrial fibrillation.[37,38] Alternatively, high-frequency atrial stimulation at rates of 500 to 2000 per minute can be used to produce atrial fibrillation, which usually will spontaneously revert to sinus rhythm.[39] However, careful attention should be paid to the technical details for achieving successful atrial stimulation, especially when intracardiac catheters are used.

Ventricular Tachycardias

Interruption of ventricular tachycardia postoperatively can be achieved by overdrive suppression.[28,40] Ventricular pacing at 10 to 20 beats faster than the tachycardia rate is usually employed (Fig. 9–3). In a few patients, seeking the appropriate overdriving rate will cause acceleration of the tachycardia; immediate discontinuation of the pacing is required in such instances. Sustained overdrive ventricular pacing at rates near or greater than 200 beats per minute may induce ventricular fibrillation. Prevention of recurrence of ventricular extrasystoles, ventricular tachycardia, or fibrillation can be achieved by overdrive atrial or ventricular pacing suppression (with or without adjunctive drug therapy) at rates 10 to 40 beats per minute faster than the spontaneous resting rate (Fig. 9–4).[41] The rate, rhythmicity, and amplitude imposed by the pacing stimulus will shorten the nonrefractory period, reduce ectopy, and prevent reentry.

Temporary cardiac pacing has not been proved useful in the treatment or prevention of ectopic atrial tachycardias due to digitalis toxicity, nonparoxysmal

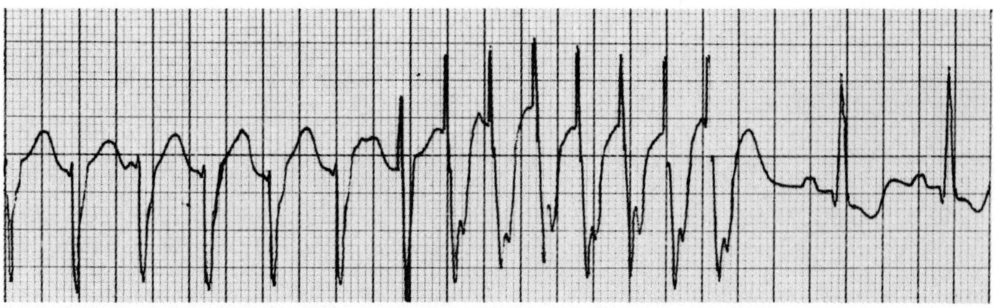

Figure 9–3. Uniform morphology ventricular tachycardia at a rate of 160 per minute is interrupted by rapid overdrive ventricular pacing, and normal sinus rhythm is restored.

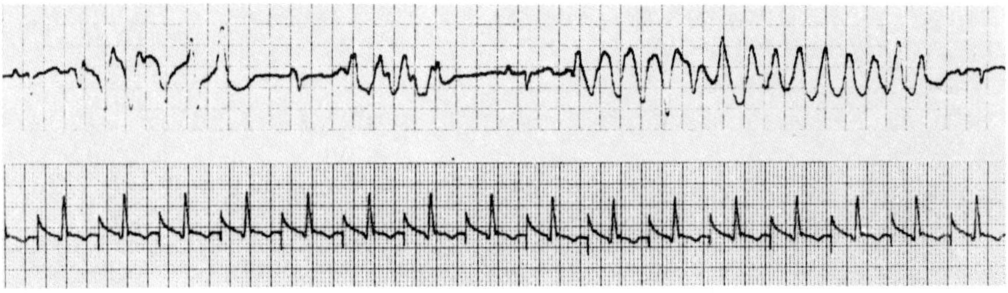

Figure 9–4. Repeated episodes of nonsustained polymorphous ventricular tachycardia (upper panel) controlled by continuous overdrive atrial pacing (lower panel).

AV junctional tachycardia, type II rapid atrial flutter (rate 340–433 beats per minute), atrial fibrillation, or ventricular fibrillation and sinus tachycardia.[26]

HEMODYNAMIC BENEFITS

Temporary ventricular pacing has often been used in the past to maintain adequate heart rate and improve a transiently depressed rate, thus increasing cardiac output postoperatively.[6] However, several investigators observed that ventricular pacing was associated with hemodynamic deterioration or was of little benefit in some patients.[42,43] This effect of ventricular pacing is attributed to the loss of a consistent atrial contribution to ventricular filling, the random atrial and ventricular contraction, and retrograde ventriculoatrial conduction.[9] Physiologic atrial or AV sequential pacing, on the other hand, preserves the atrial transport and normal AV sequencing and suppresses retrograde ventriculoatrial conduction. Several studies demonstrated an increase in cardiac output and improvement in hemodynamic parameters with atrial or AV sequential pacing compared to ventricular pacing during the period after cardiac surgery (Fig. 9–5).[7,8,42,43] The importance of these effects is more apparent in patients with poor ventricular compliance and depressed systolic left ventricular function postoperatively.[1,42,44,45]

Atrial pacing with intact AV conduction and AV sequential pacing are equally effective in improving the hemodynamic parameters after heart surgery.[7] Hartzler and colleagues,[42] however, found an 18 percent increase in cardiac output in postoperative patients by artificially shortening the AV interval using sequential pacing rather than atrial pacing. It appears that there is an optimal AV interval for sequential pacing ranging from 50 to 250 msec that is associated with the maximal cardiac output in postoperative patients. Deviation from the optimal AV interval by less than 50 msec reduced the cardiac output by as much as 33 percent in individual patients in that series.[42] These observations should be considered in preselecting the AV interval of a DVI pacing system.

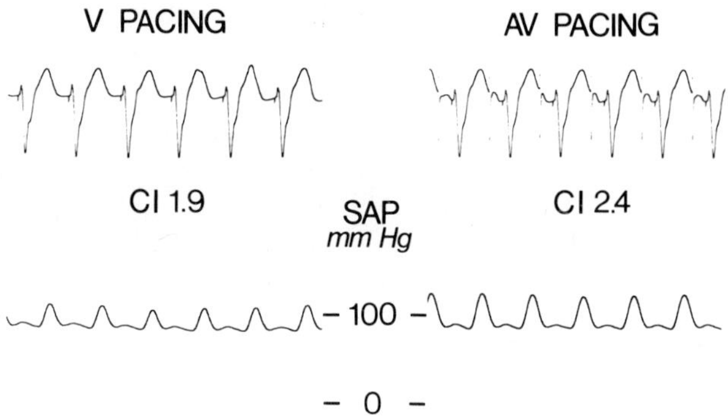

Figure 9–5. Continuous EKG monitoring (upper panel) and arterial pressure tracing (lower panel) during ventricular (V) and atrioventricular (AV) pacing. Note an increase in systolic arterial pressure (SAP) and improvement of cardiac index (CI) during AV pacing.

The presence of atrial fibrillation and flutter and certain rapid supraventricular rhythms precludes the use of atrial and AV sequential pacing after cardiac surgery but does not constitute a contraindication for affixing atrial wires, since atrial wires may provide valuable diagnostic information.

COMPLICATIONS

Sensing and pacing failures and, rarely, electrode dislodgement and perforation of a cardiac chamber, are the more common complications reported with temporary epicardial pacing.[46,47] Hemorrhage due to tissue trauma from epicardial leads may rarely be complicated by cardiac tamponade, even when the patient is receiving anticoagulation during the postoperative period. Newer techniques of insertion of the atrial electrodes and improvement in the design of the epicardial leads have minimized several of the above complications and have made temporary epicardial pacing after heart surgery a safe procedure.[10–12] Withdrawal of sutureless epicardial leads by gentle traction before the patient's discharge is also not associated with any difficulties.

SUMMARY

Implantation of epicardial leads in the right atrium and ventricle during open-heart surgery is a safe and effective procedure for the management of various rhythm and conduction disturbances in the immediate postoperative period. Temporary pacing can provide an adequate heart rate in patients with postoperative AV block or sinus node dysfunction. Treatment or prevention of certain tachycardias (supraventricular tachycardia, atrial flutter, and ventricular tachycardia) can be achieved with overdrive atrial or ventricular pacing or with adjunctive drug therapy. Atrial or AV sequential pacing preserves AV synchrony and provides improved hemodynamic parameters postoperatively, especially in patients with left ventricular dysfunction. Attachment of atrial and sometimes ventricular electrodes should be performed during open-heart surgery and used as temporary pacing whenever the need arises in the postoperative period.

Acknowledgment

We are indebted to Dr. Leonard Horowitz for providing the illustrations.

REFERENCES

1. Wisheart JD, Wright JEC, Rosenfeldt FL, and Ross JK: Atrial and ventricular pacing after open-heart surgery. Thorax 28:9, 1973.
2. MacLean WA, Cooper TB, Kouchoukos NT, and Karp RB: Use of temporarily placed epicardial atrial wire electrodes for the diagnosis and treatment of cardiac arrhythmias following open-heart surgery. J Thorac Cardiovasc Surg 76:500, 1978.
3. Sanoudos G, and Reed GE: Late heart block in aortic valve replacement. J Cardiovasc Surg 15:475, 1974.
4. Morin JE, Wynands JE, and Ralphs-Thibodeau S: Temporary cardiac pacing following open-heart surgery. Can J Surg 25:128, 1982.
5. Hodam RP, and Starr A: Temporary postoperative epicardial pacing electrodes: Their value and management after open-heart surgery. Ann Thorac Surg 8:506, 1969.
6. Litwak RS, Kuhn LA, Garboys HL, et al: Support of myocardial performance after open cardiac operations by rate augmentation. J Thorac Cardiovasc Surg 56:484, 1968.
7. Curtis JJ, Maloney JD, Barnhorst DA, et al: A critical look at temporary ventricular pacing following cardiac surgery. Surgery 82:888, 1977.
8. Fields J, Berkovits BV, and Matloff JM: Surgical experience with temporary and permanent AV sequential demand pacing. J Thorac Cardiovasc Surg 66:865, 1973.
9. Panidis I, Dreifus LS, and Michelson EL: Hemodynamic effects of cardiac pacing. *In* Dreifus LS (ed): Pacemaker Therapy. Cardiovascular Clinics. Vol. 14. Philadelphia, F.A. Davis and Co., 1983, pp. 1–12.
10. Spyrou PG: A simple technique of placing temporary atrial pacemaker electrodes. Ann Thorac Surg 31:377, 1981.
11. Breivik K, Engedal H, Segadal L, et al: New temporary pacing lead for use after cardiac operations. J Thorac Cardiovasc Surg 84:787, 1982.
12. Breivik K, Engedal H, Resch F, et al: Clinical and electrophysiological properties of a new temporary pacemaker lead after open-heart surgery. Pace 5:600, 1982.
13. Brockman SK, Webb RC, and Bahnson HT: Monopolar ventricular stimulation for the control of acute surgically produced heart block. Surgery 44:910, 1958.
14. Reemtsma K, Delgado JP, and Creech O: Heart block following intracardiac surgery; localization of conduction tissue injury. J Thorac Cardiovasc Surg 39:683, 1960.
15. Hindman MC, Wagner GS, JaRo M, et al: The clinical significance of bundle branch block complicating acute myocardial infarction. II. Indications for temporary and permanent pacing. Circulation 58:689, 1978.
16. O'Connell JB, Wallis D, Johnson SA, et al: Transient bundle branch block following use of hypothermic cardioplegia in coronary artery bypass surgery: High incidence without perioperative myocardial infarction. Am Heart J 103:85, 1982.
17. Pastore JO, Yurchak PM, Janis KM, et al: The risk of advanced heart block in surgical patients with right bundle branch block and left axis deviation. Circulation 57:677, 1978.
18. Hofschire PJ, Nicoloff DM, and Moller JH: Postoperative complete heart block in 64 children treated with and without cardiac pacing. Am J Cardiol 39:559, 1977.

19. Furman S, and Young D: Cardiac pacing in children and adolescents. Am J Cardiol 39:550, 1977.
20. Ward DE, Signy M, Oldershaw P, et al: Cardiac pacing in children. Arch Dis Childhood 57:514, 1982.
21. Bolens M, and Friedli B: Progressive atrioventricular block after total correction of Fallot's tetralogy, documented by repeat electrophysiological studies. Cardiology 69:185, 1982.
22. Schiller MS, Levin AR, Haft JI, et al: Electrophysiologic studies in sick sinus syndrome following surgery for d-transposition of the great arteries. J Pediatr 91:891, 1977.
23. Greenwood RD, Rosenthal AM, Sloss LJ, et al: Sick sinus syndrome after surgery for congenital heart disease. Circulation 52:208, 1975.
24. Bush HL, Gelband H, Hoffman BF, and Malm JR: Electrophysiologic basis for supraventricular arrhythmias following surgical procedure for aortic stenosis. Arch Surg 103:620, 1971.
25. Smith R, Grossman W, Johnson L, et al: Arrhythmias following cardiac valve replacement. Circulation 45:1018, 1972.
26. Waldo AL, Wells JL, Cooper TB, et al: Temporary cardiac pacing: Applications and techniques in the treatment of cardiac arrhythmias. Prog Cardiovasc Dis 23:451, 1981.
27. Dreifus LS, Berkovits BV, Kimbiris D, et al: Use of atrial and bifocal cardiac pacemakers for treating resistant dysrhythmias. Eur J Cardiol 3/4:257, 1975.
28. Spurrell RAJ: Use of cardiac pacemakers in the management of tachycardias. Cardiovasc Rev Rep 3:123, 1982.
29. Lurie AJ, Salel AF, Vera Z, et al: Rapid overdrive pacing for refractory tachyarrhythmias in patients after open-heart surgery. J Thorac Cardiovasc Surg 72:458, 1976.
30. Lister JW, Cohen LS, Bernstein WH, and Samet P: Treatment of supraventricular tachycardias by rapid atrial stimulation. Circulation 38:1044, 1968.
31. Cooper TB, MacLean WAH, and Waldo AL: Overdrive pacing for supraventricular tachycardia: A review of theoretical implications and therapeutic techniques. Pace 1:196, 1978.
32. Hunt NC, Cobb FR, Waxman MB, et al: Conversion of supraventricular tachycardias with atrial stimulation: Evidence for re-entry mechanisms. Circulation 38:1060, 1968.
33. Akhtar M, Gilbert CJ, Al-Nouri M, Schmidt DH: Electrophysiologic mechanisms for modification and abolition of atrioventricular junctional tachycardia with simultaneous and sequential atrial and ventricular pacing. Circulation 60:1443, 1979.
34. Waldo AL, MacLean WAH, Karp RB, et al: Continuous rapid atrial pacing to control recurrent or sustained supraventricular tachycardias following open-heart surgery. Circulation 54:245, 1976.
35. Haft JI, Kosowsky BD, Lau SH, et al: Termination of atrial flutter by rapid electrical pacing of the atrium. Am J Cardiol 20:239, 1967.
36. Zeft HH, Cobb FR, Waxman MB, et al: Right atrial stimulation in the treatment of atrial flutter. Ann Intern Med 70:447, 1969.
37. Waldo AL, MacLean WAH, Karp RB, et al: Entrainment and interruption of atrial flutter with atrial pacing: Studies in men following open-heart surgery. Circulation 56:737, 1977.
38. Wells JL Jr, MacLean WAH, James TN, and Waldo AL: Characterization of atrial flutter: Studies in man after open-heart surgery using fixed atrial electrodes. Circulation 60:665, 1979.
39. Panidis IP, Dreifus LS, and Michelson EL: Recognizing and treating supraventricular tachycardias. J Cardiovasc Med 7:1019, 1982.
40. Escher DJW, and Furman S: Emergency treatment of cardiac arrhythmias: Emphasis on use of electrical pacing. JAMA 214:2028, 1970.
41. Escher DJW, and Furman S: Pacemaker therapy for chronic rhythm disorders. Progr Cardiovasc Dis 14:459, 1972.
42. Hartzler GO, Maloney JD, Curtis JJ, and Barnhorst DA: Hemodynamic benefits of atrioventricular sequential pacing after cardiac surgery. Am J Cardiol 40:232, 1977.
43. Hilton JD, Weisel RD, Baird RJ, et al: The hemodynamic and metabolic response to pacing after aortocoronary bypass. Circulation 64(suppl II):48, 1981.
44. Hamby RI, Noble WJ, Murphy DH, and Hoffman I: Atrial transport function in coronary artery disease: Relation to left ventricular function. J Am Coll Cardiol 1:1011, 1983.
45. Reiter MJ, and Hindman MC: Hemodynamic effects of acute atrioventricular sequential pacing in patients with left ventricular dysfunction. Am J Cardiol 49:687, 1982.
46. Wolpowitz A: Perforation of the left ventricle using a sutureless screw-in epicardial electrode. J Cardiovasc Surg 22:585, 1981.
47. Schwartz DJ, Thanavaro S, Kleiger RE, et al: Epicardial pacemaker complicated by cardiac tamponade and constrictive pericarditis. Chest 76:226, 1979.

III

TROUBLESHOOTING

10

Radiographic Evaluation of Cardiac Pacemakers

LAWRENCE R. GOODMAN, M.D.

The chest x-ray is a valuable means of assessing the position of the pacing electrodes and the integrity of the leads and of detecting many mechanical complications of cardiac pacing. After a pacer has been inserted, all subsequent x-rays should be carefully scrutinized for potential or actual problems.[1–3] This chapter will first discuss the normal appearance of the more commonly used approaches to cardiac pacing and then discuss the radiographic appearance of pacer mishaps.

NORMAL APPEARANCE

Transvenous Pacing

Transvenous cardiac pacing has replaced epicardial pacing for most cardiac problems. The most frequent approach is that of transvenous stimulation of the right ventricle. Whether inserted percutaneously via a peripheral vein or surgically via a more central vein, the pacing electrode is usually guided under fluoroscopic control into the right ventricle. The tip of the electrode is ideally wedged beneath the trabeculae carneae of the right ventricular apex to ensure a stable position. On the frontal x-ray, the electrode tip should be seen in the area between the left border of the spine and several centimeters medial to the *left* heart border (Figs. 10–1 and 10–2). The tip should point caudally and to the left. Without a lateral x-ray, it is difficult to distinguish between a tip properly placed in the right ventricular apex and a tip pointed posteriorly into the right ventricle or coronary sinus (Fig. 10–3) on the frontal view. If the tip points cephalad instead of caudad, the tip may be free in the right ventricle, in the pulmonary artery, or in the coronary sinus. On the lateral x-ray the electrode tip should point anteriorly and lie at least 4 to 5 mm deep to the epicardial fat (Figs.

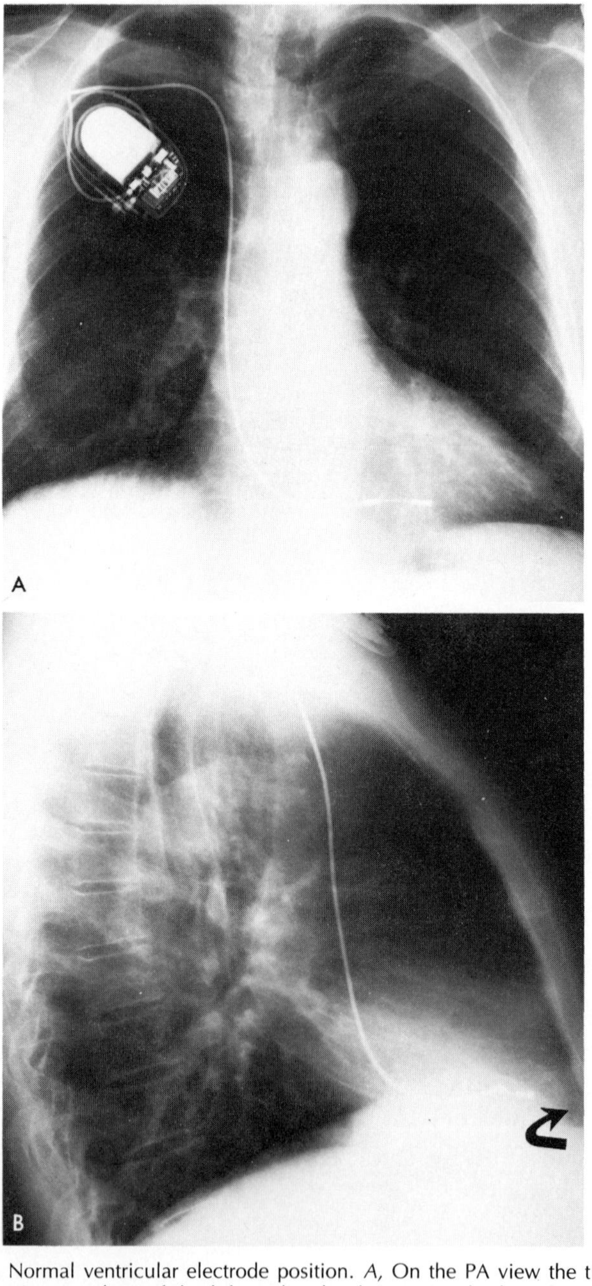

Figure 10–1. Normal ventricular electrode position. *A,* On the PA view the tip of the bipolar lead is several centimeters short of the left cardiac border. *B,* On the lateral x-ray the tip of the electrode is approximately 2 centimeters deep to the epicardial fat (arrow).

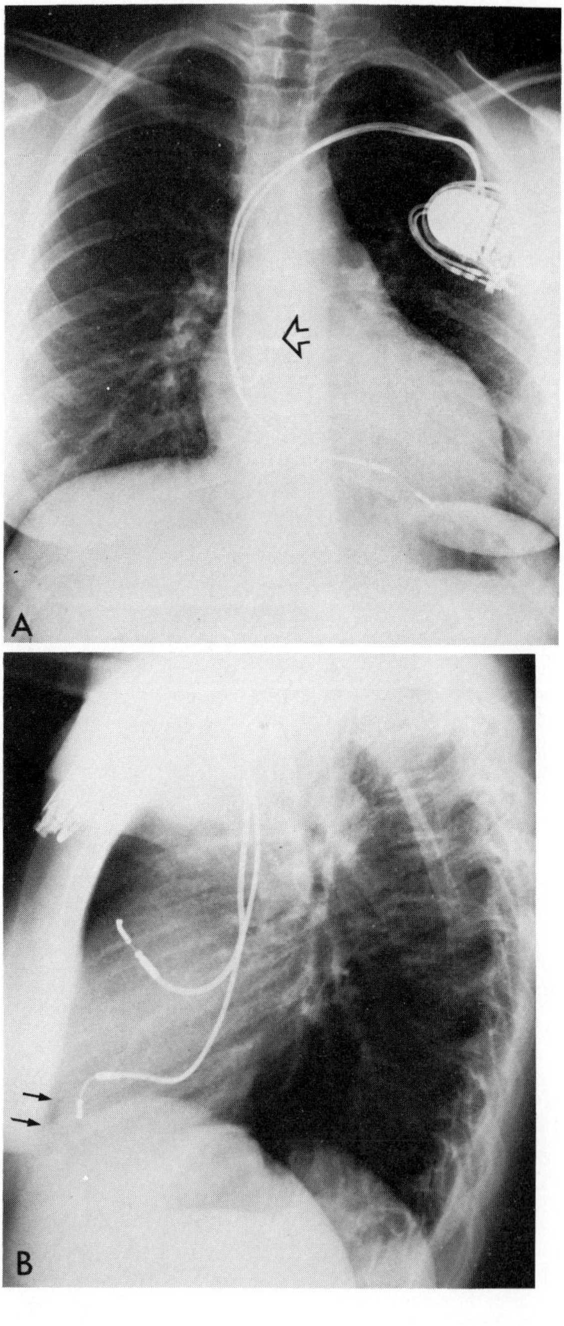

Figure 10–2. Normal AV sequential pacer. There are two bipolar electrodes. The proximal electrode is in the right atrial appendage (arrow), and the distal tip is well positioned in the right ventricular apex. Extra wire is left at the pacer-lead junction in case the pacer should migrate. On the lateral view, the apical lead stops 5 mm short of the vaguely seen epicardial fat stripe (arrows).

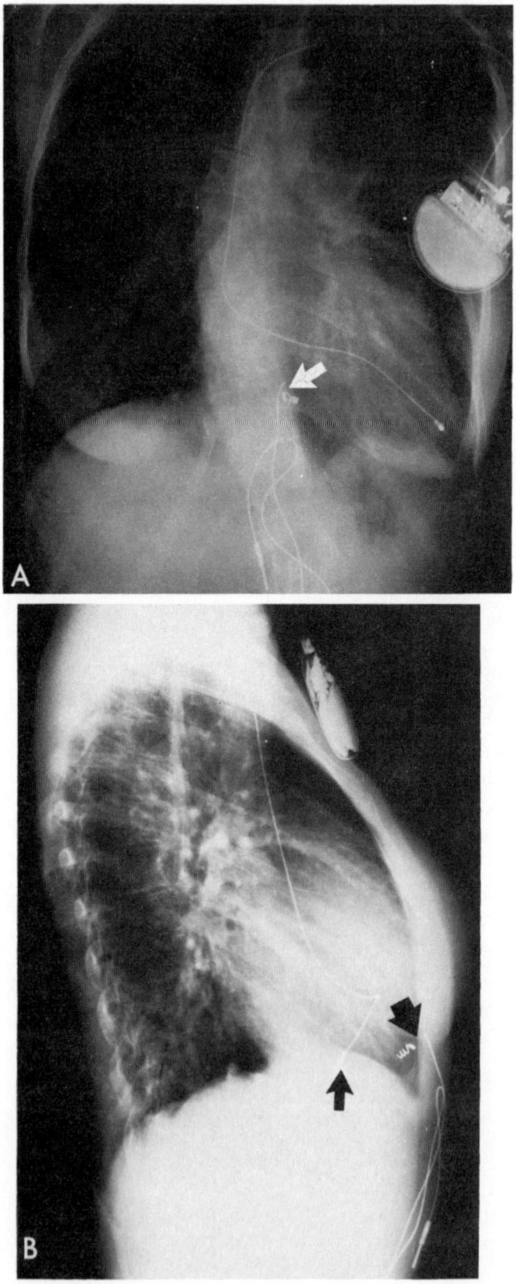

Figure 10–3. Poor electrode position, broken implanted electrode. The tip of the unipolar tranvenous electrode appears to be deep into the apex of the right ventricle on the frontal film. However, the lateral film demonstrates that the tip is pointed posteriorly (lower arrow) into the right ventricle. The pacemaker paced intermittently. Incidentally noted is an old implanted pacing electrode. Notice the break in continuity (arrow) where the wire joins the helical electrode.

10–1 and 10–2).[4] If the tip points posteriorly, the tip is in the right ventricle or coronary sinus (Fig. 10–3).[1, 2, 5, 6]

On rare occasions the coronary sinus is purposely cannulated for permanent atrial pacing.[7] As mentioned above, the pacer tip projects upward and to the left on the frontal x-ray and upward and posteriorly on the lateral film. The coronary sinus and its tributaries lie in the epicardial fat, outside the heart. Thus an electrode deep in the coronary sinus may appear on the cardiac surface, simulating myocardial perforation. In many instances, purposeful coronary sinus cannulation can be recognized by the type of lead used. Instead of the lead's ending as a blunt-tipped electrode, as is usually the case, a thin flexible piece of wire is seen beyond the electrode. This wire serves to anchor the lead deep within the coronary sinus (Fig. 10–4).[7]

When atrial pacing is desired, most physicians prefer direct atrial stimulation to coronary sinus pacing. A J-shaped lead is inserted into the atrium with the hook of the J in the right atrial appendage. When atrioventricular (AV) synchronous pacing is required, a double lead is inserted, one positioned in the right ventricular apex and one in the right atrial appendage (Figs. 10–1 and 10–2).[6, 8]

All transvenous pacer leads should be free of sharp angulations and intravascular or intracardiac redundancy or slack (a gentle curve through the veins and heart will minimize catheter recoil). In patients with permanently implanted pacers, an extra loop of lead is placed in the pulse generator pocket to minimize strain at the electrode-pacer junction (Fig. 10–2).[3, 9]

Transthoracic Pacing

In adults, permanent electrode implantation is now being used less frequently than during previous decades. The conventional technique involved direct suturing of the electrodes to the epicardium under direct vision. This has been replaced to a large extent by sutureless electrodes that can be inserted through a small incision. The electrode ends in an open-helix-type screw that is screwed into the myocardium at thoracotomy or via a smaller subxiphoid incision (Fig. 10–3). Regardless of the approach, the electrodes are brought out through the chest wall and attached to a permanent pulse generator, usually located in the left epigastric area.

Following cardiac surgery a temporary myocardial pacing wire is usually run from the right ventricular myocardium out through the chest wall. It provides emergency postoperative access to the conduction system if needed. This lead is extremely thin and barely visible on the postoperative portable x-ray. The lead is removed after the acute postoperative period.

Pacemaker Identification

The large number of pacemaker manufacturers and numerous available models have made it difficult to recognize every available pacemaker. Several

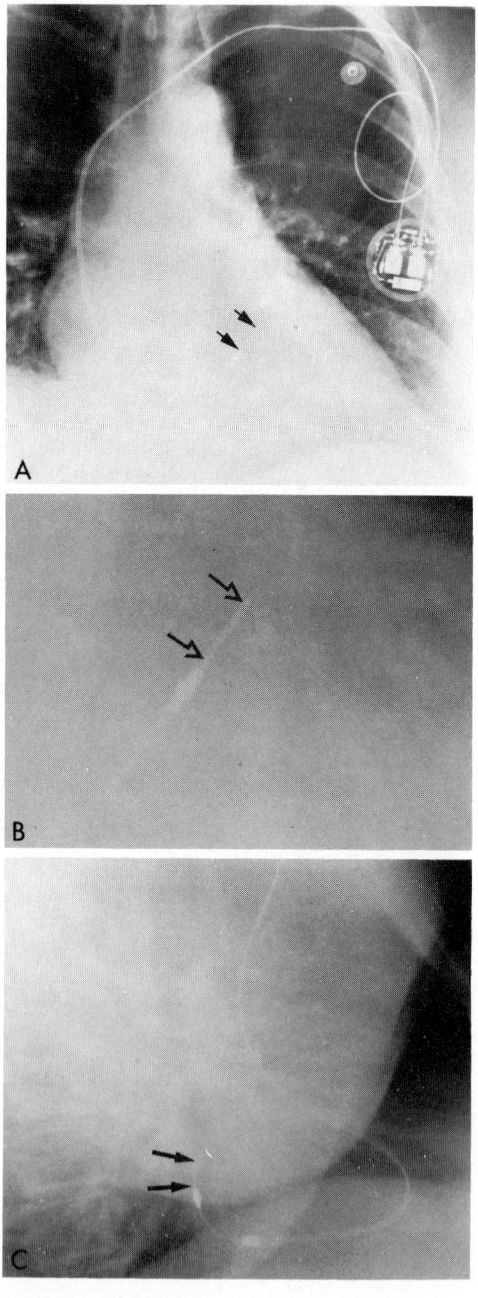

Figure 10–4. Coronary sinus pacing. The pacemaker electrode (arrows) is in the middle of the heart, pointing superiorly and to the left on the frontal film *(A)*. *A* also shows a small radio-frequency pacemaker overlying the left axilla. Unlike conventional pulse generators, this small receiver is used with an external pulse generator. In *B,* a photographic enlargement demonstrates a thin projection of wire beyond the terminal electrode to anchor the pacer in the coronary sinus (arrows). On the lateral x-ray *(C)* the tip of the electrode points posteriorly into the coronary sinus. Arrows demonstrate the anchoring wire beyond the electrode tip.

manufacturers now provide radiopaque coding of their generators. Steiner and colleagues[16] have recently published an atlas of currently available units.

COMPLICATIONS

The mortality and morbidity of transvenous pacer insertion are considerably less than with epicardial implantation.[6] Parsonnet and colleagues[10] have recently reported a 4.2 percent complication rate within a month of insertion of a transvenous pacemaker. In their series, the majority of malfunctions were caused by malposition, dislocation, or perforation, complications usually visible on an x-ray. Most required corrective intervention. In their series, patients with right ventricular dilatation or tricuspid insufficiency had the highest incidence of these types of problems.

Malpositioned Leads

Initial malposition or subsequent displacement complicates 2 to 18 percent of transvenous insertions. In the vast majority of patients displacement occurs within 4 to 6 weeks of insertion. Displacement may result in failure to pace, intermittent pacing, or continued pacing at a higher threshold, thereby hastening depletion of the energy source. The lead may float free in the right ventricle or migrate into the right atrium, vena cava, coronary sinus, right ventricular outflow tract, or pulmonary artery (Fig. 10–5). In addition to causing inadequate pacing, these misplaced electrodes may stimulate adjacent structures such as the phrenic nerve, brachial plexus, and psoas muscle (Fig. 10–6).[1, 2, 3, 10] Boake and Kroncke[5] report that diaphragmatic stimulation may occur immediately after insertion without radiographic evidence of perforation. This may disappear spontaneously or by decreasing energy output.

Migration of the pulse generator may cause the electrode to be pulled from its position in the right ventricular apex. The pacer may migrate along the chest wall if a hematoma or infection enlarges the chest wall pocket or if the skin turgor is poor. Neurotic patients who twist their pulse generators may reel in the lead as they rotate the pacer (twiddler's syndrome) (Fig. 10–7).[1, 2]

Cardiac Perforation

Cardiac perforation may occur at the time of insertion or weeks or months after uneventful placement. The complication may be asymptomatic or present with difficulty pacing, hiccups, chest wall pain, or epigastric pain from diaphragmatic stimulation. Fortunately, cardiac tamponade from hemopericardium is an

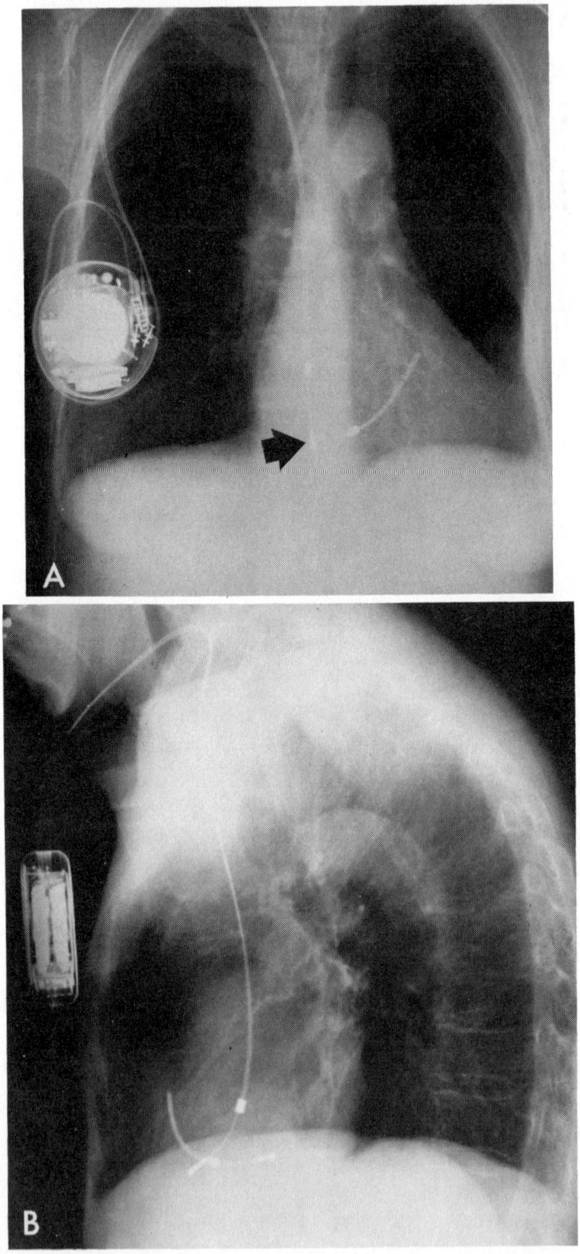

Figure 10–5. Poor electrode position, broken distal electrode. On the frontal x-ray the tip of the intact bipolar electrode is seen over the thoracic spine (arrow). On the lateral view the tip appears against the anterior right ventricular wall. The pacer functioned well despite its suboptimal position. Incidentally noted is the tip of a broken electrode in the coronary sinus. The exact circumstances surrounding this mishap could not be elicited from the patient.

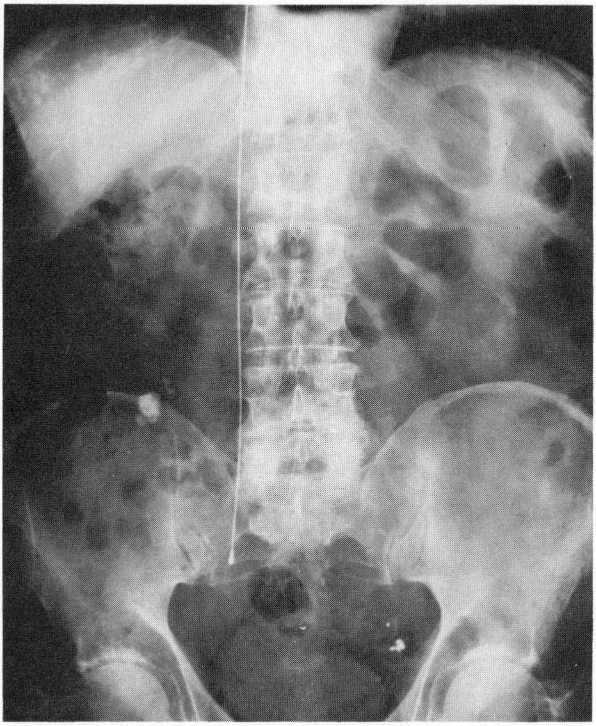

Figure 10–6. Displaced electrode. A KUB demonstrates a pacer electrode in the iliac vein. The patient complained of pain and fasciculations of the right leg. A prior chest x-ray several months earlier demonstrated the pacer wire in normal position in the right ventricular apex. Symptoms disappeared with removal of the pacemaker.

uncommon complication. On the posteroanterior (PA) x-ray the tip may be seen out to the left heart border or beyond (Fig. 10–8). Fluoroscopy is often helpful in cases of anterolateral or posterolateral perforation, when the electrode does not project beyond the heart on PA x-rays.

When the perforation is through the anterior wall of the right ventricle, the PA film is usually unremarkable.[2, 3, 9] Anterior perforation is usually diagnosed on the lateral x-ray or by lateral or off-lateral fluoroscopy. The normal pacer tip stops 4 to 5 mm short of the epicardial fat stripe. An electrode 1 to 3 mm from the stripe indicates penetration of the myocardium, whereas an electrode touching or deflecting the fat anteriorly indicates perforation (Fig. 10–9). If one can visualize the pericardium between the epicardial and anterior mediastinal fat, the presence or absence of pericardial fluid (blood) can also be evaluated. Echocardiography may also be used to locate the electrode relative to the right ventricular myocardium.[12]

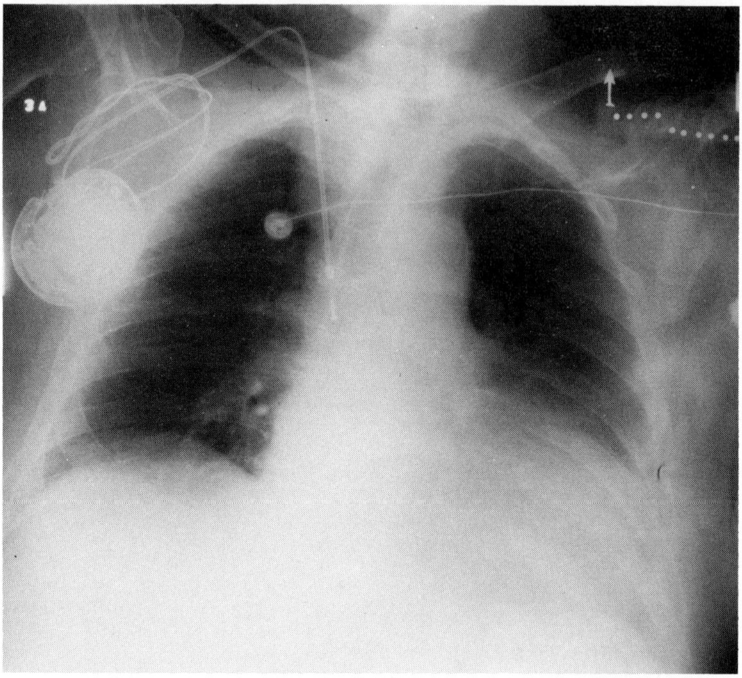

Figure 10–7. Twiddler's syndrome. The tip of the bipolar electrode is in the superior vena cava. Multiple loops of wire are in the pacemaker pouch. The electrode tip had been in normal position 4 months earlier without the redundant loops of wire. The patient admitted to manipulating the pulse generator.

Lead Fractures

With recent improvements in the manufacture of the leads, fractured electrode wires are relatively infrequent. However, with the recent improvements in the longevity of the pulse generator power source, leads will be required to remain intact for longer periods. Each x-ray should be carefully checked from the pulse generator to the electrode tip for breaks in the lead wire. Common sites of fracture include the junction of the lead and the pulse generator, the distal electrode tip, and areas of stress such as the site of entry into the vein and the area beneath the clavicle (Fig. 10–10). Most fractures are detectable on conventional x-rays, but fluoroscopy is sometimes required. If both the wire and surrounding insulation break spontaneously or at the time of attempted removal of the electrode, the fragment of electrode may remain in place in the heart or embolize into the pulmonary circulation (Fig. 10–5). These fragments may remain asymptomatic or serve as a nidus for infection, thrombosis, or perforation. Free-floating intracardiac and major pulmonary artery fragments can usually be snared with modified angiographic equipment and dragged peripherally, where they can be extracted via a peripheral venotomy.[13]

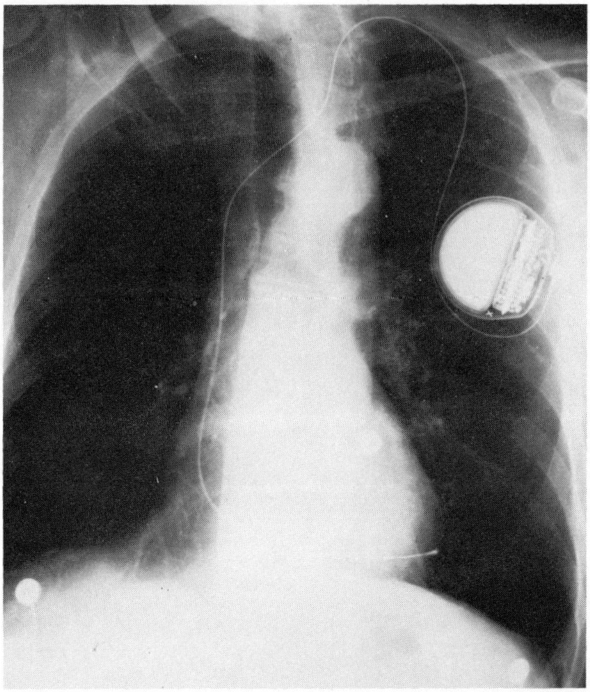

Figure 10–8. Ventricular perforation. The first x-ray after pacemaker insertion shows the unipolar electrode at the outer margin of the cardiac silhouette. Fluoroscopy confirmed that the tip was beyond the cardiac margin. The electrode was withdrawn without incident.

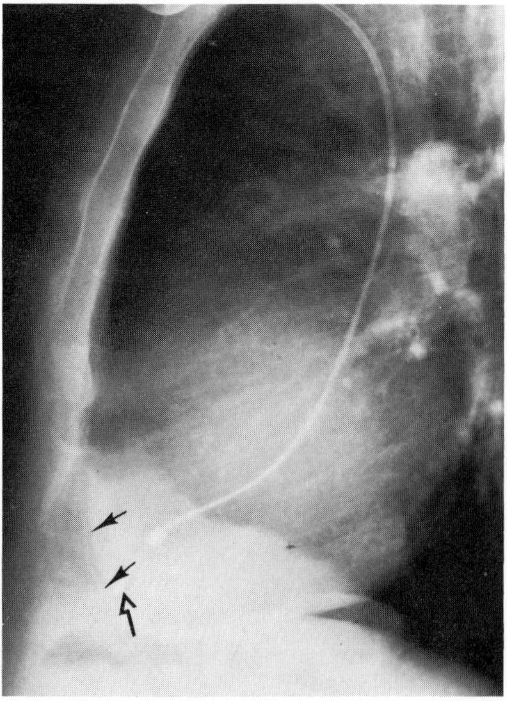

Figure 10–9. Electrode perforation. The patient presented with pain in the left anterior chest wall several months after pacemaker insertion. The pacer appeared to be functioning well. The lateral x-ray shows the tip of the bipolar electrode (open arrow) pointing anteriorly. The tip contacts the epicardial fat line (arrows), indicating myocardial perforation. The normal pericardium is vaguely seen as a fine white line between the epicardial and anterior mediastinal fat.

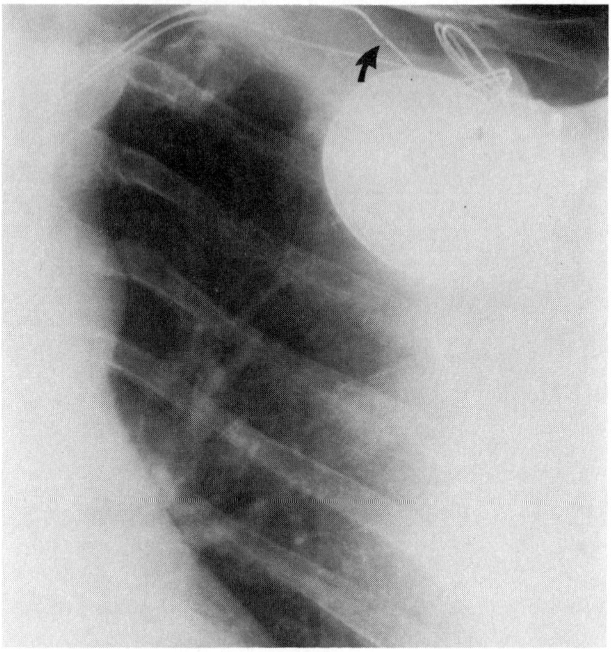

Figure 10–10. Broken electrode wire. Coned view of the pacemaker shows a break in one of the electrode wires (arrow). The pacemaker paced intermittently.

Two conditions simulate broken leads on the x-ray. Tight sutures may crimp the radiopaque insulation around the lead, giving the appearance of a lead fracture.[2] Steiner and colleagues[17] have recently reported three currently used bipolar pacemaker electrodes (Medtronic #6972 and 6990U and Pacesetter #820) that show a "pseudobreak" when viewed radiologically. This appearance is seen where a bifurcation of the dual coaxial lead requires a short straight connector section in the outer conductor before resuming its call configuration (Fig. 10–11).

Wire fatigue is much more frequent with implanted epicardial leads and is a major limitation of the transthoracic approach to cardiac pacing. Frequent fracture sites include the junction of the myocardial anchor and the wire, the entry and exit point through the chest wall, and the pulse generator connection (see Fig. 10–3).

Battery Failure

Mercury/zinc battery depletion can often be detected fluoroscopically. Normal batteries when viewed with a *perpendicular* beam have multiple sharply marginated concentric rings. With depleted batteries, the ring margins become fuzzy.[1, 2] EKG evaluation of battery dysfunction is easier and more accurate and is the procedure of choice.

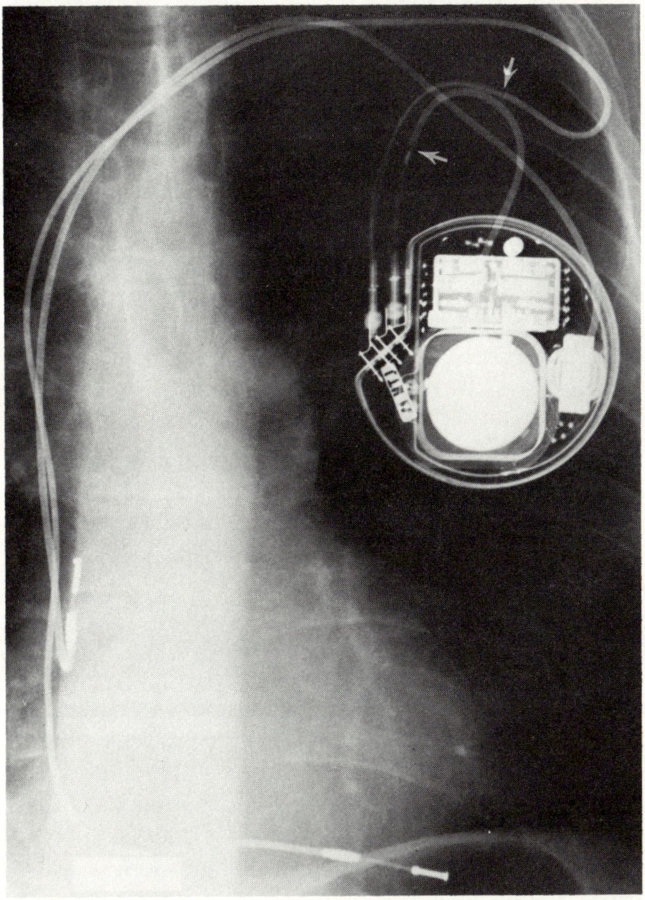

Figure 10–11. Pacemaker lead pseudofracture. Pacing electrodes are in good position in the right atrium and ventricle. There is an apparent discontinuity in each of the bipolar leads (arrows). This represents the termination of the support coil just prior to the bifurcation of the leads. On the original x-ray a thin wire, the inner distal winding of coil conductor, is seen bridging the gap. (Courtesy of Dr. Robert Steiner, Philadelphia, Pennsylvania.)

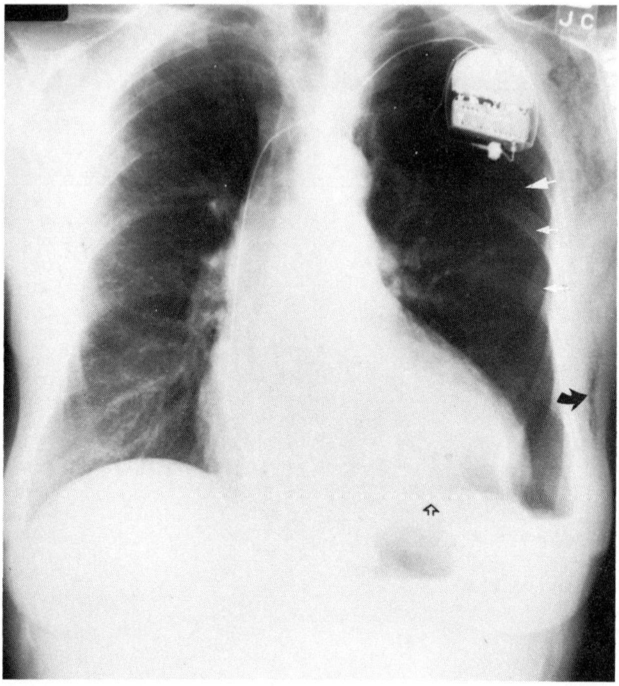

Figure 10–12. Pneumothorax. Following the subclavian insertion of the pacemaker wire, subcutaneous emphysema was noted clinically. The chest x-ray demonstrates air over the left shoulder and along the left lateral chest wall (black arrow) and a moderate pneumothorax (white arrows). The tip of the unipolar lead is barely visible in the right ventricular apex (open arrow).

Miscellaneous Complications

Clot formation along the electrode or thrombus in the vein is a frequent occurrence with both temporary and permanent pacemakers. Fortunately, serious clinical sequelae such as pulmonary embolus, septic embolus, or occlusion of the superior vena cava or tributary veins are uncommon.[14,15]

Other infrequent complications with potential radiographic manifestations include pneumothorax or hemothorax following insertion of the electrode, knotted electrode wires, chest wall infections around the pulse generator, and air embolus (Fig. 10–12).[5]

SUMMARY

PA and lateral x-rays are valuable means of diagnosing actual and potential complications of cardiac pacing. Using the guidelines outlined above, each x-ray should be evaluated for such complications.

REFERENCES

1. Ehrlich I: Cardiac pacemakers. *In* Teplick JG, and Haskin ME (eds): Surgical Radiology. Vol. II. Philadelphia, W. B. Saunders Co., 1981, pp. 1870–1904.
2. Sorkin RP, Schuurmann BJ, and Simon AB: Radiographic aspects of permanent cardiac pacemakers. Radiology 119:281, 1976.
3. Steiner RM, and Morse D: The radiology of cardiac pacemakers. JAMA 240:2574, 1978.
4. Ormond RS, Rubenfire M, Anbe D, and Drake E: Radiographic demonstration of myocardial penetration by permanent endocardial pacemakers. Radiology 98:35, 1971.
5. Boake WC, and Kroncke G: Pacemaker complications. *In* Varriale P, and Naclerio E (eds): Cardiac Pacing: A Concise Guide to Clinical Practice. Philadelphia, Lea and Febiger, 1979, pp. 229–238.
6. Smyth NPD: Cardiac pacing. Ann Thorac Surg 27:270, 1979.
7. Hewitt MJ, Chen JTT, Ravin CE, et al: Coronary sinus atrial pacing: Radiographic considerations. Am J Radiol 136:323, 1981.
8. Geddes JS, Webb SW, and Clements IP: Clinical experience with transvenous atrial pacing. Br Heart J 40:589, 1978.
9. Ravin CE: Cardiovascular monitoring and assist devices. *In* Goodman LR, and Putman CE (eds): Intensive Care Radiology: Imaging of the Critically Ill. 2nd ed. Philadelphia, W. B. Saunders Co., 1983.
10. Parsonnet V, Bilitch M, Furman S, et al: Early malfunction of transvenous pacemaker electrodes: A three center study. Circulation 60:590, 1979.
11. Bayliss CE, Beanlands DS, Baird RJ: The pacemaker-twiddlers syndrome: A new complication of implantable transvenous pacemakers. Can Med Assoc J 99:371, 1968.
12. Gondi B, and Nanda NC: Realtime two-dimensional echocardiographic features of pacemaker perforation. Circulation 64:97, 1981.
13. Glickman M: Invasive diagnostic and therapeutic procedures in the critically ill. *In* Goodman LR, and Putman CE (eds): Intensive Care Radiology: Imaging of the Critically Ill. 2nd ed. Philadelphia, W. B. Saunders Co., 1983.
14. Chamorro H, Rao G, and Wholey MH: Superior vena cava syndrome: A complication of transvenous pacemaker implantation. Radiology 126:277, 1978.
15. Williams EH, Tyers G, and Shaffer CW: Symptomatic deep venous thrombosis of the arm associated with permanent transvenous pacing electrodes. Chest 75:613, 1978.
16. Steiner RM, Morse D, and Parsonnet V: A Guide to Cardiac Pacemakers. Philadelphia, FA Davis, 1983.
17. Steiner RM, Morse DP, and Tegtmeyer CJ: Pacemaker lead pseudo-fracture. Radiology 143:793, 1982.

11

Permanent Cardiac Pacing: Complications and Management

A. HADI HAKKI, M.D., F.R.C.S.

During the past two decades we have accumulated considerable experience in the field of cardiac pacing. Recently we have expanded our indications for cardiac pacing. Thus the number of pacemaker implantations is on the rise in our institution, as well as in many other institutions across the nation.

Any surgical procedure, no matter how minor, carries some potential risks and complications. There are two time zones encountered when dealing with complications of cardiac pacing: intraoperative and postoperative.

Excellent surgical technique, sound judgment, and optimal pacing parameters are hallmark points in the prevention of pacemaker-related complications. If a complication arises postoperatively, there are three critical areas to which the focus of attention should be directed:

1. The pacemaker generator
2. The pacemaker lead
3. The host-pacemaker unit interaction

The surgeon's awareness that specific complications may occur from a variety of cardiac pacing procedures may enhance the prevention of such complications. A high index of suspicion is essential in detecting pacemaker-related problems. In a 4-year study of 1705 implanted pacemakers, Mantini reported that only 11 percent of the malfunctioning pacing systems were accompanied by symptoms.[1]

INTRAOPERATIVE COMPLICATIONS

The Transvenous Approach

This is the most widely adopted approach nationwide. At the Hahnemann University Hospital the subclavian vein puncture is the procedure of choice in the majority of patients undergoing artificial cardiac pacing. The following sections discuss complications that may be encountered using this technique.

Hemothorax

This may vary from a small collection of blood to a moderate pleural effusion. A fatal exsanguinating hemothorax was reported as a result of an attempted right subclavian vein puncture.[2] The subsequent autopsy revealed that the site of puncture was at the junction of the innominate vein and the superior vena cava. The management of this complication depends on the extent of the injury. In a small hematoma or a pleural effusion occupying less than a third of the hemithorax, close observation is all that is necessary. If the clot persists for more than 2 weeks and results in respiratory embarrassment, decortication and removal of the peel should be employed regardless of the size of the clot.[3] In rare instances when moderate or massive effusion is produced, a tube thoracostomy or an emergency thoracotomy is required.

Pneumothorax

We have observed a 40-percent incidence of pneumothorax using the subclavian vein puncture technique in females 75 years of age or older. This significant morbidity rate prompted us to resort to the cephalic vein cutdown technique as the procedure of choice for females in that age bracket. The cause of pneumothorax and its sex predilection remains unknown; however, it may be related to poor tissue integrity. It is also interesting to note that the pneumothorax may be insidious in nature, with an initial negative chest x-ray. Chest, shoulder, or interscapular pain should raise a high index of suspicion. A small pneumothorax usually resolves spontaneously without any treatment; however, serial chest x-rays should be taken to ascertain full expansion of the lung. Provided that the air leak has sealed, the rate of absorption is 1.25 percent per day. Thus the time taken for full lung expansion is directly proportional to the size of the pneumothorax.[4] In a few instances, insertion of a catheter into the corresponding pleural space and aspiration of air via a three-way stopcock has expedited resolution of the pneumothorax. Moderate or tension pneumothorax requires a tube thoracostomy. Obviously, in cases of tension pneumothorax it is an emergency procedure.[5]

Injury to the Thoracic Duct

This is an extremely rare complication that may follow left subclavian vein puncture. It is a preclusive complication if proper surgical techniques are followed.

Brachial Plexus, Phrenic Nerve, or Recurrent Laryngeal Nerve Injury

These are all potential complications of poor surgical technique during the implantation procedure. A thorough anatomic knowledge and adaptation of proper surgical technique are crucial in prevention of these complications.

Air Embolism

Whenever central veins are exposed to atmospheric pressure, the chance of air entry into the right side of the heart is increased. This is related to the negative pressure created in the major veins during phases of respiration.[6] This can be prevented by placing the patient in slight Trendelenberg's position and by requesting that the patient refrain from deep breathing and coughing. In addition, when the introducer is removed the surgeon's thumb may be applied to occlude the opening in the dilator just before the pacing electrode is inserted.

Subclavian Artery Puncture

A subclavian artery puncture with an 18-gauge needle is not an uncommon complication during pacing procedures. This however is of little consequence if recognized. It is remedied by withdrawing the needle and by repeating the puncture, angling the needle more anteriorly. If unrecognized and the introducer and dilator are inserted into the artery, a major hemorrhage may develop, requiring emergency surgical repair. Unless there is a proximal arteriovenous fistula, the bright red color of the arterial blood and its pulsating nature are fairly good indicators that the artery was tapped.

Subclavian Vein Thrombosis

The thrombosed vein usually extends down the axillary vein distally and may involve the superior vena cava proximally. It may even produce pulmonary embolism.[7,8] Management depends on the extent of the thrombosis. If no contraindications exist, streptokinase therapy is the treatment of choice.[9,10] In the event of contraindications, heparin therapy should be instituted instead.

Other Rare Complications

These include infraclavicular bone spicule formation, damage to the tricuspid valve,[11] and endocarditis.[12] In cases of endocarditis, treatment with intravenous antibiotics should commence as soon as cultures are taken.

The Transthoracic Approach

Because the vast majority of patients undergoing the transthoracic approach are placed under general anesthesia, atelectasis is the most common complication.[13–15] Other problems include pleural effusion, pneumothorax, pneumonitis, and, rarely, empyema. The incidence of cardiac arrhythmias and pericarditis is also significant.[16] In patients with chronic obstructive pulmonary disease a transxiphoid approach (usually under general anesthesia but occasionally under local anesthesia), without entering the pleura, may be a suitable alternative to an unsuccessful transvenous procedure. There is evidence of increased pulmonary shunting following open-heart surgery if the pleura was inadvertently entered.[17]

If proper surgical techniques are not followed some serious complications may arise, such as ventricular laceration and injury to the coronary vessels. Overtorquing the screw-in electrodes or excessive compression and penetration of the myocardial wall into the cardiac chamber may lead to exit block.

A pacing electrode should be placed at least an inch away from the left phrenic nerve when the pericardium is closed, otherwise stimulation of the nerve can cause hiccups synchronous with cardiac pacing.[18, 19] When bipolar epicardial leads are inserted, adequate distance between the implantation sites is needed to prevent undersensing.

POSTOPERATIVE COMPLICATIONS

In a 4-year study of 1705 implanted pacemakers Mantini reported 340 malfunctions. Of these, 41 percent were a result of battery depletion (mercury/zinc units), 50 percent were pacemaker lead-related problems, and 9 percent were generator component failures and non–pacing-related arrhythmias.[1]

With the introduction of lithium batteries and active-fixation pacemaker leads, there has been a significant reduction of pacemaker-related complications.[20–25]

There are a number of troubleshooting categories that can emerge following cardiac pacing procedures (Table 11–1). Furman outlined a protocol to follow in investigating suspected pacemaker malfunctions.[26] As most patients are asymptomatic, an ideal follow-up should include a thorough history and physical examination and the use of certain diagnostic tools. The latter include EKG, Holter monitoring, pacing system analysis, and electronic studies. If a problem cannot be identified and resolved noninvasively, surgical intervention is mandatory.

Table 11–1. Major Troubleshooting Categories in Cardiac Pacing

Failure of pacing	Rate difficulty
Failure of sensing	Muscle stimulation
Undersensing	Pacemaker generator erosion and/or migration
Oversensing	Infection
	Others

Failure of Cardiac Pacing

This may be seen in the early or late postoperative period and can be associated with either a continuous or intermittent loss of capture. Nonpacing is caused by lack of capture or lack of current delivered from the pacemaker generator (Table 11–2).

Lead Dislodgement

The importance of proper positioning of the pacemaker lead and obtaining the best possible parameters at the time of initial implantation cannot be overstressed. The high initial threshold associated with poor lead placement is compounded by normal acute threshold increase to chronic values.[27] Although lead dislodgement can occur at any time in the postoperative period, it is most common in the first 48 hours following implant. The incidence in one series was 5 percent;[28] however, it could range anywhere from 2 to 18 percent. With the advent of active-fixation leads, the incidence is close to 1 percent. The

Table 11–2. Failure of Cardiac Pacing (Nonpacing)

Etiology	Management
Lack of Capture	
Dislodged lead	Reposition or replace with an active-fixation lead
Lead insulation break	Replace the lead Repair if minor and accessible
Ventricular perforation	Lower output strength Try to program bipolar lead to unipolar Reposition lead
Exit block	Correct metabolic imbalance Increase the generator output Use high-output pulse generator Reposition lead or replace with a different type of lead
Lack of Current	
Lead is disconnected or connector set screws are improperly tightened	Reconnect properly
Lead fracture without insulation break	Replace lead
Battery depletion	Replace the battery

diagnosis can be confirmed by EKG. Gross lead dislodgement is revealed on x-ray, whereas microdislodgement can masquerade as normal lead positioning. The analyzer may show increased pacing current and voltage with normal resistance or high and varying threshold, if obtainable. Some cases of late lead dislodgement were attributed to twiddler's syndrome, in which the patient twists and turns the pulse generator until the lead dislodges and winds around it. The management of lead dislodgement usually consists of either repositioning the lead or replacing it with an active-fixation lead. In addition, the pulse generator must be transfixed with suture at two points in cases of twiddler's syndrome.

Lead Insulation Break

This tends to occur in polyurethane leads, in which the transfixing stitch is tied directly on the lead itself instead of applying it on the protective sheath. The diagnosis is suspected if the pacing spikes on EKG are seen at regular intervals with no capture, or if they vary in size on the same EKG strip. It can be confirmed by visualizing the analyzer reading a normal voltage, increased current, a low resistance (usually less than 250 ohms) and a decreased rate. At operation, the diagnosis may be erroneously labeled as an exit block if the insulation break was in the air and not in contact with the body tissues during lead parameter measurements. Unless the insulation break is tiny and accessible, the lead should be replaced.

Ventricular Perforation

Since the diagnosis of ventricular perforation is not easily confirmed, it probably occurs more frequently than is realized. The incidence of ventricular perforation ranges from 2 to 20 percent, but only rarely do hemopericardium and cardiac tamponade result.[29, 30] The diagnosis may be suspected if there is a change in the axis of paced beats compared to earlier records, or sensing or capturing is lost or intermittent on EKG. Right bundle branch block of the paced complexes strongly suggests perforation of the ventricle and particularly of the septum. However, this may be seen in coronary sinus or right ventricular pacing in the absence of perforation.[31] Intercostal muscle contractions, hiccups caused by diaphragmatic stimulation, pansystolic murmur, or a pericardial friction rub are other signs of possible ventricular perforation. X-ray study may be helpful in certain cases. When this situation requires surgical correction the analyzer may show an increased pacing current and voltage with normal resistance. Barold and Center reported disappearance of the current of injury (ST-segment elevation) on the intracardiac electrogram as the lead is pulled back into the right ventricle.[32] Although cardiac tamponade is a rare occurrence following lead withdrawal and repositioning, close monitoring in the immediate postoperative period is highly recommended.

Exit Block

Normally, it takes 2 to 3 weeks for an acute threshold to rise to a stable chronic threshold value. The threshold scale is relative, as voltage thresholds are usually dependent on the lead surface area (Fig. 11–1). Theoretically, pacing electrodes with larger surface area should display better sensing characteristics.[33] Amundson suggested that the increased surface area of the totally porous electrode should improve its performance.[34] However, the sensing ability of the porous-surfaced electrode with a smaller total surface area (if the surface area due to porosity was included) was superior to that of the totally porous regular-sized electrode.[35] Furman reported that 19 percent of patients experienced an average 14-percent increase per year over the initial thresholds because of poor initial lead placement.[26]

X-ray is not helpful in diagnosis of exit block, since the position of the lead is essentially unchanged from the time of the initial implant. The pacing threshold is increased because of high fibrotic buildup at the electrode site. High doses of some antiarrhythmics, such as quinidine, lidocaine, or procainamide may produce an abnormally high pacing threshold. Hypokalemia and hypocalcemia also increase the pacemaker threshold. Obviously myocardial infarction in the area of the pacemaker lead would markedly affect the pacing threshold. EKG will show a regular spike-to-spike interval with no capture. Management depends on the cause, but usually operative intervention is required to reposition the lead. The use of a high-output generator is optional. In other situations, the original lead may be replaced.

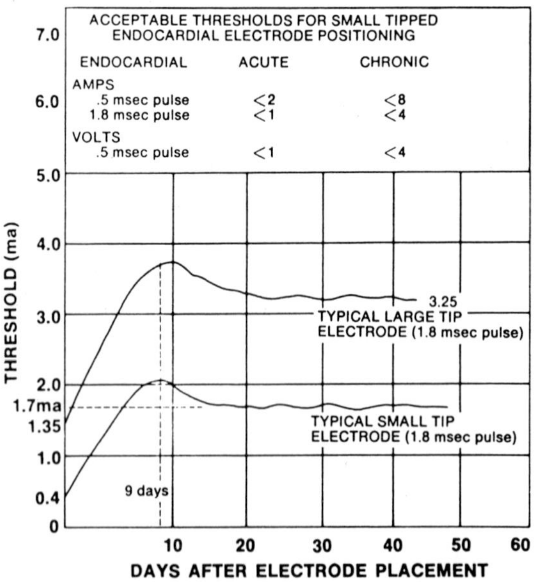

Figure 11–1. Alteration of endocardial stimulation threshold (in milliamps) versus time (in days). Insert illustrates acceptable thresholds for small-tip endocardial electrode positioning.

Lead Fracture

Complete lead fracture usually occurs at stress-point areas and at sharp angulation sites and can cause intermittent pacing (Table 11–3). It can be easily differentiated from pseudofracture of the lead, in which the only abnormality present is the evidence of what appears to be a fractured lead on x-ray.[36] Nonpacing may also occur when there is a conduction defect in the pacing electrode that totally blocks the current derived from the generator. External manipulation of the pacemaker unit while watching an EKG strip for resumption of intermittent pacing may aid in establishing the diagnosis. X-ray may be helpful in detecting gross fractures. Magnet application will show no response in cases of complete lead fracture without insulation break. However, it will cause multiples of the spike-to-spike interval, which does not reach the electrode if the wire is separated in cases of intermittent touching of a completely fractured lead. Intraoperatively, traction on the lead (without dislodging it) confirms the diagnosis of a completely fractured lead. The analyzer would show large variations in the pacing current values. In patients with lead fracture but with intact insulation, the EKG shows no tracing. The analyzer would show high or normal pacing voltage, decreased current, and increased resistance. Replacement of the lead is the treatment of choice for pacemaker lead fractures.

Lead Connection Problems

In cases of loose connection between the pacing electrode and the pulse generator, external manipulation of the pacemaker unit while observing the EKG strip for resumption of pacing may give a clue to the diagnosis. Magnet application would show multiples of the spike-to-spike interval, which does not reach the electrode if the connector is separated. X-ray can show only gross

Table 11–3. Failure of Cardiac Pacing (Intermittent Pacing)

Etiology	Management
Intermittent Current With Capture	
Completely fractured lead	Replace lead
Intermittent connection of lead pin and battery	Reconnect lead pin and battery
Intermittent Capture	
Borderline thresholds	Correct metabolic imbalance Increase generator output and lower sensing if possible Reposition lead
Ventricular perforation	With bipolar lead program to unipolar Reposition lead
Dislodged and floating lead	Reposition lead or change to an active-fixation lead
Lead insulation break	Replace lead Repair if minor and accessible

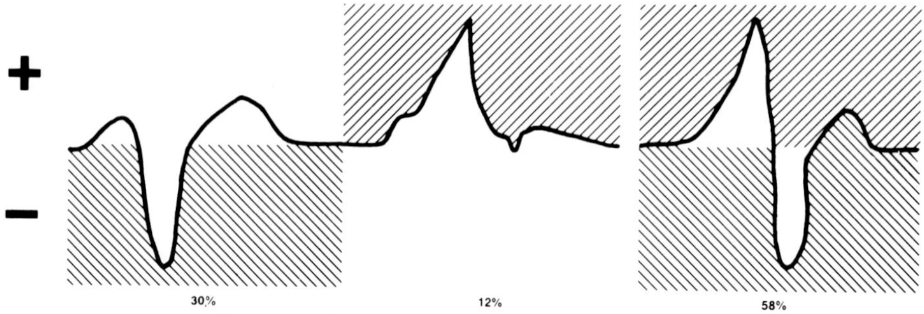

Figure 11–2. R-wave polarities.

disconnection. Intraoperatively, application of traction on the lead or connector will confirm the problem. Management is by proper connection of the pacing electrode to the generator.

Failure of Sensing

Although this may be an isolated feature, it is usually associated with failure of pacing.

Furman reported three types of acute intracardiac signals: 58 percent are biphasic, 30 percent are monophasic negative, and 11 percent are monophasic positive (Fig. 11–2).[37]

Most pacemaker units have bidirectional sensing, although some do not sense equally in positive and negative directions. Thus they may not consistently inhibit even with a large amplitude R wave.

R-wave amplitude usually ranges from 5 to 15 mV. We recommend 6 mV as the minimum acceptable acute value, since chronically there is approximately a 15-percent decrease in amplitude, which may be compounded by a decrease in the chronic slew rate. Most pacemaker generators exhibit a current sensitivity that can be programmed to 1.5 mV or lower, thus a 6.0-mV R-wave measurement at the time of implantation allows a very comfortable margin of safety.

The pacing electrode surface area may affect amplitude transmission to the pulse generator, and the smaller the surface area the smaller the amplitude transmission.[38]

Undersensing

In the acute phase most patients' R waves are biphasic, but the R wave may chronically change polarity. If a pacemaker unit senses less effectively in one direction, undersensing is apt to develop because of inability to detect full peak-to-peak voltage (Table 11–4). The incidence of undersensing is less than 1

Table 11–4. Failure of Sensing (Undersensing)

Etiology	Management
Normally Functioning Battery that Receives Inadequate Cardiac Signals	
Lead dislodgement	Lower pacemaker sensitivity if applicable Reposition or replace with a different type of lead
Lead fracture	Replace lead
Lead insulation break	Repair if minor or accessible Replace lead
Excessive body fluid within the connector or missing silicon cap on the Allen screws	Disconnect lead, dry it, and reconnect Apply silicon cap on the Allen screws if missing
Good lead position with inadequate shape or amplitude of cardiac signals	Adjust metabolic imbalance Lower pacemaker sensitivity, if applicable Reposition or replace with different type lead
Normal Cardiac Signals and Lead with Pulse Generator Malfunction	
Reed switch stuck in the closed position	Wave magnet over the pulse generator in an attempt to loosen the Reed switch Replace battery if asynchronous pacing not applicable
Circuitry failure	Replace the pacemaker battery

percent and is more frequently seen in epicardial bipolar systems because of an inadequate distance between the implanted leads.

Obvious or microdislodgement of the pacing electrode is the most common cause of undersensing. Chest wall stimulation may be attempted to verify whether the pulse generator is inhibiting.[39, 40] EKG reading is usually diagnostic when the pacemaker output pulse is not inhibited by the intrinsic R wave. An x-ray may be of benefit in diagnosing cases of major dislodgement. Intraoperatively, in addition to the analyzer measurements, an electrogram may show decreased slew rate indicating distance from the endocardium. Management is initially by lowering the sensitivity of the pacemaker generator. If that is not possible or is ineffective, then repositioning the lead or replacing it with a different type of lead is the next alternative.

A fractured electrode may lead to failure of sensing per se or be combined with failure of pacing, depending on the extent of the contact between the two fractured ends. Diagnosis and management are identical to that in lead fractures causing failure of pacing.

With good lead positioning, a low amplitude or a changing shape of the cardiac signal may cause intermittent undersensing. This may also be due to metabolic imbalance, drugs, or myocardial infarction at the electrode site.

Excessive body fluid within the connector, insulation break, or loss of a Silastic plug over the Allen screws in pacemaker units can reduce or short-circuit

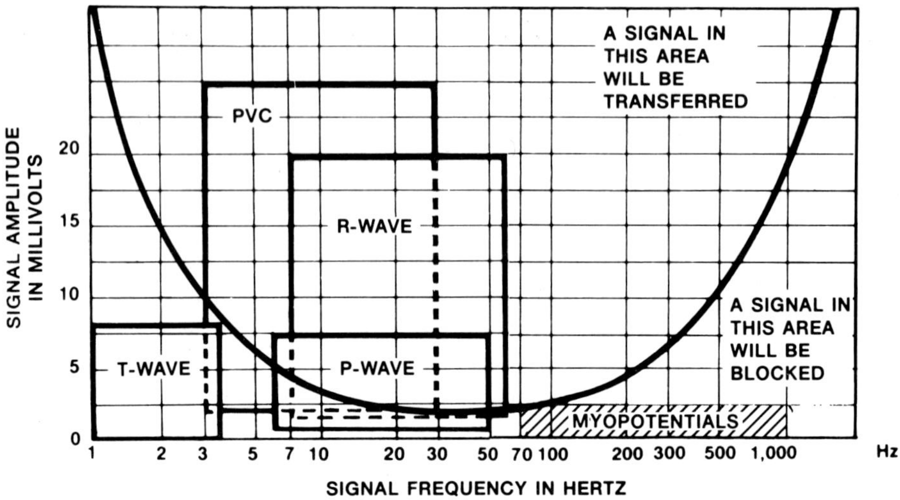

Figure 11–3. Sensitivity curve for sensing R waves.

Undersensing may also be related to pulse generator failure. The Reed switch may be stuck in a closed position; thus, in the presence of a magnetic field the sensing amplifier is prevented from resetting the timing circuit. Waving a magnet may occasionally loosen the Reed switch and correct the problem. If this is unsuccessful the decision must be made whether to leave an asynchronous unit or to replace it. In rare cases of circuitry failure the pulse generator should be replaced.

Oversensing

Only signals with both appropriate amplitude (1.5 mV or more) and frequency activate the refractory generator, which implements the preset refractory period (Fig. 11–3). Oversensing occurs when the pacemaker generator senses signals that should be ignored. These unwanted signals may be skeletal muscle potentials, electromagnetic interference,[41] pacemaker afterpotentials, and T or P waves (unless pacing atrially). In spite of the sophisticated bandpass filters of contemporary pacemakers, the problem of oversensing, although significantly reduced, still exists.[42]

Studies have shown that skeletal myoinhibition may be present in 85 percent of patients with unipolar pulse generators and is usually preventable by using a bipolar system, unless there is an associated insulation break.[43–46] The diagnosis can be reached by exercising the muscle in question during an EKG recording.[47, 48] In symptomatic patients with sufficient underlying rhythm who are not willing to restrict certain activities, the treatment of choice would be to change to a bipolar system. New versions of some pulse generators are equipped with a revision circuit that recognizes some myopotentials and rejects them as noise. Waving a magnet over the pulse generator can open and close the Reed switch, causing inhibition of the pacemaker, and some physicians use this method to detect the patient's underlying rhythm. Other electromagnetic interference may be caused by such devices as microwave ovens, radar, electrical generators, sabre saws, hair dryers, and electric razors. Generally, household appliances will not influence today's pacemaker functioning.

A T wave of sufficient amplitude and shape would be sensed if it occurred after the refractory period. For newly implanted leads, this may resolve spontaneously within 24 hours; otherwise, the lead should be repositioned. Pulse generator refractory periods offer some protection against T-wave sensing, and adjusting the refractory period may infrequently solve this problem.

P-wave sensing in ventricular pacing systems is rarely seen, and it usually denotes improper lead placement either in the coronary sinus or near the tricuspid valve area. Although rare, a lead insulation break in the atrial area may also produce P-wave sensing. If the lead is intact the treatment of choice is lead repositioning.[49]

Oversensing may also be attributed to lead-related problems such as intermittent lead fracture or insulation break, the diagnosis and treatment of which have already been discussed.

Pacing afterpotential is the residual energy that dissipates through tissue after high-energy pulse has been delivered. Afterpotential sensing occurs following the refractory period, when the remaining T wave and the afterpotential itself are picked up by the pulse generator as a combined voltage burst. Although afterpotential sensing has been associated with high current[50] or long pulse-width stimuli,[51] it also has been seen with nominal output pulses of 5.5 volts and 0.5 msec.[52] Large-capacitance electrodes,[53] close apposition of bipolar epicardial leads,[52] long battery output circuit recovery time,[53, 54] and a relatively short refractory period are incriminatory factors enhancing afterpotential sensing. EKG will show prolongation of the interval to exactly the paced interval plus the refractory period. Treatment consists of lowering the pacemaker generator output, provided that safety margin for pacing is adequate. It may also be abolished noninvasively by increasing the refractory period duration or decreasing the sensitivity of multiprogrammable models.[55] Occasionally, increasing the rate and masking the T wave within the refractory period may be helpful; otherwise, the lead should be repositioned.

Pulse generator failure of electronic components, including battery depletion with sensing circuit changes, can cause oversensing, and replacing the pacemaker battery is the recommended treatment.

Rate Difficulty

These problems, although usually pulse generator related, may not indicate failure and are not caused by changes in the patient or lead conditions.

Fast Rates. Presently, cases of runaway pacemakers are rare, because most circuits incorporate some protective device, minimizing the likelihood of ventricular capture at rates above 150 paced beats per minute. Some lithium pulse generators are designed to operate at certain rates at room temperature and will increase in speed by about ½ paced beat per minute per degree Celsius. In other words a rate increase is expected after implantation and during the course of a febrile illness. Excessive rate increase is most likely caused by component failure of the pulse generator, requiring immediate replacement.

Slow Rates. T-wave sensing and afterpotential sensing after the refractory period can lead to a rate decrease. If it is feasible to program the pulse generator sensitivity or refractory period, the problem can be solved; otherwise, repositioning the lead is a suitable alternative. Rarely does a break in lead insulation subject the pacemaker battery to an extreme load and cause a reduction in pacemaker rate. A slow rate can also be caused by component failure, in which case replacement of the battery should be performed.

Muscle Stimulation

Diaphragmatic muscle stimulation can be caused by either pacing the phrenic nerve or the diaphragm itself, causing hiccups synchronous with pacemaker rate.[56] Pacemaker electrode perforation or insulation break can cause skeletal muscle stimulation leading to subtle or marked contractions of the rectus abdominis, the pectoralis, the intercostals, or the muscles of the diaphragm. This complication is most commonly associated with a unipolar pulse generator; however, it may occur infrequently in bipolar lead systems. Loss of a Silastic cap over the Allen screws that secure the electrode to the battery may produce stimulation of the pectoral or abdominal muscles. Lead dislodgement has been incriminated as a cause of focal motor seizure.[57]

Pacemaker Migration or Erosion

Different factors have been blamed as causes of pacemaker migration and subsequent erosion. These include pacemaker pocket hematoma, gravitational force, poor tissue turgor, and excessive weight of the pulse generator. Either the pulse generator or the pacing electrode may migrate if there is little fibrotic tissue to protect against muscle flexion and shearing motion.[26]

The use of artificial pouches is to be discouraged, since they represent a foreign body material. If proper surgical techniques are exercised this complication is preventable. With faulty development of the pacemaker pocket at the time of the initial implantation, migration into the lower chest and axilla can be a troublesome problem for both patient and physician. There has been a significant decline in the incidence of this complication because of the marked reduction in size, mass, and physiologic shape of the pulse generator along with improved surgical expertise.

Migration may or may not lead to erosion. At the same time, erosion can develop with or without migration. Skin erosion is more of a serious problem, as it points to the possibility of infection.[58] When erosion is imminent (the overlying skin is still intact), the treatment should be urgent repositioning of the pacemaker battery beneath the pectoral muscle. When the integrity of the skin is broken, with or without evidence of infection in the pocket area, removal of the unit and insertion of a new unit at another site is the procedure of choice.

Infection

Previous reports show the incidence of this complication to be approximately 5 to 6 percent with a mortality rate of about 2 percent. The most common infecting organisms are *Staphylococcus aureus, Staphyloccus epidermidis,* and *Staphylococcus albus,* although gram-negative infection has also been reported.

A study of 24 patients showed that infection involving the battery developed an average of 2½ weeks after implantation, whereas catheter infection occurred an average of 33 weeks following implantation and was related to erosion of the lead in the neck region.[58] It was observed that there was an increased risk of battery infection with subsequent replacement. The study concludes that removal of the entire septic pacemaker unit with insertion of a new unit in a different location should be undertaken, and that antibiotic therapy with or without conservative surgery is unsatisfactory.

In another study of five patients with staphylococcal bacteremia 2 weeks to 10 months following initial implantation, it was concluded that antibiotics alone were helpful in only one patient who did not have any evidence of pocket infection.[60]

A third study, in which local signs of infection developed in nine patients with epicardial pacing systems during a period from less than 2 weeks to more than 6 months following surgery, *S. epidermidis* was isolated in seven out of nine patients. The report concludes that since the extent of infection is difficult to determine at the time of operation, initial removal of the entire pacing system is recommended.[61]

A fourth study described three late pacemaker pocket infections 18, 32, and 47 months postimplantation that were caused by *S. epidermidis.* The study concluded that, in view of the insidious nature of the *S. epidermidis* infection, regular inspection of the pocket by both the patient and the physician is mandatory and that the infected pacemaker unit should be explanted.[62]

Others

Other, rare complications include pacemaker sounds[63, 64] and fractured leads that perforate the atrial and bronchial walls, compounded with infection and subsequent bronchocutaneous fistulae. The tricuspid valve may be damaged during pacemaker lead insertion, predisposing to bacterial endocarditis. Arrhythmias may include ventricular fibrillation, which may be pacer-related or may follow external defibrillation.[65–69] In patients with unipolar units, incomplete conduction at the anode (sometimes referred to as "dry" or "gas" pocket) may be corrected by an attempt to aspirate gas from the pocket with a syringe.[70] Dentritic spur in the substrate of the programming circuit is an extremely rare cause of pacemaker malfunction.[71]

There are also some new but rare complications that are encountered with the use of active-fixation leads.[72, 73] Pacemaker syndrome[74, 75] is an important complication following demand ventricular pacing or P-wave synchronous pacing.[76] In this syndrome hypotension, dizziness, fatigue, effort intolerance, and presyncope result secondary to lack of atrial contribution. Patients with this syndrome can be effectively treated by replacing their pacemaker units with dual-chamber physiologic pacemakers (DDD). It is thus apparent that physiologic pacemaker units are capable of preventing pacemaker syndrome.

Physiologic pacing restores atrioventricular synchrony and promotes improved cardiac performance and hemodynamics. Some of the newer physiologic pacing units have the ability to control a variety of atrial and ventricular arrhythmias. In view of this fact, we tend to insert DDD pacemakers in all of our patients requiring cardiac pacing whenever indicated.

REFERENCES

1. Mantini EL, Majors RK, Kennedy JR, and Lebo GR: A recommended protocol for pacemaker follow-up: Analysis of 1,705 implanted pacemakers. Ann Thorac Surg 24:62, 1977.
2. Vander Salm TS, Haffajee CI, and Okike ON: Transvenous insertion of double sets of permanent electrodes through a single introducer: Clinical application. Ann Thorac Surg 32:307, 1981.
3. Kirsh MM, and Sloan H: Blunt Chest Trauma: General Principles of Management. Boston, Little, Brown and Co, 1977.
4. Kircher LT, and Swartzel RL: Spontaneous pneumothorax and its treatment. JAMA 155:24, 1954.
5. Borrie J: Management of Thoracic Emergencies. 3rd ed. New York, Appleton-Century-Crofts, 1980.
6. Rotem CC, Greig JH, and Walters MB: Air embolism to the pulmonary artery during insertion of transvenous endocardial pacemaker. J Thorac Cardiovasc Surg 53:562, 1967.
7. Wertheimer M, Hughes RK, and Castle CH: Superior vena cava syndrome—complication of permanent transvenous endocardial cardiac pacing. JAMA 224:1172, 1973.
8. Pauletti M, Di Ricco G, Solfanelli S, et al: Venous obstruction in permanent pacemaker patients: An isotopic study. Pace 4:36, 1981.
9. Marder VJ, and Bell WR: Fibrinolytic therapy. *In* Colman RW, Hirsh J, Marder VJ, and Satzman EW (eds): Hemostasis and Thrombosis: Basic Principles. Philadelphia, JB Lippincott Co., 1982, pp. 1037–1057.
10. Mich RJ, and Bell WR: Thrombolytic therapy of deep-vein thrombosis. Practical Cardiol 8:43, 1982.
11. Freidberg HD, and D'Cunha, GF: Adhesions of pacing catheter to tricuspid valve: Adhesion endocarditis. Thorax 24:498, 1969.
12. Schwartz IS, and Perez N: Bacterial endocarditis associated with a permanent transvenous cardiac pacemaker. JAMA 218:736, 1971.
13. Morris JJ, Whalen RE, McIntosh HD, et al: Permanent ventricular pacemakers: Comparison of transthoracic and transvenous implantation. Circulation 36:587, 1967.
14. Chardach WM, Gage AA, Federico AJ, et al: Clinical experience with an implantable pacemaker. Ann NY Acad Sci 3:1075, 1964.

15. Elmquist R, Landergren J, Pettersson SO, et al: Artificial pacemaker for treatment of Adams-Stokes syndrome and slow heart rate. Am Heart J 65:731, 1963.
16. Brenner AS, Wagner GS, Anderson ST, et al: Transvenous, transmediastinal, and transthoracic ventricular pacing. A comparison after complete two-year follow-up. Circulation 49:407, 1974.
17. Burgess GE 3rd, Cooper JR Jr, Marino RJ, et al: Pulmonary effect of pleurotomy during and after coronary artery bypass with internal mammary artery versus saphenous vein grafts. J Thorac Cardiovasc Surg 76:230, 1978.
18. Sprinkle JP, Takard T, and Scott SM: Phrenic nerve stimulation as a complication of the implantable cardiac pacemaker. Circulation 28:114, 1963.
19. Peleska B, and Buda J: Stimulation of the phrenic nerve as a complication of implanted pacemaker: Management without thoracotomy. J Thorac Cardiovasc Surg 6:477, 1965.
20. Perrin EJ, Sutton R, Kaesic B, et al: Modern atrial and ventricular leads for permanent cardiac pacing. Br Heart J 46:196, 1981.
21. Bilitch M, Hauser RG, Goldman BS, et al: Performance of cardiac pacemaker pulse generators. Pace 4:607, 1981.
22. Snow N: Elimination of lead dislodgements by the use of tined transvenous electrodes. Pace 5:571, 1982.
23. Brievik K, Engedal H, and Ohm OJ: Electrophysiological properties of a new permanent endocardial lead for uni- and bipolar pacing. Pace 5:268, 1982.
24. Hirshorn MS, Holley LK, Hales JRS, et al: Screening of solid and porous materials for pacemaker electrodes. Pace 4:380, 1981.
25. Hakki A, Horowitz L, Reiser J, and Mundth ED: Improved pacemaker fixation and performance using a modified finned porous tip lead. Int Surg, 1984. In press.
26. Furman S: Cardiac pacing and pacemakers. VI: Analysis of pacemaker malfunction. Am Heart J 94:378, 1977.
27. Furman S, Hurzeler P, and Mehra R: Cardiac pacing and pacemakers. IV: Threshold of cardiac stimulation. Am Heart J 94:115, 1977.
28. Boake WC, and Kroncke GM: Pacemaker Complications, Cardiac Pacing. Philadelphia, Lea and Febiger, 1979.
29. Nathan DA, Center S, Pina RG, et al: Perforation during indwelling catheter pacing. Circulation 33:128, 1966.
30. Bassan MM, and Merin G: Pericardial tamponade due to perforation with a permanent endocardial pacing catheter. J Thorac Cardiovasc Surg 74:51, 1977.
31. Chung EK: Artificial Cardiac Pacing. Baltimore, Williams and Wilkins Co, 1978.
32. Barold SS, and Center S: Electrographic diagnosis of perforation of the heart by pacing catheter electrode. Am J Cardiol 24:274, 1969.
33. Amundson DC: Sensing properties of pacemaker electrodes (abstract). 78th ACEMB, p. 83.
34. Amundson DC, McArthur W, and Mosharrafa M: The porous endocardial electrode. Pace 2:40, 1979.
35. Bobyn JD, Wilson GJ, Mycyk TR, et al: Comparison of a porous-surfaced with a totally porous ventricular endocardial pacing electrode. Pace 4:405, 1981.
36. Witte AA: Pseudo-fracture of pacemaker lead due to securing suture: A case report. Pace 4:716, 1981.
37. Furman S, Hurzeler P, and Decaprio V: Cardiac pacing and pacemaker. III. Sensing the cardiac electrogram. Am Heart J 93:794, 1977.
38. Hughes HC, Brownlee RR, and Tyers GFO: Failure of demand pacing with small surface area electrodes. Circulation 54:128, 1976.
39. Hakki HI, Goel IP, and Mundth ED: Pacemaker inhibition in cardiac surgery. Ann Thorac Surg 33:295, 1982.
40. Barold SS, Pupillo GA, Gaidula JJ, and Linhart JW: Chest wall stimulation in evaluation of patients with implanted ventricular-inhibited demand pacemakers. Br Heart J 32:783, 1970.
41. Furman S, Parker B, Krathamer M, et al: The influence of electromagnetic environment on the performance of artificial cardiac pacemakers. Ann Thorac Surg 6:90, 1968.
42. Taniguchi K, Takaoka T, Fujiwara H, et al: Clinical experiences and experimental studies of false sensing with demand pacemakers. *In* Watanabe Y (ed): Cardiac Pacing. Amsterdam, Excerpta Medica, 1977, p. 333.
43. Berger R, and Jacobs W: Myopotential inhibition of demand pacemakers. Pace 2:596, 1979.
44. Barold SS: Current problems with demand pacemakers. Eur J Cardiol 1:339, 1974.
45. Widlansky S, and Zipes DP: Suppression of a ventricular-inhibited bipolar pacemaker by skeletal muscle activity. J Electrocardiol 7:371, 1974.
46. Secemsky SI, Hauser RG, Penes P, and Edwards LM: Unipolar sensing abnormalities: Incidence

and clinical significance of skeletal muscle interference and undersensing in 228 patients. Pace 5:10, 1982.
47. Anderson ST, Pitt A, Whitford JA, and Davis BB: Interference with function of unipolar pacemaker due to muscle potentials. J Thorac Cardiovasc Surg 71:698, 1976.
48. Ohm OJ, Bruland H, Pederson OM, and Woerness F: Interference effect of myopotentials of function of unipolar demand pacemakers. Br Heart J 36:77, 1974.
49. Barold SS, and Gaidula JJ: Evaluation of normal and abnormal sensing functions of demand pacemakers. Am J Cardiol 28:201, 1970.
50. Beller BM, and Pupillo G: Potentially dangerous rate and amplitude control interaction in an external battery-powered demand pacemaker. Am Heart J 81:717, 1971.
51. Gould L, Reddy CVR, Singh BK, et al: Inappropriate slowing of the pacemaker rate with programmable demand pacemaker. Pace 2:370, 1979.
52. Taniguchi K, Takaoka T, Fujiwara H, et al: Clinical experience and experimental studies of false sensing in the demand pacemakers. *In* Watanabe Y (ed): Cardiac Pacing. Amsterdam, Excerpta Medica, 1977, p. 333.
53. Barold SS: "Double reset" of demand pacemakers. Am Heart J 84:276, 1972.
54. Keller JW, Gosselin AJ, Nathan DA, et al: Rhythm anomalies in contemporary demand pacing. Am J Cardiol 29:572, 1972.
55. Hauser RG, and Susmano A: After-potential oversensing by a programmable pulse generator. Pace 4:391, 1981.
56. Wicks J, Davidson R, and Belk N: Malfunction of a demand pacemaker caused by phrenic nerve stimulation. Chest 74:303, 1978.
57. Catherwood G, Elzwahry MKH, Kotler MN, and Adam A: Dislodgement of pacemaker electrode simulating focal motor seizure. Chest 75:627, 1979.
58. Imparato A, and Kim G: Electrode complications in patients with permanent cardiac pacemakers. Arch Surg 105:705, 1973.
59. Kennelly BM, and Piller LW: Management of infected transvenous permanent pacemakers. Br Heart J 36:1133, 1974.
60. Corman LC, and Levison MG: Sustained bacteremia and transvenous cardiac pacemakers. JAMA 233:264, 1975.
61. Choo MH, Holmes DR Jr, Gersh BJ, et al: Infected epicardial pacemaker systems. Partial versus total removal. J Thorac Cardiovasc Surg 82:794, 1981.
62. Wohl B, Peters RW, Carliner N, et al: Late unheralded pacemaker pocket infection due to Staphylococcus epidermidis: A new clinical entity. Pace 5:190, 1982.
63. Kluge WF: Pacemaker sound and its origin. Am J Cardiol 25:362, 1970.
64. Korn M, Schoenfeld CD, Ghahramani A, and Samet P: The pacemaker sound. Am J Med 49:451, 1970.
65. Das G, and Eaton J: Pacemaker malfunction following transthoracic countershock. Pace 4:487, 1981.
66. Gould L, Patel S, Gomes GI, and Chokshi AB: Pacemaker failure following external defibrillation. Pace 4:575, 1981.
67. Spielman SR, Farshidi A, Horowitz LN, et al: Ventricular fibrillation during programmed ventricular stimulation: Incidence and clinical implications. Am J Cardiol 42:913, 1978.
68. Palac RT, Hwang MH, Klodnycky ML, and Loeb HS: Delayed pulse generator malfunction after DC countershock. Pace 4:163, 1981.
69. Tolentino AO, Javier RP, Byrd C, and Samet P: Pacer-induced tachycardia associated with an atrial synchronous ventricular inhibited (ASVIP) pulse generator. Pace 5:251, 1982.
70. Lasala AF, Fieldman A, Diana DJ, and Humphrey CB: Gas pocket causing pacemaker malfunction. Pace 2:183, 1979.
71. Comer TP, Saxena N, and Salzman SH: The case of the two-timing pacemaker. Pace 4:465, 1981.
72. Furman S, Pannizzo F, and Campo I: Comparison of active and passive leads for endocardial pacing. II. Pace 4:78, 1981.
73. Ong LS, Barold SS, Craver WL, et al: Partial avulsion of the tricuspid valve by tined pacing electrode. Am Heart J 102:4, 798, 1981.
74. Miller M, Fox S, Jenkins R, et al: Pacemaker syndrome: A non-invasive means to its diagnosis and treatment. Pace 4:503, 1981.
75. Nishimura KA, Gersh BJ, Vlietstra et al: Hemodynamic and symptomatic consequences of ventricular pacing. Pace 5:903, 1982.
76. Levine PA, Seltzer JP, and Pirzada FA: The "pacemaker syndrome" in a properly functioning physiologic pacing system. Pace 6:279, 1983.

12

Flap Coverage for Exposed Pacemakers

HANI S. MATLOUB, M.D.

Exposure and extrusion are not rare complications of implantable pacemakers. Sowton and colleagues[1] demonstrated in a series of 372 patients that during a 10-year period 10 percent of the pacemakers had to be removed. Excessive friction, pressure, trauma, and infection are all incriminating factors in pacemaker erosion. Other studies have reported less than 5 percent of soft-tissue complications over the implantable pacemaker.[2, 3]

Some of the factors that precipitate problems may be related to the advanced age of the majority of candidates for cardiac pacing. In this group nutritional debilitation, skin changes, and scanty subcutaneous tissue offer poor coverage for the pacing system.

There are certain technical guidelines that during pacemaker insertion may reduce the risk of future complication.[4, 5] These include

1. Placing the skin incision as remotely as possible from the implanted material.
2. Avoiding the use of braided sutures for fixation of leads or pulse generators, as they may produce foreign body reaction.
3. Placing lead loops horizontally and as deeply as possible.
4. Subclavian vein insertion with infraclavicular placement of the pacemaker.
5. Meticulous surgical technique, avoiding unnecessary injury to the surrounding tissue.

LOCAL SKIN FLAP

Preceding surgical repair of an exposed pacemaker wound, local infection must be eradicated by debridement of all nonviable tissue, appropriate systemic

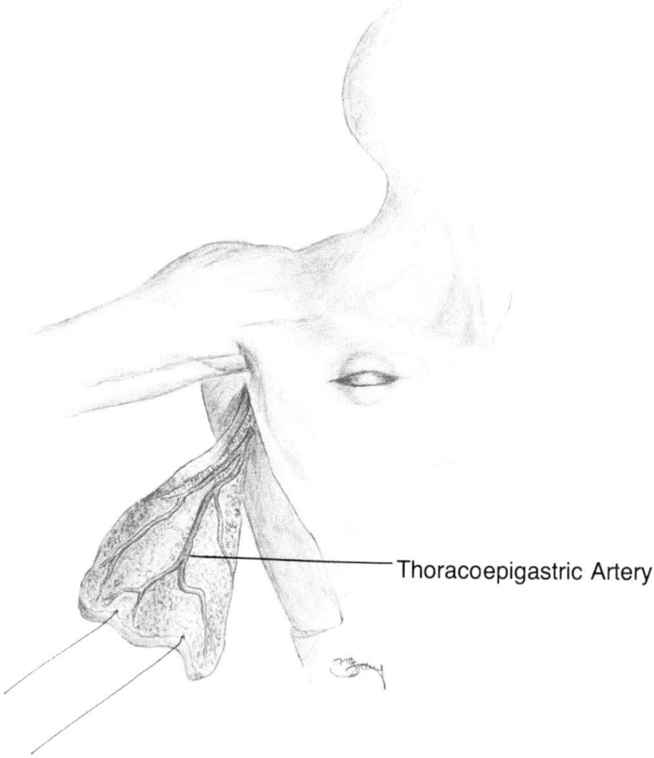

Figure 12–1. Axillary flap with intact vascular supply is elevated before being rotated to cover the defect.

antibiotics, and wound irrigation with antibiotic solution. Skin flaps used for coverage of the pacemaker have the advantage of being technically simpler than muscle flaps.[6] Chari and Suri[7] reported the use of a skin flap based on the deltopectoral region transplanted inferiorly to cover the base of the defect with application of a split-thickness skin graft to the donor area. In 1979, Baudet described the use of the axillary flap.[8] The advantage of this axillary flap, which is widely preferred, is the presence of a direct cutaneous artery and vein, which should assure complete survival and excellent blood supply. This flap is based on the thoracoepigastric artery and vein, a branch of the thoracodorsal artery. With the aid of a directional flow Doppler, the artery is located and outlined preoperatively. The flap may be raised under local anesthesia. After thorough debridement of the wound, the flap is elevated, carefully avoiding injury to the vascular supply (Fig. 12–1). The flap is then rotated to cover the defect, and the wound edges are sutured in layers. The donor site may be closed primarily by local undermining of the surrounding skin (Fig. 12–2).

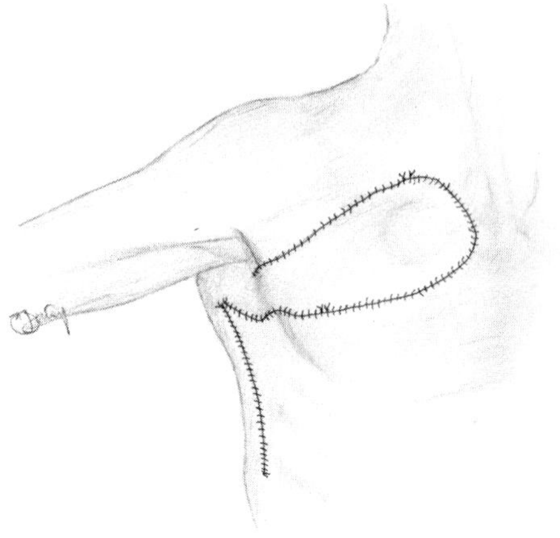

Figure 12–2. Axillary flap is in place; the donor site is primarily closed.

MUSCLE FLAP

Muscle flaps have been used in difficult cases in which local skin flaps proved unsuitable for coverage. One advantage of muscle flaps is that they give a greater increase in local blood supply to the recipient area than do skin flaps. In this manner they enhance healing and aid in the control of local infection.[9] Another advantage is that muscle adds an extra amount of bulk or cushion over the implanted area, thereby reducing the incidence of exposure secondary to breakdown of tissue overlying the pacemaker. The disadvantage of this procedure is that the operation is rather lengthy and may require general anesthesia.

There are basically two types of muscle flaps that may be utilized for coverage of exposed pacemakers.

The Pectoralis Major Muscle Flap

The most common muscle flap used for anterior chest wall defects is the pectoralis major. The muscle is isolated on its major vascular pedicle, the thoracoacromial artery and vein. In covering small defects, a pocket is formed between the pectoralis major and minor, and the pulse generator is placed between these two muscles.

In cases of larger defects, the entire origin of the muscle may be detached and elevated, with its vascular supply intact. The generator is then covered by the pectoralis major muscle (Fig. 12–3). The elevated muscle is sutured back to the adjacent tissue, and the wound is closed in layers.

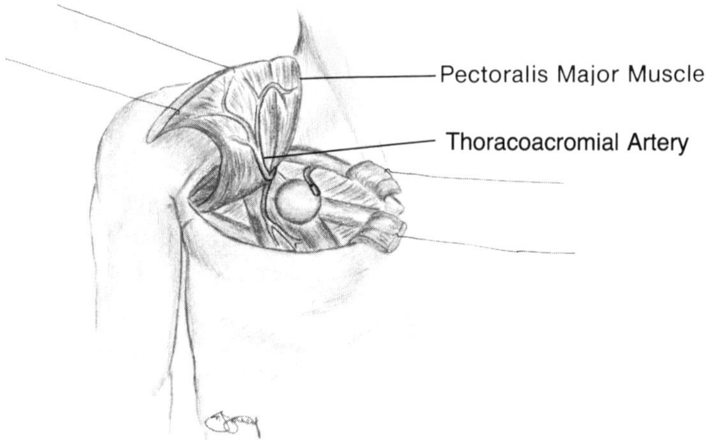

Figure 12–3. Pectoralis major flap elevated with neurovascular bundle. Note the detached origin of the muscle and placement of the pulse generator.

The Latissimus Dorsi Muscle Flap

The latissimus dorsi muscle flap is a large flap arising from the midline of the back and from the lower sixth thoracic vertebra down to the posterior crest of the ilium. From its very broad origin, it narrows and inserts into the intertendinous sulcus of the humerus. The neurovascular supply is through the thoracodorsal branch of the subscapular artery and the thoracodorsal nerve. The neurovascular pedicle enters the muscle near the axillary insertion.

This muscle may be elevated from its origin either as a muscle flap or as a myocutaneous flap (muscle and skin) and rotated to cover any anterior chest

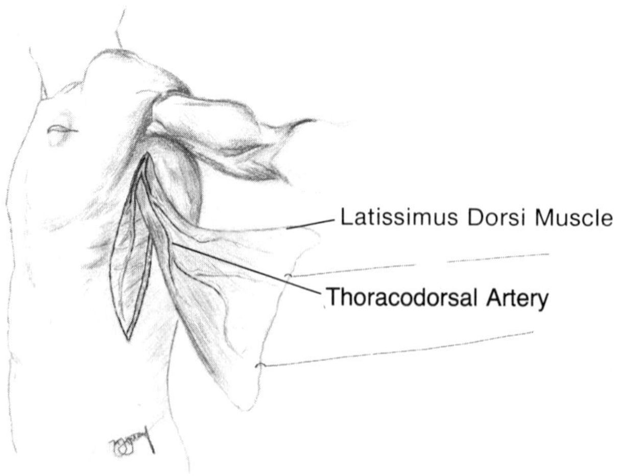

Figure 12–4. Latissimus dorsi muscle flap elevated with intact neurovascular bundle.

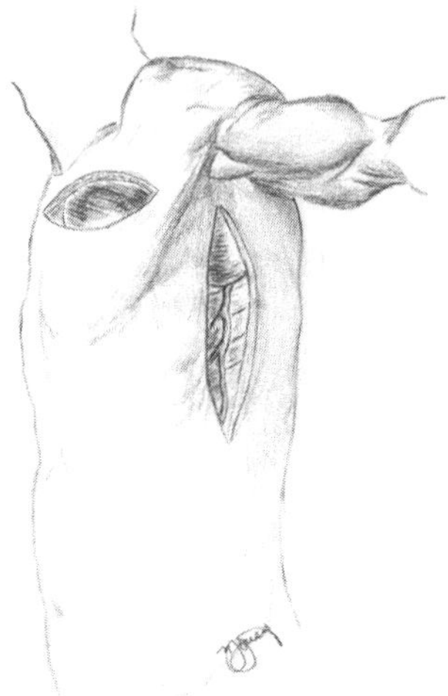

Figure 12–5. Muscle rotated and tunneled under the skin, covering the pulse generator.

wall defect.[3] An incision is made near the lateral margin of the muscle. The muscle is then partially or totally freed from its origin (Fig. 12–4). The origin and neurovascular bundle are left intact and the flap is passed through a tunnel in the subcutaneous tissue and brought onto the anterior chest wall (Fig. 12–5). The muscle may be sutured to the adjacent tissue, and the wound may then be closed in layers.

Acknowledgment. The author wishes to thank N. John Yousif, M.D., for the production of the illustrations and for his help in preparation of this chapter.

REFERENCES

1. Sowton E, Hendrix G, and Roy P: Ten year survey on treatment with implanted cardiac pacemaker. Br Med J 3:155, 1974.
2. Coburn RJ, Blank HL, and Campbell RM: Covering an exposed pacemaker. Plast Reconstr Surg 50:622, 1972.
3. Mathes J, and Stephen F: Clinical Applications for Muscle and Musculo-cutaneous Flaps. St. Louis, C. V. Mosby, 1982.
4. Chait LA, and Ritchie B: Methods of treating the exposed cardiac pacemaker. Br J Plast Surg 32:281, 1979.
5. Borie J, and Lichter I: Surgical management and problems of heart pacing. Br J Surg 62:186, 1975.
6. Barrett BM Jr, Hallman G Jr, and Mullins C: Groin flap coverage for an infant's exposed cardiac pacemaker in complete heart block. Ann Plast Surg 4:227, 1980.
7. Chari PS, and Suri RU: Skin cover for exposed cardiac pacemakers. Br J Plast Surg 30:231, 1977.
8. Baudet J: Axillary Flap, Microsurgical Composite Transfer. St. Louis, C. V. Mosby, 1979.
9. Azuma H, Kondo T, et al: Treatment of chronic osteomyelitis. Acta Orthoped Scand 47:271, 1976.

13

Pacemaker Follow-Up

RONALD PENNOCK, M.D., and
STUART SNYDER, M.D.

PACEMAKER FOLLOW-UP

Presently the number of implanted pacemakers is growing very rapidly and is already greater than 2,000,000. All pacemaker units contain electronic components: a source of energy and some form of wire system. The latter is incorporated in a catheter, which conducts bidirectionally the electrical stimulation and cardiac signals between the power pack and the heart itself.

The pacemaker batteries will eventually be exhausted, and the electronic components and circuits may suddenly or gradually fail. The electronic section of the pacemaker is subject to the same type of failure that any electronic system may develop. Furthermore, the catheter or wire system used to transmit the electric current and cardiac signals is subject to prolonged and rather strenuous forces and may mechanically fail. In addition there may be an unpredictable deterioration of the conductive wire's components. Even the most modern pacemaker systems sooner or later will undergo deterioration and failure in one or all of their components. The result of this failure in patients may range from the patient's total absence of any knowledge of the failure, to dizziness, syncope, or even sudden death in a patient who may be totally pacemaker-dependent.

Since most pacemaker patients have had some form of bradyarrhythmia, it is expected that with pacemaker failure this same bradyarrhythmia will emerge. Furthermore, with the lapse of time and the progression of the intrinsic heart disease that usually occurs, these same bradyarrhythmias may actually be worse when unmasked by failure of the pacemaker system.

It is obvious that all patients with pacemakers need some form of follow-up to predict any deterioration of the pacemaker function. Ideally, this deterioration should be observed before any symptoms or risks are encountered by the patient. If prediction is not possible in any patient who suddenly develops pacemaker failure, at least the follow-up system should allow the earliest possible detection of this type of failure while the patient is still asymptomatic. Various studies of patients who have had pacemakers show a change in the natural history of bradyarrhythmias that necessitate pacemaker implantation. Patients with Stokes-Adams disease due to heart block usually will have abolition of symptoms and prolongation of survival. Of course, many patients not only have severe conduction system disease but also have myocardial and coronary artery disease, and their survival, even after implantation of a permanent pacemaker, often is rather limited. In these cases, the causes of death seem to be related to tachyarrhythmias, congestive heart failure, or ischemic heart disease, none of which are affected by a permanent pacemaker.

In young adults who had a permanent pacemaker because of heart block with significant symptoms such as syncope or dizziness, all have shown marked improvement in symptoms, although some have died of causes unrelated to the pacemaker.

A study by Van Hemel and colleagues of patients who had pacemaker implantation because of sick sinus syndrome showed approximately a 50 percent survival rate after 5 years.[3] However, much of the mortality seemed related to chronic heart disease (which was partially the basis of the sick sinus syndrome), the advanced age of the patients, or their susceptibility to other degenerative diseases. These workers concluded that the pacemaker implantation did appear to influence the quality of life but not necessarily the length of life.

There are a number of modalities by which permanent pacemakers may be followed. Patients may frequent a doctor's office or a pacemaker clinic for EKG or electronic monitoring of the pacemaker. As the pacemakers age, the visits become as frequent as weekly. Some practitioners feel that this is a great overuse of outpatient facilities. For these reasons, systems for monitoring patients outside a doctor's office or clinic have been developed. The most successful of these systems has been transtelephonic pacemaker analysis. Some of the transtelephonic monitoring systems measure only the pacemaker spike. Pacemaker failure may be attributable to either battery or electronic catheter malfunctions. Thus it is necessary to monitor the cardiogram as well as the pacemaker spike. This has been done in many different countries and is often computerized. The overall cost has been variable but seems to add a relatively small amount to the cost of the pacemaker—perhaps $50.00 to $100.00. The various alternatives that have been mentioned, including frequent visits to an outpatient clinic or elective removal of the pacemaker at a stipulated time, seem to overuse medical facilities and underuse the pacemaker itself, since many units would be removed prematurely, before malfunction is detected.

Various characteristics of the pacemaker may be followed (Tables 13–1 to 13–3). Rate change seems to be a most significant parameter in pacemaker follow-up. Early after pacemaker implantation there may be small increases or decreases of pacemaker rate over several weeks. With normal pacemaker function this generally will plateau, and very little change in rate should occur. As the pacemaker battery fails, the interval between pacemaker spikes will increase and continue to increase in an exponential fashion. The ideal time for replacement is when there is a significant increase of the pacemaker spike interval. This is not emergent and allows the patient several weeks to plan for pacemaker replacement.

Table 13–1. Criteria Used by a Typical Telephone Monitoring Service, Cardiac Data Incorporated, to Report on Various Pacemaker Malfunctions

Pacer Function	Amount	Classification	Apply Magnet	Cover Sheet
Loss of capture (atrial or ventricular)	Causing symptoms or ventricular rate <50 BPM	Emergency	Yes	Yes
Loss of output or oversensing	Causing symptoms or ventricular rate <50 BPM	Emergency	Yes	Yes
Loss of capture or oversensing	Causing >3 BPM missed	Urgent	Yes	Yes
	Causing <3 BPM missed	Unusual	Yes	Yes
Loss of sensing or competition with a VOO pacer	Causing ventricular rate >100 BPM	Emergency	Yes (except VOO)	Yes
	Causing ≥5 BPM missed	Urgent	Yes (except VOO)	Yes
	Causing <5 BPM missed	Unusual	Yes (except VOO)	Yes
Rate increase or erratic rate changes	Exceeding pacer spec if available or ± 2 BPM from baseline or ± 5 BPM from normal	Urgent	Yes	Yes
Rate declines	Due to reprogramming	Urgent	Yes	Yes
	Possibly due to reprogramming	Urgent	Yes	Yes
	Exceeding spec sheet EOLI or 5 BPM for lithium or nuclear	Urgent	Yes	Yes
	15 msec per week or 25 msec per month for mercury/zinc	Urgent	Yes	Yes
	Exceeding ½ spec sheet EOLI or 2½ BPM for lithium or nuclear or 8 msec per week or 15 msec per month for mercury/zinc	Unusual. Use "pacer suspect" sticker.	Yes	Yes

Table 13–2. Criteria Used By a Typical Telephone Monitoring Service, Cardiac Data Incorporated, to Report on Symptoms with Normal Pacer Function

Symptoms	Classification	Apply Magnet	Cover Sheet	Comments
Suggesting cardiac involvement and present at time of call (≤ 1 hr prior to contacting CDI)	Emergency	No	Yes	
Suggesting cardiac involvement but not present at time of call (>1 hr prior to contacting CDI)	Urgent	Only if necessary to determine pacer function	Yes	Contact during business hours. Instruct patient to contact his physician immediately.
May or may not be of cardiac origin	Use supervisory judgment	Only if necessary to determine pacer function	Yes	If supervisor feels notification is warranted, use URGENT classification.
Definitely not cardiac symptoms	Unusual	Yes	No	Instruct patient to contact his physician. No phone notification necessary; send written notification.

If pacer function is abnormal, refer to pacer malfunction section.

Other characteristics of the pacemaker spike may be measured, including the shape of the pulse, amplitude, and impulse duration. However, none of these characteristics seems to be as specific a mark of pacemaker depletion as does the rate change. In addition to the characteristics of the pacemaker spike itself, the patient's EKG or pulse can be determined telephonically, and pacemaker sensing and capture function is determinable. Depending on which pacemaker battery the patient has, initial transtelephonic monitoring usually takes place weekly for about a month after pacemaker implantation. This frequency has been judged necessary to detect that frequently occurring early period of electrode failure. After the first month, monitoring is monthly for 30 months. After 30 months, weekly surveillance is recommended during the period when pacemaker battery failure becomes more likely. Most of these measurements are taken spontaneously, but occasionally the pacemaker may be detected in the magnetic mode. This technique is most valuable in patients who have demand pacemakers that are inhibited at the time of the telephone call.

Table 13–3. Criteria Used By a Typical Telephone Monitoring Service, Cardiac Data Incorporated, to Report on Arrhythmia with Normal Pacer Function

Arrhythmia	Frequency	Classification	Apply Magnet	Cover Sheet	Comments
Tachycardia (supraventricular)	13 beats in 6 sec (sustained and regular)	Emergency	No	Yes	Increase limit by 6 BPM for each battery year less than 12 yr old.
Ectopic ventricular beats (single focus random)	<10 per min	Normal	Yes	No	
	<15 but >10 per min	Unusual	No	No	Physician can be called if supervisor feels it is warranted.
	>15 per min	Urgent	No	Yes	Contact physician for first occurrence only. When calling physician, request instruction for magnet application. Also notify physician that we will no longer contact by phone for this arrhythmia. Send letter regarding discontinuation of telephone notification.
Multifocal, bigeminal, or trigeminal	<10 per min	Unusual	No	No	
	<15 but >10 per min	Unusual	No	Yes	Contact physician at supervisor's discretion.

	>15 per min	Urgent	No	Yes	Contact physician for first two occurrences. Request instruction for magnet application. Also notify physician that we will no longer notify by phone for this arrhythmia. Send letter regarding discontinuation of telephone notification.
Pairs or couplets	2 or more pairs per min	Urgent	No	Yes	Contact physician for first two occurrences as above.
	1 pair per min	Unusual	Yes	Yes	Phone notification unnecessary.
Tachycardia (ventricular)	≥3 PVCs in a row	Emergency	No	Yes	**Always notify physician of ventricular tachycardia.**
Supraventricular extra systoles	Any	Normal	Yes	Yes	
Atrial fibrillation or flutter with VVI, VOO, or AAI pacer	<150 BPM	Normal	Yes (except VOO)	No	
Atrial fibrillation or flutter with VVI, VOO, or AAI pacer	Average >150 BPM	Urgent	Yes	Yes	
Atrial fibrillation or flutter (with two-chamber pacer)	Any	Urgent	Yes	Yes	Contact physician for first occurrence only. If pacer has been programmed to single-chamber mode, follow instruction for single-chamber system.

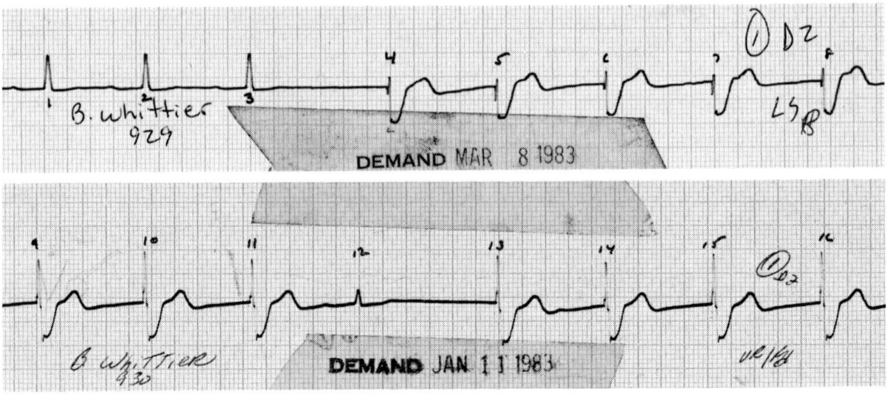

Figure 13–1. A VVI (R wave–inhibited) pacemaker. Complexes 1, 2, and 3 are the patient's own QRS. There is no pacemaker spike or pacemaker-induced QRS until beat 4. Twelve hundred milliseconds elapse between beat 3 and beat 4. However, between beats 4 and 5, both paced beats, there are only 930 milliseconds. Similarly, between beats 5, 6, 7, and 8, there are only 930 milliseconds. The reason for this is called hysteresis, a phenomenon that allows the patient's own rhythm to occur, i.e., beats 1, 2, and 3 occur without any pacemaker activity until an interval of 1200 milliseconds, in this case, elapses. Following this long interval, the pacemaker will start pacing at a quicker rate. Similarly, in the lower strip, pacing occurs at approximately 920 milliseconds between beats 9, 10, and 11. When beat 12 occurs sooner than a paced beat can, it inhibits the pacemaker. The QRS sensed by the pacemaker inhibits the firing cycle, and pacemaker activity is no longer seen until 1200 milliseconds elapse between beats 12 and 13, and the pacemaker resumes stimulating. Beats 14, 15, and 16 then occur at the previous pacing rate, that is, 930 milliseconds. This allows the patient's own rhythm, with its atrial "kick," to occur for as long a period as possible. Following hysteresis, pacing starts at a faster rate.

These methods of monitoring not only detect pacemaker malfunction more economically and conveniently than in the office, but actually can detect small drops in pacemaker rate that cannot be ascertained by an ordinary EKG. The newer types of batteries appear to be lasting longer than the older mercury/zinc cells, as shown by transtelephonic monitoring. The mercury/zinc batteries lasted an average of 30 months; lithium types are expected to last for 5 to 15 years. There have also been implantations of nuclear pacemakers, which seem to be expensive and encumbered by numerous regulatory problems. The chargeable systems seem to have a reasonably good life span but do not seem to have been well accepted by physicians or patients. About 20 percent of the lithium pacemakers malfunctioned within the first 5 years because of catheter failure, electrode migration, or failure of other components. Because of the many common causes of failures after 3 years of implantation, even lithium pacemakers should be monitored frequently.

In a study of 1,705 pacemakers by Mantini and colleagues, approximately 10 percent of the failures occurred within the first month of implantation and were usually the result of catheter migration or displacement, fractures, or problems with the wound or pacemaker pocket.[2] Of the total 340 malfunctions detected in these pacemaker systems, 41 percent appear to be caused by battery exhaustion (mercury/zinc units), and the rest to other causes. The results of this study show the necessity for early frequent pacemaker follow-up by monthly checks for approximately 24 to 30 months and then weekly checks until pacemaker failure. The causes of pacemaker failure were not only battery depletion but also some electronic failure in the pacemaker pack. The most common cause of lead failure is distraction or dislodgement of pacemaker catheters, usually in the right atrium or ventricle. In rare instances, the pacemaker electrode may puncture the interventricular septum and migrate into the left ventricle. In the latter instance, the pacemaker may continue to pace normally. Lead failure may be attributed to high threshold, which causes failure to capture or failure to sense. Pacemakers may undersense, but this may simply be functional.

Other studies have confirmed that various types of batteries actually may not be as similar as is thought. There are different types of lithium batteries with different anionic ions from different anionic sources, and they may have quite variable durations of longevity. In spite of the fact that battery survival has increased substantially with the advent of lithium pacemakers, one-third of the explants were still attributable to rate decline, with a small number removed because of loss of capture, failure to sense properly, fractured lead, erosion, or other less common causes.

There are extensive data in Philadelphia concerning almost 20,000 pacemaker implantations. Most of the older mercury/zinc-powered pacemakers began to fail within 36 to 48 months. Approximately one-half of the pacemakers failed in approximately 36 months. By 48 months, approximately 80 percent of these pacemaker battery sources failed. In contrast to these older batteries, the newer

Text continued on page 194

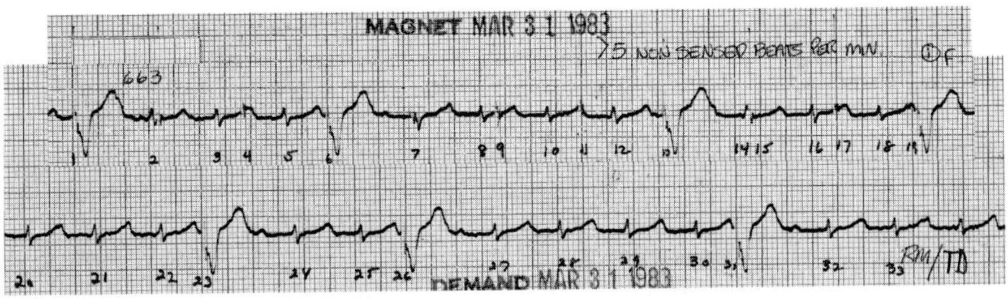

Figure 13–2. The function of a VVI (R wave–inhibited) pacemaker both in the magnet or induced rate mode *(upper strip)* as well as in the demand mode *(lower strip).* Beat 1 shows the pacemaker firing and capturing the ventricle. Beat 2 shows the pacemaker firing, but because the QRS has already occurred, the ventricle is refractory. Beat 3 is the patient's own intrinsic rhythm. Beat 4 shows the pacemaker firing without capturing the refractory ventricle. Beat 5 is the patient's own intrinsic rhythm. Beats 6, 13, and 19 show the ventricle being captured by the pacemaker. Pacemaker beats 7, 9, 11, 15, and 17 do not capture the refractory ventricle. The lower strip shows the patient's own intrinsic rhythm, beats 20, 21, and 22, but beat 23 is due to the pacemaker firing at a point at which it can capture the ventricle after the "T" wave. The pacemaker should not have fired at this point nor in beat 26 or 31, since the intrinsic rhythm is faster than the pacemaker rate. This demonstrates intermittent lack of sensing. The lack of sensing is intermittent in that it does not always occur. If it did occur without intermittency, it would appear the same as the magnetic mode in the top strip, where the magnet has turned off the sensing mode, and the pacemaker is operating as a fixed rate pacemaker. In the lower strip, the magnet has not been applied and, therefore, the pacemaker is firing inappropriately.

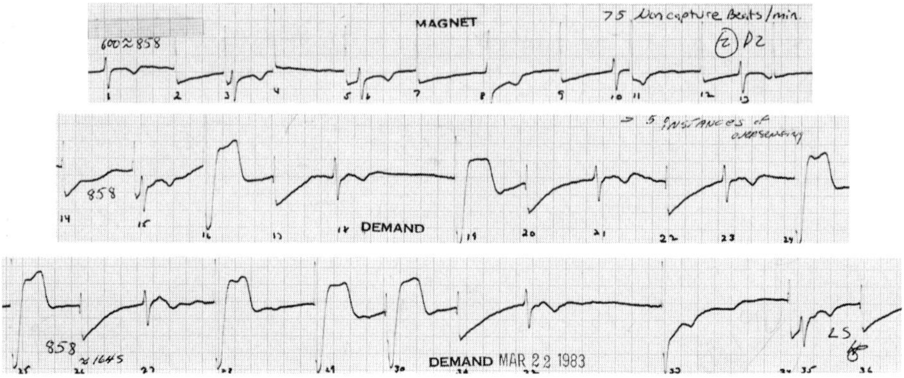

Figure 13–3. A VVI pacemaker at approximately 70 beats per minute. The top strip shows the magnet-induced rhythm. Beats 2, 3, 4, 5, 7, 8, 9, 11, and 12 are pacemaker spikes which do not capture the ventricle. This is made especially clear by beat 6, which is the patient's own intrinsic rhythm, and is able to capture the ventricle right after beat 5—the pacemaker spike. If the pacemaker spike had captured the ventricle, the patient's own beat 6 could not have occurred following such a short coupling interval. The middle strip continues to show lack of capture in beats 14 and 15. This is demonstrated in beat 15, with the patient's own rhythm able to occur right after the pacemaker-induced beat. Beat 16, however, shows capture as well, as do beats 19 and 24. There is also significant variability in the magnet and demand pacing rates, indicating battery failure. Because of the combination of irregular pacing rates and lack of capture, a battery problem with the pacemaker is indicated.

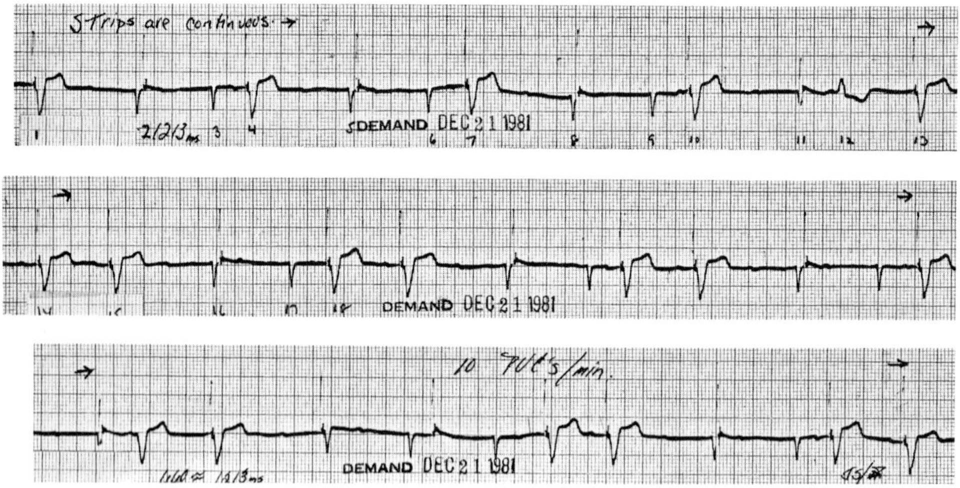

Figure 13–4. A VAT pacemaker. This is a two-catheter pacemaker with the sensing circuit in the atrium and the capturing circuit in the ventricle. Beat 1 shows the pacemaker firing to cause a QRS spike. In beat 2, the spike occurs but does not capture because the patient's own intrinsic rhythm has occurred. Similarly, beats 5, 8 and 11 also occur when the ventricle is refractory and do not cause depolarization. The pacemaker in the top strip is, therefore, actually firing in a fixed rate mode, although it is supposed to be sensing the atrium and, after a preset P-R interval, stimulating the ventricle, as is seen in beats 14 and 15, where the pacer-induced QRS follows the "P" wave. After beat 15, however, one can see a "P" wave but no pacemaker spike, and the pacemaker once again starts firing in the fixed rate mode, with approximately 1200 milliseconds between each beat as in the upper strip. This is an example of intermittent loss of atrial sensing. Capture is appropriate at all times when the ventricle is not refractory.

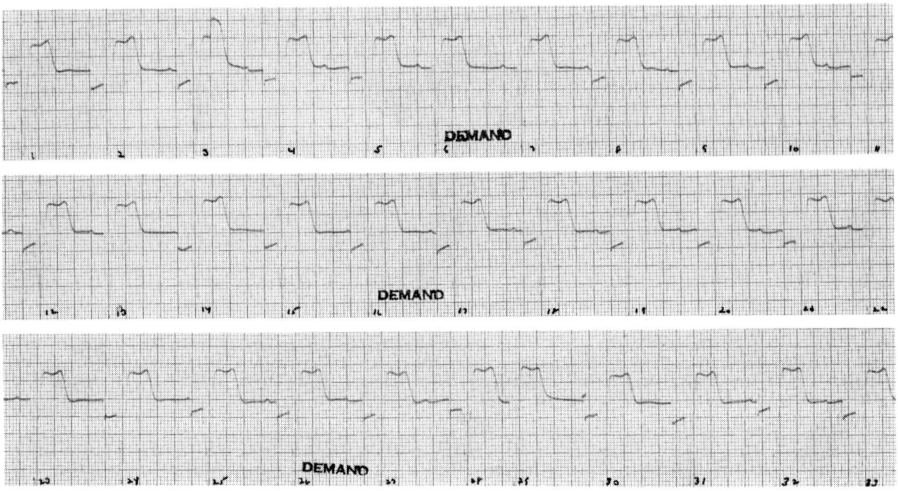

Figure 13–5. A DDD pacemaker. It can be seen on the top strip, especially in beats 3 to 5, that there is a pacemaker spike that occurs after the "P" wave. In this DDD pacemaker, the "P" wave should have been sensed and the atrial pacemaker spike no longer should have occurred as in beats 6 and 7, where the "P" wave is sensed. An appropriate ventricle spike occurs, which causes a QRS to occur. However, in beat 8 the "P" wave occurs, but is not sensed, and there is an atrial pacemaker spike which should not have occurred. Similarly, beats 9, 10, and 11 demonstrate lack of "P" wave sensing. Beat 13 in the middle strip shows "P" wave sensing with appropriate lack of pacemaker "P" wave spike, but with a spike causing a QRS. The end of the middle strip shows lack of "P" wave sensing until the 22nd and 23rd beat, which show sensing. The pacemaker stops atrial sensing again in beats 25, 26, 27, and 28. Beat 29 comes early, most likely because a "P" wave was sensed and caused premature depolarization of the ventricle at that time. This figure clearly demonstrates intermittent lack of atrial sensing in a DDD pacemaker.

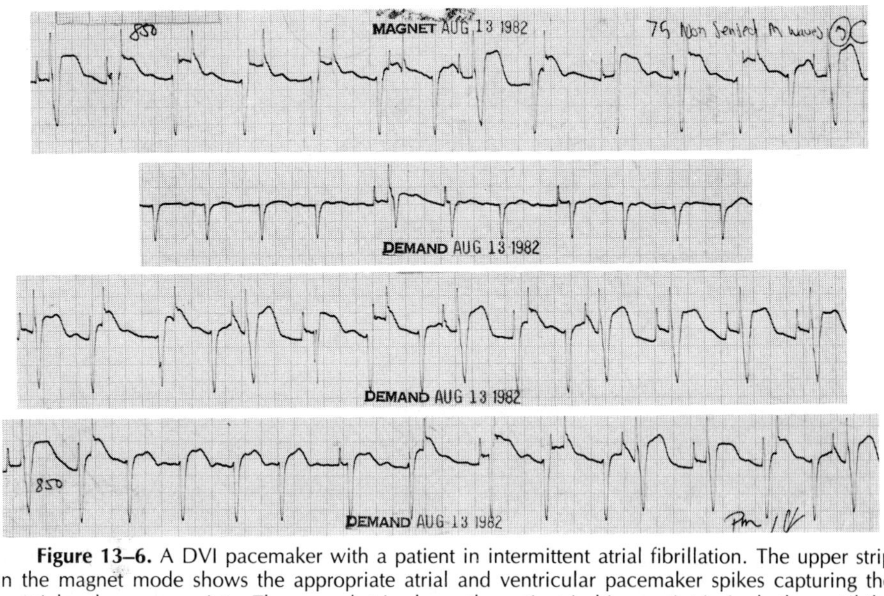

Figure 13–6. A DVI pacemaker with a patient in intermittent atrial fibrillation. The upper strip in the magnet mode shows the appropriate atrial and ventricular pacemaker spikes capturing the ventricle when appropriate. The second strip shows the patient in his own intrinsic rhythm until the 5th beat, which is appropriately paced with this pacemaker set in the demand rate of 70 per minute. The third and fourth strips, however, show the pacemaker to be firing, with loss of ventricular sensing at times. This, thus, demonstrates intermittent loss of ventricular sensing in a DVI pacemaker.

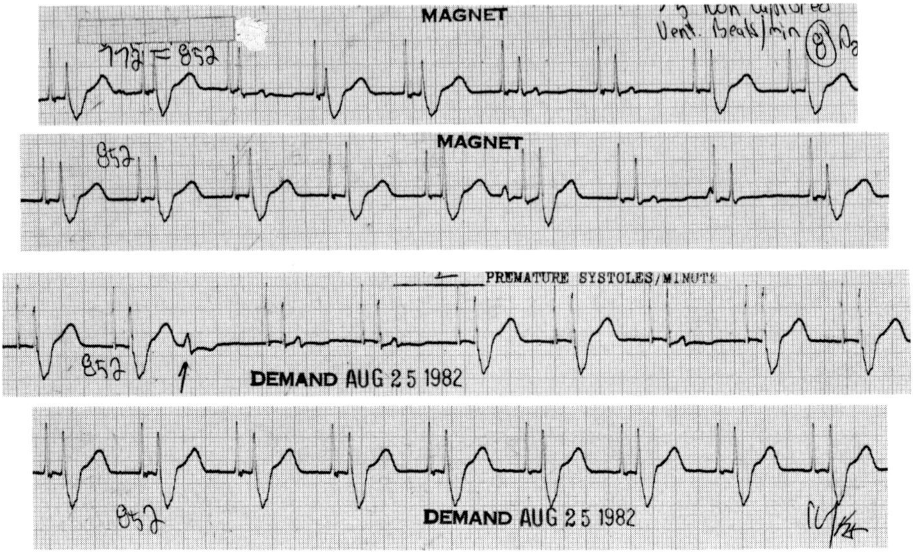

Figure 13–7. A DVI pacemaker which shows noncapture in the magnet as well as in the demand mode. In the lower strip, sensing appears appropriate, but when the pacemaker ventricular spike occurs, it only intermittently captures the ventricle.

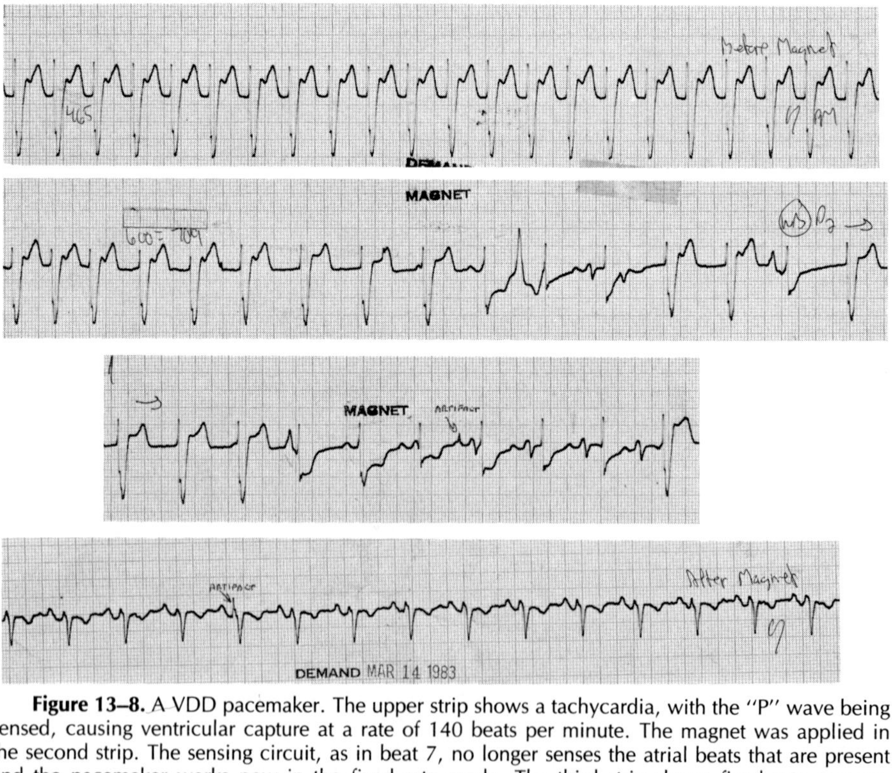

Figure 13–8. A VDD pacemaker. The upper strip shows a tachycardia, with the "P" wave being sensed, causing ventricular capture at a rate of 140 beats per minute. The magnet was applied in the second strip. The sensing circuit, as in beat 7, no longer senses the atrial beats that are present and the pacemaker works now in the fixed rate mode. The third strip shows fixed rate magnet-induced beats. In the fourth strip when the magnet is removed, sinus rhythm has been restored. This demonstrates pacemaker atrial tachycardia due to sensing of retrograde "P" waves.

CARDIAC DATACORP, INC.
CARDIAC MANAGEMENT SYSTEMS
1280 BLUE HILLS AVE., BLOOMFIELD, CT. 06002 (203) 243-2986

Patient Information/Please enroll this patient on your service. Date ____________

℞ First Name Middle Name Last Name

Mr. □ Mrs. □ Miss □ ____________

Address ____________ Soc. Sec. # ____________

City ____________ State ____________ Zip ____________ Date of Birth ____________

Home Phone ( ) ____________ Degree of pacer dependancy: Minimal ______ Moderate ______ Severe ______

Diagnosis (underlying rhythm): ____________

Physician Information

____________ Name of Prescribing Physician ____________ Signature of Prescribing Physician

Address ____________ Implanting Hospital Name: ____________

City ____________ State ____________ Zip ____________ Phone ( ) ____________

In case of a PACER EMERGENCY NOTIFY Dr. ____________ Phone ( ) ____________

In case of a NON-PACER PROBLEM NOTIFY Dr. ____________ Phone ( ) ____________

Send Additional Report to:
Physician ____________
Address ____________
City ____________ State ____________ Zip ____________
Primary Specialty ____________ Phone ( ) ____________

Pacemaker System Information

Pulse Generator Manufacturer ____________ Model # ____________ Serial # ____________

Lead Manufacturer ____________ Model # ____________

Chamber Paced (A, V or D) ____________ Chamber Sensed ____________ Action (Triggered, Inhibited, Other) ____________

Date of Implant ____________ Rate at Implant or Last Programmed Rate ____________

Location of Pacemaker ____________

Monitor in accordance with the following schedule (approved Medicare parameter):

New Implant	0 - 4 weeks - weekly	5 weeks to failure - every 4 weeks
Reimplant	0 - 2 weeks - weekly	3 weeks to failure - every 4 weeks

Special Instructions: ____________

CR 64 (R1/81)

Figure 13–9. The approved Medicare schedule for telephone follow-up of pacemaker patient should be weekly for the first month and then every four weeks to failure. If it is a re-implantation, follow-up is weekly for two weeks and then every four weeks to failure.

lithium, nickel/cadmium, or nuclear pacemakers all had relatively similar survivals, and approximately 50 percent of the lithium power sources were projected to survive about 8 years. Furthermore there was not a great deal of difference between the nuclear power source, the nickel/cadmium source, and the lithium power source.

Some of these more advanced power sources, though apparently somewhat similar, actually are greatly dissimilar. Various anionic compounds of lithium, including compounds of lead, silver, copper, and iodine, have rather different survival periods. In data collected by Cardiac Datacorp, covering almost 20,000 pacemakers with lithium anodes and almost 500,000 pacemaker months, there was a marked variation in pacemaker survival depending on the exact anionic source.

It therefore can be concluded that all pacemaker systems will eventually fail. Failure rate is high in the first months after implantation, often because of a mechanical problem. After this there seems to be approximately a 2-year period in which failure is relatively infrequent, eventually followed by a gradual increase in failure rate. Transtelephonic monitoring for pacemaker failure seems to be a most economical and expedient way of following pacemakers.

Figures 13–1 to 13–8 are examples of various types of pacemaker malfunction as detected by a typical monitoring service.

REFERENCES

1. Dreifus SL, Ohm OJ, and Pennock RS: Long-term monitoring of patients with implanted pacemakers. Heart and Lung 1:2, 227, 1972.
2. Mantini EL, Majors RK, Kennedy RK, and Lebo GR: A recommended protocol for pacemaker follow-up: Analysis of 1,705 implanted pacemakers. Ann Thorac Surg 324:62, 1977.
3. Van Hemel NM, Schaepkens van Riempast ALE, Bakema H, and Swenne CA: Long-term follow-up after pacemaker implantation in sick sinus syndrome. PACE 4:8, 1981.
4. Bilitch M, Hauser RG, Goldman S, Furman S, and Parsonnet V: Performance of cardiac pacemaker pulse generators. PACE 5:465, 1982.
5. Frank G, Tyers O, and Brownlee R: Power pulse generators, electrodes and longevity. Prog Cardiovasc Dis 23:421, 1981.
6. Parsonnet V, Myers G, and Manhardt M: A pacemaker follow-up clinic for analysis of detection of signs of impending pacemaker failure. *In* Sarnet P, and Elsherif N (eds): Cardiac Pacing. Second edition. New York, Grune & Stratton, 1980.
7. Furman S: Cardiac pacing and pacemakers. No. VIII—The pacemaker follow-up clinic. Am Heart J 94:795, 1977.
8. Shaw GB, Evans AL, Brewster GM, Groden BM, and Murdoch WR: Telephone monitoring of patients with pacemakers in the west of Scotland. Br Med J 283:127, 1981.
9. Hansen JS, and Grant ME: Comprehensive cardiac pacemaker information system: Basis for a regional follow-up network. PACE 1:327, 1978.
10. Besley DC, McWilliams J, Moodie DS, and Castle LW: Long-term follow-up of young adults following permanent pacemaker replacement for complete heart block. Am Heart J 103:332, 1982.

14

Cardiac Pacing: A Nursing Perspective

SUSAN J. FRYE, R.N., M.S.N., and
LINDA A. YACONE, R.N., B.S., CCRN

Cardiac pacing has been practiced for more than three decades, and technological strides offer a growing variety of techniques and new indications for its use. Common to all types of pacing is the patient's realization that an artificial device is assisting the heart. This knowledge may enrich the physical benefits of a pacemaker only if the patient is well informed and not hindered by the presence of the unit.

The nurse's goals and responsibilities in pacing are determined by the patient's physical dependence on the pacemaker, the physical or emotional distress related to it, and the potential for pacemaker malfunction or failure.

Nurses from several specialties may be required to participate in some phase of the patient's care. These personnel may be drawn from the emergency services, the operating room, the coronary and surgical intensive care units, and the cardiac catheterization laboratory. Basic nursing education in electrocardiography, electrophysiology, and pacing techniques and complications is necessary in all of these areas. It is ideal for the nurse who is primarily responsible for patient teaching to work closely with the cardiologist, surgeon, and other nurses to facilitate the patient's progress.

This chapter will focus on the nurse's responsibilities and considerations in temporary epicardial and transvenous endocardial pacing as well as permanent, transvenous endocardial pacing.

TEMPORARY EPICARDIAL PACING AFTER OPEN-HEART SURGERY

Temporary Epicardial Electrodes

Temporary epicardial electrodes provide access for diagnostic recording and therapeutic electrical stimulation of the myocardium in the postoperative cardiac patient. During open-heart surgery, pacing wires are attached to the right atrium and also the right ventricle, usually two electrodes on each chamber. The use of two wires is preferred over the use of a single wire, since two wires make bipolar pacing possible. Bipolar pacing is more resistant to interference by external electrical fields.[1] The wires either are made of stainless steel with a Teflon coating or are plastic-insulated. The Teflon-coated stainless steel wires are used more commonly. They are placed prior to sternal closure. After they are sutured onto the myocardium, they are brought out through the anterior upper abdominal wall.

Temporary epicardial wires are used to (1) record distinct atrial and ventricular electrograms to facilitate accurate diagnosis of arrhythmias in the postoperative cardiothoracic patient, (2) provide reliable temporary pacing for symptomatic bradyarrhythmias, and (3) provide overdrive pacing for termination of sustained atrial tachyarrhythmias, primarily flutter rather than fibrillation.

Arrhythmias that commonly occur in the postoperative cardiothoracic patient include sinus bradycardia, junctional rhythms, atrial arrhythmias, and heart block. Heart block is common after operative repairs of atrial septal defects, ventricular septal defects, and valvular replacements due to edema and suture placement.[2] In the presence of intact atrioventricular (AV) conduction, atrial pacing increases cardiac output since the atrial contraction is coordinated with ventricular filling and contraction.[2] Otherwise, temporary AV sequential pacing may be utilized.

Complications that may be encountered with the use of temporary epicardial pacing include dislodgement, infection (local and systemic), myocardial irritation producing arrhythmias, cardiac tamponade, and microshocks.

Microshocks may initiate ventricular fibrillation. They are caused by very small currents from environmental sources and pass through the heart via catheters and wires.[3] It is therefore imperative that the patient's environment be electrically isolated. The biomedical engineering department should inspect the patient's bed area and perform safety checks on a routine basis. The same safety precautions used for temporary transvenous cardiac pacing should be employed.

Nursing care of the patient with temporary epicardial pacing wires should include daily cleansing utilizing sterile technique. Iodine or 70% isopropyl alcohol can be used. The area around the wire insertion should be cleaned and an antibiotic ointment applied. The insertion site should then be covered with a gauze pad and taped securely. Nonallergic tape is preferred for taping, to minimize skin irritation. After inspection of the site for signs of infection or irritation, the findings should be recorded in the progress notes.

If the wires are not to be connected to an external pulse generator, coil them loosely, wrap them in a gauze pad, and tape them to the dressing. The ends of the wires must be kept visible so that rapid access may be achieved if necessary.

The atrial and ventricular wires must be identified. The atrial wires are usually shorter and are on the patient's right side. The ventricular wires are usually longer and are on the patient's left side. Rubber gloves should be worn whenever handling the exposed wires.

Dysrhythmias are common in the postoperative cardiothoracic patient and occasionally can only be correctly diagnosed by atrial electrograms. Atrial electrograms show the relationship of the activation sequence between the atrium and the ventricle. In order to perform an atrial or ventricular electrogram, a portable 12-lead EKG machine should be used. Use of a portable machine allows for better amplification of the recording and will provide a hard-copy recording. The patient should never be disconnected from his bedside monitor. The portable unit must be properly maintained for safe use in patients with indwelling cardiac catheters.[2] Attach the ends of an insulated alligator clamp to the metal end of the atrial wires. The opposite end of the alligator clamp should be attached to the chest lead of the EKG machine. Record the strip in the V-lead mode. When two atrial wires are present, the electrode that offers a better electrogram should be used. The electrogram recordings should be taken initially after the surgical procedure to provide a baseline. They may then be repeated whenever necessary.

Temporary epicardial electrodes are removed when the time for frequent arrhythmias has passed, usually 5 days after surgical intervention. After removal, the patient's blood pressure and heart rate should be checked every 15 minutes for 1 hour and then at least every hour for 4 hours. Observe closely for signs of hemorrhage, hemopericardium, and cardiac tamponade. These include hypotension, distended neck veins, an elevated central venous pressure, distant heart sounds, and the presence of pulsus paradoxus. Examine the wires to make sure they are intact. An elastic bandage may be applied to the site.

TEMPORARY TRANSVENOUS PACING

Temporary transvenous cardiac pacing is a medical modality with potentially lifesaving benefits. Today's nurse plays an important role in the use of this technique. Through patient and family education, she can make this experience an extremely positive one. By her understanding, she can provide a safe, therapeutic environment, thereby preventing potential complications.

Indications for temporary cardiac pacing may be either prophylactic or therapeutic (Table 14–1).

Bradyarrhythmias are the most common indication for temporary cardiac pacing.[4] Bradyarrhythmias and bifascicular or actual heart block may complicate the course of an acute myocardial infarction. Temporary transvenous pacing can be lifesaving in these situations. Temporary cardiac pacing may be used for termination or overdrive suppression of tachyarrhythmias.

The insertion of a temporary pacemaker usually is an urgent or semi-emergency situation. There is often little time for preparation. The nurse must be familiar enough with the procedure so that she may prepare the patient quickly and safely.

Table 14–1. Indications for Temporary Cardiac Pacing

Therapeutic
Bradyarrhythmias if the patient is hemodynamically compromised
Second- or third-degree heart block
Termination of supraventricular tachycardias
Termination or overdrive suppression of ventricular tachycardias
Prior to permanent pacemaker implantation
Prophylactic
During cardiac catheterization for protection against potential bradyarrhythmias
After open-heart surgery for use in diagnosis of arrhythmias and protection against potential heart block
During an acute myocardial infarction when bifascicular block is present

Preparation

Explanations to the patient and family depend on the clinical situation. If time permits, the nurse may review the procedure with the patient and family. Demonstration of actual temporary pacemaker generators and catheters may facilitate comprehension. The benefits of temporary pacing as it pertains to the individual patient should be reinforced. In addition to providing reassurance, the nurse should describe subsequent nursing management, including movement restrictions and safety precautions. Emphasis should be placed on the temporary nature of the device. The decision for permanent pacing can be discussed after a few days of observation. Witnessed, informed written consent is necessary prior to insertion of a temporary pacemaker. If the patient is compromised by the clinical situation, the family will be required to give consent.

The patient should have a functioning intravenous line other than the antecubital, femoral, jugular, or subclavian veins as they may be necessary for pacemaker insertion. The site selected for temporary pacemaker insertion should be shaved and prepped. Preoperative sedation is rarely required. If sedation is needed during the procedure, a low dose (2 to 4 mg) of intravenous diazepam may be administered.

In addition to a routine preoperative check list, pertinent laboratory data must be assessed prior to the procedure. This should routinely include coagulation screening (prothrombin time, partial thromboplastin time, and platelet estimates) and determinations of electrolytes and hemoglobin or hematocrit. Any abnormalities should be reported to the physician. A 12-lead EKG should be posted on the patient's chart. If a rhythm strip documenting the arrhythmia is available, it should also be included to clarify the indication for the pacemaker.

Insertion

Insertion of a temporary pacemaker should be performed under fluoroscopy, if at all possible. This may occur at the bedside (with portable fluoroscopy), in a special procedures room, or in the cardiac catheterization or electrophysiology laboratory.

Since the critical care nurse may be called on to assist with the insertion, she should be familiar with the procedure and necessary equipment.

Sterile gowns and drapes must be used. An emergency cart equipped with drugs and resuscitation equipment should be at the bedside. Continuous EKG monitoring must be employed during the procedure.

Equipment

A temporary pacemaker insertion tray is a convenient way to ensure that all necessary instruments are sterile and readily accessible. It should include the following items:

scalpel and blade (#15)
syringes, 10 ml (2)
21-gauge needle ⅝″
25-gauge needle 1½″
4 × 4 gauze pads (10)
curved mosquito hemostats (2)
straight mosquito hemostats (2)
sterile basin
sterile medicine cups (2)
towel clips (4)
eye forceps (1)
plain forceps, fine (1)
toothed forceps, fine (1)
towels (4)
needle holder (1)

The following items should also be available:

local anesthetic agent
introducer #7F
2″ needle with obturator (i.e., Potts-Cournand needle)
sterile gloves
heparinized saline (1 unit heparin to 1 ml saline ratio)
iodine antiseptic solution
1-ml syringe (if balloon-tipped catheter used)
electrode catheter #6F
external pulse generator
arm board
gauze wrap
3–0 silk or 4–0 Prolene suture on a straight needle
antibiotic/germicidal ointment
transparent surgical dressing (e.g., Op-Site)
nonallergic tape

There are two types of temporary pacemaker electrode catheters available:

1. Woven Dacron catheters: These are firm catheters with platinum or stainless steel electrodes. Because of their stability, they are preferred for routine use.

2. Flexible or balloon-tipped catheters: This single-lumen balloon-tipped catheter is used to provide a rapid means of ventricular pacing only in a crisis situation. It is not intended to be inserted under fluoroscopy. It is used for immediate emergency support of the patient until a more stable means of pacing can be instituted.

Bipolar (two-electrode) catheters are preferred over the use of unipolar (one-electrode) catheters. Most standard catheters are bipolar. However, there is a new unipolar catheter available that makes DDD pacing possible. When the bipolar catheter is used a skin electrode is not required. The two electrodes provide better contact with the myocardium.[5] The unipolar catheter is more sensitive to extraneous stimuli and intercostal myopotentials, which may interfere with pacemaker functioning.[1] The bipolar catheter may be converted into a unipolar mode if necessary. New catheter designs provide multielectrodes with various interelectrode distances from which AV sequential pacing may be performed.

The external pulse generator is a small portable unit powered by either a 9-volt alkaline battery or a lithium battery. It is insulated and is available as a single-channel (for use in the atrium or ventricle) or dual-channel (AV sequential) model.

The essential functions of each external generator are similar, with only slight variations between manufacturers. Most pulse generators include the following features:

1. On/off mechanism: This may be a dial or a switch. It must have a safety lock feature in order to safeguard against accidental discontinuation or initiation of pacing activity.

2. Indicators: Each portable unit has an indicator light or needle. It indicates that the temporary unit has generated a pacing stimulus. There may be an indicator for both pacing and sensing. In an AV sequential pulse generator, the sensing indicator is for the ventricle. This will coincide with R-wave sensing.

3. Stimulus output or ma dial: This adjusts the pulse amplitude present in the output terminals. Its range is from 0.1 to 20.0 ma. This pacing output should be set at five times the minimum intensity pacing stimulus that is needed to produce adequate capture of the heartbeat.

4. Sensitivity dial: This adjusts the pacemaker to sense the patient's own electrical signal. It is recorded in millivolts. Its range is from 1.0 to 20.0 mv. If it is set to the highest sensitivity (beyond 20 mv) it will operate in the asynchronous or fixed mode; otherwise, it operates as a demand pacemaker, with the sensitivity decreasing as the millivolts are increased beyond 1.0.

5. Rate control or stimulus frequency control: This determines the rate of the pacemaker, which ranges from 30 to 150 or 180 beats per minute. It may be used for atrial, ventricular, or dual-chamber pacing, depending on the generator model.

6. AV interval control: This adjustment is present on the dual-chamber models. It adjusts the interval between the atrial stimulus and the subsequent ventricular stimulus to insure proper AV synchrony.[6] Its range is between 0 and 300 msec.

Procedure

The temporary pacemaker is inserted under local anesthesia percutaneously or by venous cutdown. The percutaneous method is more commonly used. In order of relative safety of insertion, the veins that may be used include the antecubital, the femoral, the jugular, and the subclavian.

If atrial pacing is desired the catheter may be positioned high in the right atrium or in the coronary sinus. Ventricular pacing is performed with the pacing catheter placed in the right ventricular apex.

The specified parameters should be listed in the nurse's note. These should include the pacing mode, the rate, and the milliamperes.

In the immediate postoperative period, the insertion site should be observed for hematoma, swelling, and drainage. EKG monitoring should continue. Obtain a 12-lead EKG to document function and position. The vital signs should be checked more frequently for the first few postoperative hours. Obtain a portable chest x-ray to document catheter position and rule out the possibility of pulmonary complications. Complications of temporary pacing that must be considered include thrombophlebitis, myocardial perforation, cardiac tamponade, pneumothorax, hemothorax, catheter-induced arrhythmias, infection (local and systemic), pulmonary embolization, and local hematoma.

Continue to offer reassurance to both the patient and family. Mild analgesics may be given if the patient complains of discomfort.

The temporary pacemaker site should be inspected, cleaned, and dressed daily. Sterile technique should be used. Observe the site for the presence of any signs of infection and inflammation (redness, swelling, discharge, or local heat). Clean the site with an antiseptic solution and apply an antibiotic/germicidal ointment. Your initials, the date, and the time of the dressing change should be written on the outside of the dressing if possible. Document your observations in the nurse's note. The dry dressing may be composed of either sterile gauze pads or a clear adhesive material (e.g., Op-Site). It is imperative that the temporary wire not be pulled out or maneuvered during the dressing change. The catheter should be sutured in place after insertion, to prevent dislodgement.

In order to prevent catheter movement, the external pulse generator must be stabilized. This will require restriction of the patient's movement appropriate to the insertion site. The generator should be secured to either the forearm or the thigh. Pad the limb with surgical gauze pads and then place the pacemaker generator on the padding. Make sure there are no creases or wrinkles in the padding to cause skin irritation. The faceplate of the pacemaker box must be exposed for viewing and easy adjustment of the settings. The dials themselves may be covered with transparent tape in order to prevent accidental manipulation. The generator itself may be equipped with a plastic shield and strap supports; if it is not, gauze wrap may be used to secure the generator by threading it through strap holders (if present) or encircling it at its end. An arm band may be used for extra support when the antecubital approach is used. If the femoral route is used, extra care must be exercised to avoid extreme hip flexion. By limiting the patient's mobility, the risk of catheter dislodgement is decreased.[7] We do not recommend mobilization to a chair for patients with femoral catheters.

When pacemaker cables are used, ensure that the external pulse generator is secured to some fixed position in the patient's bed. If the patient is uncooperative or confused, light restraints are indicated, as pulling on the catheter or manipulating the dial may cause serious consequences.

The pacing parameters should be checked at the beginning of each shift. The pacing threshold and sensitivity should be determined daily by the physician. If any changes are noted, be sure to record them in the patient's chart and on the nursing care plan.

Daily chest x-rays and EKGs are recommended. Compare the EKG to the postinsertion tracing to check for signs of pacemaker malfunction. Pacing of the right ventricle produces a complete left bundle branch block pattern on the EKG.[8]

Malfunctions

Some of the problems encountered with the use of temporary transvenous cardiac pacing are described in Table 14–2. Elimination of potential electrical hazards is a primary nursing responsibility. The temporary pacemaker catheter creates a direct low-resistance pathway to the myocardium. Leakage of alternating current that comes in contact with the catheter can induce ventricular fibrillation. Precautionary measures to be considered include the following:

1. All line-powered equipment in the patient's environment should be properly grounded. Each piece of equipment should have a three-wire power cord and a three-wire power plug.[3] This grounding carries the leakage current away from the equipment and the patient. Do not have any physical contact with the patient while operating any electrical devices.

2. If the patient is lying on an electrically operated bed, keep it disconnected. It should be plugged in only to effect the necessary positional change.

3. Use only battery-powered external pulse generators.

4. If you must handle the exposed pacing wire terminals, wear rubber gloves. If they are not to be connected to an external pulse generator, wrap them in a rubber glove. Today's external pulse generators have insulated terminals for better electrical safety.

5. Avoid the use of extraneous electrical devices and equipment in the patient's environment (e.g., electric shavers, televisions, portable radios, diathermy, and electrocautery).

Table 14–2. Problems Associated with Temporary Transvenous Pacing

Problem	Cause	Intervention
Failure to sense or inappropriate sensing	Low battery voltage	Change battery
	Ineffective sensing setting or T-wave sensing	Adjust sensitivity control
	Inadequate catheter position	Confirm with chest x-ray and reposition catheter
	Fractured lead	Confirm with chest x-ray and replace catheter
	Pacemaker generator failure	Test against alternate generator and replace if necessary
	Extraneous electrical activity	Inspect electrical environment for leakage and inappropriate equipment use
Failure to capture (intermittent or continuous)	Fractured lead	Confirm with chest x-ray and replace catheter
	Generator failure	Test against alternate generator and replace if necessary
	Poor connections between generator, catheter, and/or lead cables	Inspect all connection sites for appropriate fit and insertion
	Inadequate catheter position	Confirm with chest x-ray and reposition catheter
	Low battery voltage	Change battery
	Myocardial perforation	Confirm with chest x-ray and reposition; observe for signs of cardiac tamponade
Alteration in pacemaker artifact		
Increase in bipolar pacemaker artifact (Note: Bipolar artifact is ⅛ to ½ the size of the QRS. Unipolar artifact is larger.)[9]	Defective pacemaker output circuit	Change external generator
Decrease in pacemaker artifact	Decline in pacemaker output	Change external generator
Absence of pacemaker artifact on ECG	Fractured lead	Confirm with chest x-ray and replace lead
Stimulation of the diaphragm or phrenic nerve	Catheter improperly positioned (with or without myocardial perforation)	Confirm position with chest x-ray and reposition
Failure of the indicators to move (flash or jump)	Low battery voltage	Replace battery
Catheter-induced dysrhythmias	Catheter in improper position, which produces myocardial irritation	Reposition catheter (Note: All catheter repositionings must be performed under fluoroscopy)

6. Protect the generator from wetness. Be especially careful when bathing the patient and removing a bedpan or urinal.

7. If defibrillation is necessary, turn the temporary pacemaker off. Disconnect it if time permits, even though most units can withstand an electrical shock as great as 400 watts/second.[5] After defibrillation, the pacemaker should be inspected by responsible personnel, usually the biomedical engineering department. They should verify proper functioning of the unit.

Before a temporary pacemaker generator is reused on a new patient it should be properly cleaned and sterilized. Gross contamination may be removed with water or alcohol. It may then be gas sterilized (ethylene oxide). An external pulse generator should never be immersed for cleaning purposes.

A supply of fresh batteries and extra external pulse generators should be available. Each time a temporary pacemaker is used a new battery should be inserted. It is best to perform the battery change when the generator is not being used.

A temporary pacemaker should be removed under fluoroscopy. The rate should be decreased gradually, since abrupt cessation may result in periods of asystole.[6] Once the catheter has been removed, inspect the site for bleeding, discharge, and hematoma.

PERMANENT TRANSVENOUS ENDOCARDIAL PACING

New indications for pacing, a greater variety of pacer units, and a growing patient population over 65 years of age have resulted in an increasing number of people living with pacemakers. Transvenous endocardial implantation of permanent pacemakers with local anesthesia has largely replaced transthoracic placement and is now performed in most hospitals.[10] Myocardial implantation via limited thoracotomy is the approach used in 10 to 15 percent of the procedures.[1] This small percentage includes those patients who have had repeated failure with the transvenous method and those for whom open-heart surgery was already planned. It is also a frequently preferred route in infants and children.

Preoperative Management

Once the decision for implantation has been made, the cardiologist and surgeon will discuss with the family the indications for and benefits of a pacemaker and will explain the risks and obtain consent. After the physician has informed the nurse of the type of unit chosen and implantation time, the nurse reviews this information with the family. Teaching aids such as pictures, diagrams, or models may augment preoperative instruction, but they are overwhelming to some people. The patient's age, intelligence, and prognosis should be considered, and the teaching should be tailored to the individual's needs and ability to understand. Consider also that people vary in what they need and want to know.

In explaining the basics of pacing, it is important to stress the positive aspects but also to allow the patient to understand what pacing cannot do for the heart. The impact of this information may not be felt until sometime after the procedure and should be reinforced later. Other points that may help and comfort the patient are summarized below:

1. If a temporary pacemaker was previously used, explain how a permanent one differs.
2. Fasting and the insertion of an IV preoperatively are indicated for precautionary reasons.
3. Preoperative sedation is helpful and often necessary.
4. Inform the patient of the time and length of the procedure (½ to 3 hours).
5. Explain to the patient where the operation will be performed and who will participate.
6. Local anesthesia is used; the patient will not be unconscious and should be encouraged to tell the staff if there is any discomfort.
7. There will be some postoperative pain and stiffness, for which the patient can receive medication.
8. Describe the size of the unit and where it will be placed. Emphasize that this is not open-heart surgery: A lead is placed through a vein and guided with fluoroscopy into the heart; a small incision is made in the chest, where the generator will be placed in a pocket under the skin.
9. Internal sutures are used, and a dressing is worn for a few days. The scar will usually be small and faint.
10. Describe the early postoperative activity and limitations.
11. The length of the hospital stay is usually 3 to 5 days if there are no complications.
12. Tell the patient what will be reviewed before discharge: precautions, exercise, medications, implications for work, and clinical follow-up.

Generally the pacemaker is placed on the nondominant side, but a job requirement, hobby, or old orthopedic injury may preclude use of that side. This information should be communicated to the physician. Although the majority of patients can return to their work, the physician should be made aware of an occupation that involves the use of heavy equipment or exposure to electromagnetic fields, as these factors may influence the type of unit chosen. Interstate truck drivers and airline pilots usually are not permitted to return to their work with a pacemaker.[1] Obviously, permanent pacing in such patients may have serious impact.

The patient fasts for 6 to 8 hours preoperatively. Anticoagulation is stopped prior to implantation (4 to 6 days for warfarin and 6 hours for heparin), and the first dose of prophylactic antibiotic is given just before the procedure. Initial skin preparation is helpful before sending the patient to the operating facility; it is then completed in the laboratory. The chest and axilla are shaved to the posterior axillary line (laterally), medial to the opposite sternal border (medially), over the clavicle (superiorly), and below the nipple (inferiorly). Laboratory values should be obtained the day of the procedure, and the results should be placed in the chart. These determinations should include hemoglobin and hematocrit, prothrombin time, partial thromboplastin time, serum potassium, and platelet count. An EKG rhythm strip documenting the sinus node dysfunction, arrhythmia, or any variant of heart rhythm is placed on the chart. Any associated symptoms are also described in the preoperative note. If there is a primary rhythm disturbance that is not the indication for pacing, this must be noted. For example, a patient may have a history of chronic tachyarrhythmia that is being treated with a drug that has caused a bradycardia—which is the indication for the pacemaker. Or a patient may be considered for a dual-chamber pacemaker and have a history of atrial fibrillation or flutter, conditions in which dual-chamber pacing is contraindicated.

The Pacemaker Laboratory

Unless there is a special facility, transvenous pacemakers are generally implanted in the operating room, the cardiac catheterization laboratory, or the electrophysiology laboratory. These facilities are already equipped for cardiac emergencies and have fluoroscopy, image intensifiers, and television viewers. When the laboratory is used it should also be equipped with a thoracostomy tray and drainage system for complications of pneumothorax, hemothorax, and hemopneumothorax. Instruments that are used during the procedure are listed in Tables 14–3 and 14–4. The laboratory must meet the infection control specifications of an operating area, including gowning and hand-washing techniques.

All of the pacemaker company manuals offer guidelines for the sterilization and handling of the units, and the Inter-Society Commission for Heart Disease Resources (ICHD) offers additional guidelines for the operation of a pacemaker facility.[11] The technician or biomedical engineer is responsible for equipment maintenance and prevention of electrical hazards.

Table 14–3. Additions to an Equipped Cardiac Catheterization Laboratory

Pacemaker		
Leads		
Pacemaker accessory kit (supplied by manufacturers for specific pacemaker model)		
Programmers		
Stylet kit:	0.016-in diameter, 58 cm 0.014-in diameter, 58 cm	(lengths may vary)
Introducer systems		
Magnet		
Pacemaker Systems Analyzer (PSA)		

Table 14–4. Pacemaker Tray Equipment

2 #3 knife handles	1 Weitlander retractor
1 #7 knife handle	2 Beckman retractors
2 small Russian forceps 6″	1 DeBakey forceps
2 Hudson Adsons forceps	1 Cyd Mayo scissor
2 medium Potts forceps	2 sponge sticks
1 curved Mayo scissor suture 6¾″	2 silin hooks (single)
1 gold-handled Metzenbaum curved scissor	2 sarot needle holders
1 fine-tip Metzenbaum scissor 7″	6 towel clips 5½″
4 curved mosquito hemostats	2 prep cups
4 straight mosquito hemostats	1 tray
2 fine right-angle hemostats	1 prep basin
1 Army-Navy retractor	1 small eye basin

Final skin preparation is completed in the laboratory or operating room. Because the face is mostly covered with sterile drapes, it is advisable to give low-flow oxygen during the procedure. Diazepam may be given intravenously in small (2 to 4 mg) divided doses, but narcotics should be avoided. During the implant either the nurse or the technician monitors and reassures the patient while the other assists in the procedure. Complaints of sudden chest or shoulder pain or shortness of breath are suggestive of pneumothorax. This type of pain must be differentiated from angina. During the procedure someone must watch the monitor at all times. After suturing, the wound is covered with a sterile, occlusive dressing. Incisions that have been reopened for battery or lead replacement or repositioning often develop friable skin edges, and butterfly sutures on the wound surface may be beneficial. At this time pacemaker parameters are rechecked, and a 12-lead EKG (perhaps with a magnet) is taken. Accurate record keeping is essential for later reference to a patient registry. After the procedure the laboratory record is placed in the patient's chart, and a copy is kept in the clinic file. An example of a pacemaker record is given in Table 14–5. Most programmers have a computerized printout sheet, and it is helpful to place the list of parameters in the patient's chart. The programmed mode described is the ICHD letter code (e.g., VVI or DDD): chamber paced, chamber sensed, and mode of response;[12] fourth and fifth letters to indicate degree of programmability and tachyarrhythmia functions have recently been added.[13]

Postoperative Phase

The goals of postoperative management are (1) a properly functioning pacemaker with maintenance of cardiac output and hemodynamic stability, (2) physical rehabilitation and a healed wound free of infection, and (3) a well-informed patient who understands the signs of pacemaker malfunction and what to do if a problem occurs. Complications following transvenous lead installation that occur early tend to result from lead displacement,[1, 10] increased endocardial stimulation threshold,[1] and problems associated with the lead and generator. These can cause pacemaker failure to capture and sense and can contribute to the development of arrhythmias.

Table 14–5. Sample Pacemaker Laboratory Record

Date of implant:	Biographical data:
Allergies:	
Insurance:	
Side of implant:	
Fluoroscopy time:	
Physician:	
Pacemaker implantations:	Reposition of lead:
Battery change:	Pacemaker removal:
Pertinent history:	
Medications:	
Indication for pacemaker:	
Laboratory values:	
Company:	Pulse generator model number:
Hysteresis mode:	Serial number:
Pacing threshold:	Battery type:
Pulse widths:	Electrode model number:
Generator output:	Serial number:
AV interval:	Model number:
R-wave amplitude:	Serial number:
Mode and rate:	

Time	Rate	Rhythm	BP	Medication

Pacer rhythm strip

The lead may migrate from the right ventricular apex to the right atrium, vena cava, pulmonary artery, coronary sinus, or another region of the right ventricle, resulting in loss of capture. Less common but very serious complications include perforation of the interventricular septum with movement of the catheter into the left ventricle, or myocardial perforation with cardiac tamponade. It is important to listen for a friction rub in the event of a hemopericardium. An echocardiogram may be ordered to detect a pericardial effusion. Loss of capture is also caused by increases in stimulation threshold from metabolic changes (hypocalcemia or hypokalemia) and some antiarrhythmic agents (lidocaine, quinidine, and procainamide).[1] Failure of the sensing function is evidenced by undersensing or oversensing and is caused by malfunction or malposition of the lead-generator system. Extraneous sources such as skeletal muscle stimulation or electromagnetic interference can cause the pacemaker to oversense. Undersensing can be extremely dangerous if the pacemaker begins firing randomly—that is, not sensing the QRS complexes, which may result in atrial or ventricular tachyarrhythmias.

The development of ventricular premature depolarizations or an increase in the frequency of ectopy may suggest lead movement and the need for repositioning.

Upon return to the intensive care unit, the patient is monitored for 24 to 72 hours, especially if there is a prior history of arrhythmias or if the patient is pacer dependent. EKGs are obtained daily. Posteroanterior and lateral chest x-rays are taken 24 hours postoperatively to document lead position and for later reference.

In observing the patient and analyzing the rhythm strip, the following points should be considered:

Clinical assessment

1. Blood pressure
2. Peripheral pulse
3. Comparison of apical rate to radial pulse rate
4. Auscultation for friction rub; questioning the patient concerning palpitations, chest pain, shortness of breath, dizziness, light-headedness, discomfort with pacing (thumping, diaphragmatic pacing, and hiccups)

Identifying the features of paced rhythm

1. Is the pacemaker atrial, ventricular, or both, and what is the mode (e.g., DDD, DVI)?
2. What does the pacing stimulus artifact look like?
3. Differentiate between the stimulus artifact and the QRS.
4. Differentiate a paced P and QRS from spontaneous beats.
5. Know the AV interval.
6. Know what bundle or axis morphology is expected. (Right ventricular pacing produces a left bundle branch block morphology. Right bundle branch block pattern during pacing implies movement of the lead into the coronary sinus or left ventricle.)
7. Know the determined rate; compare this to the patient's apical rate and rapid pulse. Rate increases or decreases greater than 10/minute from the programmed rate should be reported.

Analyzing the paced rhythm

1. Note complete, incomplete, or loss of capture.
2. Note changes in sensing.
3. Observe for competitive rhythms.
4. Identify ectopic beats and note their effect on pacer activity.
5. Note increases or decreases in the amplitude of the spike and QRS.
6. Observe for arrhythmias.
7. Observe for changes in axis due to fusion or ectopic beats or patient movement.

Pacemaker sites are generally closed with absorbable sutures, and the wound is cleaned and occlusively dressed with sterile technique for 2 or 3 days. Surgical drains are not routinely indicated, as collected blood and fluid in the pocket are slowly absorbed. Drains also serve as a portal for bacterial entry. In the early postoperative period the wound should be inspected for bleeding and a developing seroma or hematoma. These usually subside spontaneously but very rarely may necessitate needle aspiration or reopening of the site. Although unlikely, body rejection phenomena and infection can occur as a result of several predisposing factors. The reported incidence of infection in permanent pacemakers varies from 0 to 15 percent and averages approximately 4 percent.[14] Predisposing patient factors contributing to infection include advanced age, debilitation and poor nutrition, immunity-compromising diseases or drugs, and an existing focus of infection elsewhere in the body. The erosion of the generator or lead through the skin, hematoma formation, and acute reopening for reposition or replacement of the generator or lead all potentially contribute to infection. Infections of the generator pocket tend to occur within the first month after implantation, whereas those associated with the electrode tend to occur later.[14] In one study of 46 infected patients, 17 percent of the infections were early onset (less than 2 weeks), 37 percent were intermediate (onset between 2 weeks and 6 months), and 46 percent developed 6 months following implantation or later.[15] Fever, redness, swelling, erosion, or persistent drainage of the site indicates the need for further investigation. Although the value of antibiotic prophylaxis remains unestablished, it is common practice in many institutions to use broad-spectrum antibiotic therapy before the procedure and for 1 to 2 days after.

The 24 hours of flat bed rest prescribed for few patients postoperatively are uncomfortable for most patients, and analgesics or sedatives are usually necessary. Those patients may need help with feeding. There is no evidence in the literature or in our experience that immobilization of patients following permanent pacemaker insertions will prevent pacemaker lead dislodgement. Bed rest is poorly tolerated in this age group of patients and may predispose to venous complications among others. Thus the majority of our patients are allowed out of bed the same day of operation and gradually resume preoperative activity. Gentle range of motion exercise is instituted on the first postoperative day to prevent complications from immobility.

Discharge planning should center on helping the patient become comfortable with the new pacemaker and teaching about pacer malfunction and what to do in the event of its occurrence. In most cases this means emphasizing the reliability and longevity of the newer units without instilling false hopes. Patients should have a basic understanding of the difference between electrical and mechanical heart function, why a pacer was necessary, and what it is doing for the heart. The components of the system can be described with visual aids or by using a model of the pacemaker. Patients should know the name of the manufacturer and model, the expected battery life of the generator, and, in simple terms, the unit's operating mode (e.g., AV sequential, ventricular demand). All of the manufacturers have heart and pacemaker models that can be used in patient and staff education, and most companies have designed their own instruction booklet for patient use. The American Heart Association has a pamphlet for patients entitled "Living With Your Pacemaker."* If a hospital has a large volume of implantations per year, it is advisable for the staff to write their own patient booklet with instructions for home and work. The manufacturer also provides an identification card with pacemaker model and serial numbers. It must be stressed to the patient that this card should be carried at all times, in the event of an emergency. Many patients arrive at the emergency room with an acute condition and no pacemaker identification with them. This situation creates a variety of problems. For a patient arriving with pacemaker malfunction, lack of identification causes delay in treatment or reprogramming. Since many of these people are elderly or have other heart disease, they may present to an emergency room unconscious or needing resuscitation. In such cases the presence of a pacemaker might go unnoticed, and there are potential complications if defibrillation is carried out. Newer pulse generators have greatly improved resistance to the effects of external defibrillation, but damage can occur—especially if anterior paddles are placed directly over the generator or lead. Anterior paddles should be placed at least 4 to 5 inches from the generator and lead system, with confirmation of pacer function following cardioversion or defibrillation. To minimize risk, Furman recommends the use of anterior-posterior paddles to direct the output vector of the defibrillator at right angles to the sensing vector of the generator.[16]

Emergency room staff awareness of a pacemaker is easily accomplished if the patient is wearing Medic Alert[17] jewelry. There is room on the necklace or bracelet for the model and pacing mode and the telephone number of the implanting physician.

Before discharge, patients are given a written procedure (which may be part of a booklet) identifying signs or symptoms of pacer malfunction and describing how to obtain appropriate care in an emergency. If the cardiologist wants the patient to use daily pulse counting as a way of assessing proper function, the family is taught the technique, the characteristics of the intrinsic heart rate, and an acceptable pulse range. They are specifically instructed regarding the symptoms or abnormal pulse rate that would warrant notifying the physician. The dates and locations of their follow-up visits are also included in these instructions.

Much has been written about electromagnetic interference (EMI) and the various power sources that potentially alter (by triggering or inhibiting) pacemaker function. People can be advised with certainty regarding some sources of EMI, but with many sources the effects are variable and depend on the individuals, their proximity to EMI, and the duration of exposure. Safe and unsafe machines and devices and potential sources of interference are summarized in Table 14–6.

A guideline to follow in counseling patients about possible EMI is the need for caution and supervision when first returning to work. Industrial supervisors and nurses must be informed. Patients who experience symptoms or changes in pacemaker function should avoid the EMI source.

---

*American Heart Association, 7320 Greenville Avenue, Dallas, Texas 75231.

Table 14–6. Extrinsic Sources of Electromagnetic and Radio-frequency Interference

Devices that **do not** affect pacemaker function:

- Household appliances
- Household tools
- Theft-prevention equipment (pacemaker may activate the alarm)
- Magnetometer weapon detectors (pacemaker may activate the alarm)
- Garage door openers

Devices that **may** affect pacemaker function (depending upon model, proximity to device, and duration of exposure):

- Electric razors
- Ultrasonic dental instrument cleaners
- Car, tractor, and boat engines (if the person is working on the motor, not operating the vehicle)
- Microwave ovens (most manufacturers still recommend staying at least 2 feet away)
- High-energy electromagnetic fields such as:
  - Industrial arc-welding units (resistance welding)
  - Smelting induction furnaces
  - High-energy radar, television, and radio transmitters; CB radios with high-powered amplifiers
  - Radio-frequency–activated fuses for explosives

Devices that **do** affect pacemaker function:

- Therapeutic electrocautery
- Diathermy
- Electrosurgical units

Generally patients can return to the same or a greater level of activity, although the physician may have specific instructions about aerobic sports or isometric exercise (at the time of discharge the effects of sinus tachycardia and muscle contractions on pacing should have been determined). Medications and diet are reviewed before discharge, and it is important to reassure the patient that bathing, restrictive clothing, and shoulder straps will not affect pacemaker function. However, injury may occur at the pacemaker site from trauma such as shooting a rifle or shotgun that is positioned on the affected side.

Outpatient Care

Pacemaker malfunction is frequently detected before symptoms can occur. In many institutions, pacemaker surveillance and follow-up care consist of outpatient clinics supplemented with transtelephonic monitoring, a technique that has been used for more than ten years.[1, 10, 18] The frequency of clinic visits depends on the type and age of the pacemaker, condition of the patient, and the philosophy of the institution. Generally, as the pacemaker ages, clinic visits and telephone monitoring become more frequent with impending battery failure. Transtelephonic monitoring is handled through physicians' offices or private companies. It is a 24-hour service that gives basic pacemaker parameters as well as an EKG rhythm strip. The monitors are simple to operate, and most people learn to use them quickly. The patient places electrodes on both wrists (the electrodes are connected to a transmitter box), places his telephone receiver on the transmitter, and a recording is then taken over the telephone. The nurse or technician may question the patient regarding symptoms or request another recording with the patient placing a magnet over the site for approximately 30 seconds. A report is then sent to the physician; it identifies the type of pacemaker, its operating status, and any arrhythmias. The value of transtelephonic surveillance is significant but limited and must not substitute clinical evaluation. Patients need to understand the importance of regular office visits, which provide the opportunity for a clinical examination, patient interview, and complete evaluation of pacemaker function.

The Patient With an Antitachycardia Pacemaker

Established techniques in clinical cardiac electrophysiology have recently led to the development of a variety of antitachycardia pacing systems. Automatically triggered and manually activated pacemakers are in limited use to control or terminate recurrent ventricular and supraventricular tachycardias.[19–22] These investigational devices are alternative therapy in patients whose arrhythmias have proved refractory to more conventional forms of treatment (surgery or drugs), or in those who have suffered intolerable side effects from drug therapy.

Initially, the tachycardia is evaluated in the electrophysiology laboratory. In this setting, programmed electrical stimulation is used to control (reduce the rate of) the tachycardia or terminate it. Control or termination is achieved with either overdrive (burst) or competitive underdrive pacing of the atria (for supraventricular tachycardia) or ventricles (for ventricular tachycardias), or with the delivery of timed single or multiple ventricular extrastimuli (for ventricular tachycardia). A complication of pacing is acceleration of the tachycardia. The demonstration of this arrhythmia in the laboratory precludes the use of an antitachycardia pacemaker.[19] Also of critical importance is the hemodynamic response of the patient during the arrhythmia and whether or not it is life-threatening. Automatically triggered units may be chosen if the arrhythmia produces syncope or seizure activity. It has been suggested that for the successful use of patient-activated pacemakers, the following criteria be met: (1) The patient is able to recognize the onset and termination of the arrhythmia, (2) the tachycardia does not compromise ventricular and cerebral function to the extent that the patient cannot trigger the unit, and (3) the patient is capable of properly using the pacemaker.[19]

Patient-activated pacing is performed with a magnet held over the implantation site, to induce slow competitive or underdrive pacing, or by means of a radio-frequency unit that has programmable rates for underdrive or overdrive pacing. The patient applies the radio-frequency transmitter to the chest over the implanted receiver and presses a button to activate it.

Patients with antitachycardia units are a small population receiving a very individualized type of therapy. Although all patients with permanent pacing need education, those with manually triggered systems require extensive support and education. The patient must be intelligent and stable. Anxiety is to be expected, especially in people with chronic ventricular tachycardia who probably have experienced multiple hospitalizations and cardioversions and failed several drug regimens. During electrophysiologic testing and after pacemaker implantation until discharge, the tachycardia is induced and terminated repeatedly. This demonstrates reproducibility, allows the cardiologist and the staff to ensure that the patient can identify and properly terminate the arrhythmia, and increases the patient's confidence in his ability to recognize the arrhythmia. Blood pressure, peripheral pulses, and symptoms are assessed during this time. The following points should be reviewed with the patient:

1. If a magnet is used, it is applied correctly and left on for an appropriate period of time.
2. If a radio-frequency transmitter is used, the patient knows the effective rate for underdrive or overdrive pacing, if the rate should be changed and under what conditions, how long the button should be depressed (usually 1 to 3 seconds), the number of bursts necessary (usually one or two), and how to change the batteries.
3. What emergency room or physician to contact if reprogramming or disabling the pacemaker is necessary.
4. Medications, especially if antiarrhythmic drugs are used with the pacemaker for arrhythmia control.

Return visits to the clinic are similar to those recommended for other pacemaker patients, except that special attention should be given to patient concerns and complaints, the frequency and duration of tachycardia, and any symptoms or problems.

REFERENCES

1. Varriale P, and Naclerio EA: Cardiac Pacing. Philadelphia, Lea and Febiger, 1979, pp. 33–317.
2. Wulff KS: Use of temporary epicardial electrodes for atrial pacing and monitoring. Cardiovasc Nursing 18:1, 1983.
3. King OM: Care of the Cardiac Surgical Patient. St Louis, CV Mosby Co, 1975, pp. 199–200.
4. Hauser RG: Indications for pacing bradyarrhythmias. Medtronic News, September, 1981.
5. Winslow EH, and Marino LB: Temporary cardiac pacemakers. AJN 75:587, 1975.
6. A-V sequential demand pulse generator. Model 5330. Medtronic Inc, 1981.
7. Weinstein J, Gnoj J, Mazzara JT, et al: Temporary transvenous pacing via the percutaneous femoral vein approach. Am Heart J 85:703, 1973.
8. Castellanos A, Ortiz JM, Pastis N, and Castillo C: The electrocardiogram in patients with pacemakers. Prog Cardiovasc Dis 13:192, 1970.
9. Furman S, and Escher DJW: Principles and Techniques of Cardiac Pacing. New York, Harper and Row, 1970, p. 227.
10. Friedberg HD: Follow-up care after artificial pacing. *In* Chung EK (ed): Artificial Cardiac Pacing: Practical Approach. Baltimore, Williams and Wilkins Co, 1979, p. 305.

11. American Heart Association Inter-Society Commission for Heart Disease Resources, 7320 Greenville Avenue, Dallas, Texas 75231; see also Parsonnet V, Furman S, Smyth NPD, and Bilitch M: Optimal resources for implantable cardiac pacemakers. Circulation 68:236A, 1983.
12. Parsonnet V, Furman S, and Smyth NPD: Implantable cardiac pacemakers. Am J Cardiol 34:489, 1974.
13. Parsonnet V, Furman S, and Smyth NPD: A revised code for pacemaker identification. Pace 4:400, 1981.
14. Beeler BA: Infections of permanent transvenous and epicardial pacemakers in adults. Heart and Lung 11:152, 1982.
15. Choo MH, Holmes DR, Gersh BJ, et al: Permanent pacemaker infections: Characterization and management. Am J Cardiol 48:560, 1981.
16. Furman S: External defibrillation and implanted cardiac pacemakers. Pace 4:485, 1981.
17. Medic Alert Foundation International, P.O. Box 1009, Turlock, CA 95381.
18. Furman S: Transtelephone pacemaker clinic. J. Thorac Cardiovasc Surg 61:827, 1971.
19. Josephson ME, and Seides SF: Clinical Cardiac Electrophysiology: Techniques and Interpretations. Philadelphia, Lea and Febiger, 1979, p. 304.
20. Peters RW, Shafton E, Frank S, et al: Radiofrequency triggered pacemakers: Uses and limitations. Ann Intern Med 88:17, 1978.
21. Fisher JD, Kim SG, Furman S, and Matos JA: Role of implantable pacemakers in control of recurrent ventricular tachycardias. Am J Cardiol 49:194, 1982.
22. Griffin JC, Mason JW, and Calfie RV: Clinical use of an implantable automatic tachycardia terminating pacemaker. Am Heart J 100:1093, 1983.

IV

NEW FRONTIERS

15

New Advances in Cardiac Pacemaking

SCOTT R. SPIELMAN, M.D.

INTRODUCTION

During the past 15 years we have witnessed an astounding increase in the rate of pacemaker implantation.[1, 2] Recent surveys by Parsonnet and colleagues show 115,000 new implants in the United States in 1981, equivalent to 513 new implants per million population (Fig. 15–1). This represents a 12-year growth rate of more than 600 percent. At the same time, pulse generator replacements have diminished by more than 30 percent coincident with a changeover to lithium battery sources. Looked at in another way, 1 out of every 460 Americans now has an implanted pacemaker.

Along with the proliferation of devices has come a technological explosion in their complexity and potential application to both bradyarrhythmias and tachyarrhythmias.[3–35, 57–69] Although in current practice more than 90 percent of all implanted generators are single-chamber ventricular demand units, during the next few years it is likely that dual-chamber devices or devices based on some physiologic variable for control will ultimately account for 25 to 45 percent of new implants (Fig. 15–2).[11] Moreover, in the absence of ideal antiarrhythmic drug therapy and the increased salvage rate for patients with ventricular arrhythmias by rescue squads, coronary care units, and other emergency interventions, antiarrhythmic pacemakers will also account for an increasing proportion of implantations.

Like most new technological advances in medicine, such as CAT scanning and Nuclear Magnetic Resonance that develop from concepts that make "physiologic sense," it remains for us to understand the need for the devices in question, to master their use, to develop scientific proofs for their value, and to determine the patient population appropriate to individual units. In this chapter we will examine each of these areas for the new anti-bradycardia and anti-tachycardia pacemakers that are now available.

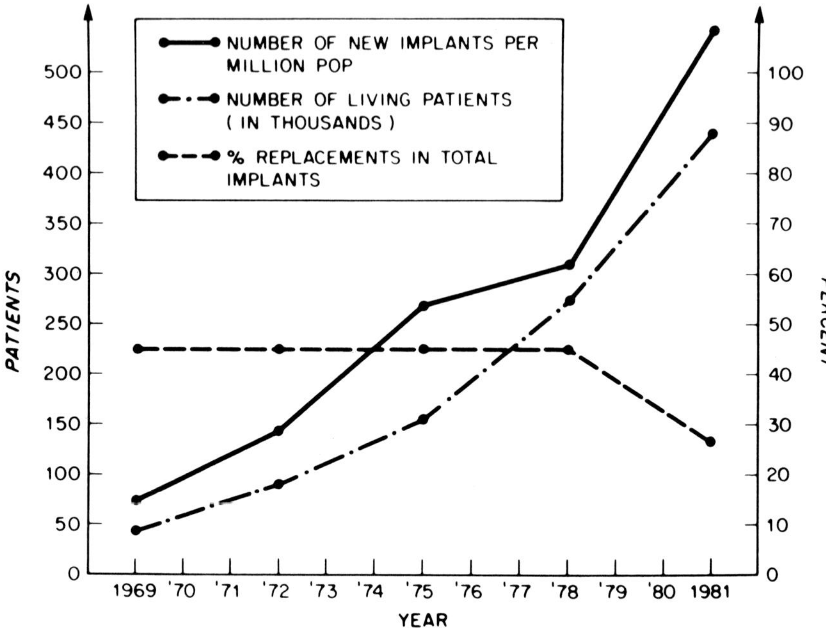

Figure 15–1. Total implants and pulse generator replacements plotted over a 12-year period together with the number of living pacemaker patients. Note the marked decrease in the proportion of replacement units. (Reproduced from Parsonnet and Bernstein: JACC 1:340, 1983, by permission of Elsevier Science Publishing Co., Inc.)

PHYSIOLOGIC PACING

Theoretic Considerations

Ryden has sensibly suggested that the purpose of physiologic pacing is to pace each patient to obtain the optimal level of function for his demands, no more and no less.[36] Since what is technically achievable is not always medically needed, a pacing system should not be more advanced than is medically justifiable. Ventricular demand pacing may be an inadequate technique for many patients, leaving them with a system that performs at less than the actual demand. Many paced patients, satisfied with the absence of Stokes-Adams attacks, may not complain of symptoms associated with a nonphysiologic pacing mode. The attending physician may believe that a patient's advanced age is responsible for such symptoms as dizziness, fatigue, and palpitations, which may occur with loss of atrioventricular (AV) synchrony, 1:1 retrograde conduction, or inability to increase rate during exercise. Worse yet, these symptoms may not be elicited by the physician, who is himself satisfied that the patient is no longer syncopal. It has been estimated that as many as 20 percent of patients with ventricular demand pacers will suffer such symptoms of the so-called

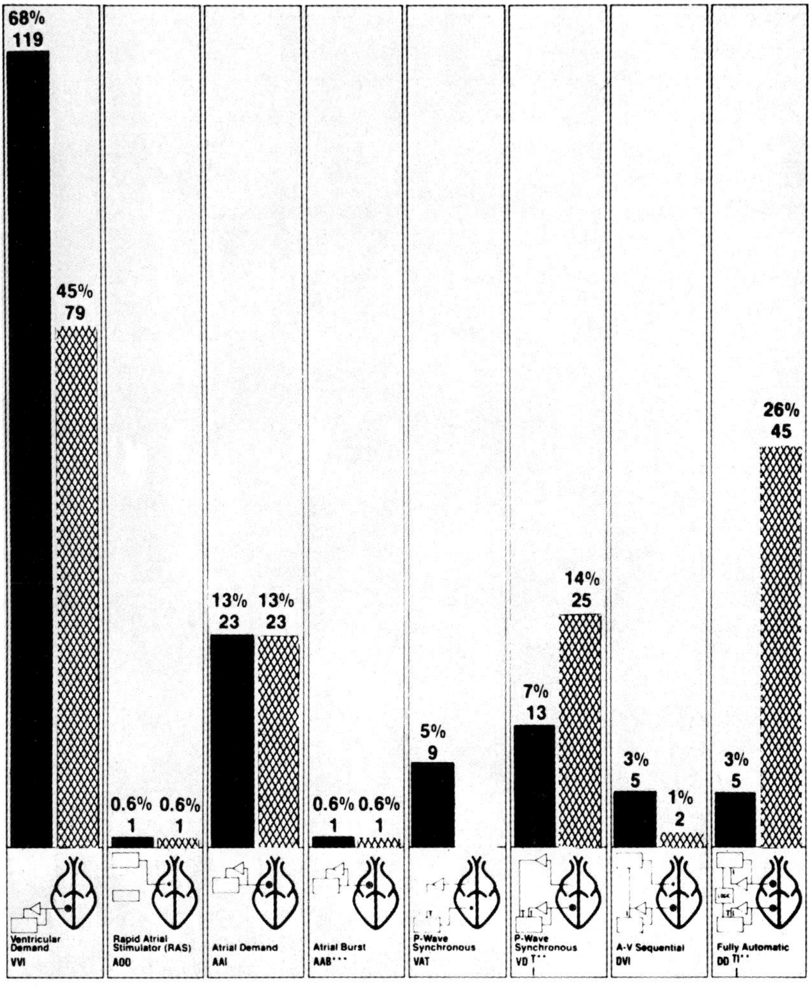

Figure 15–2. Comparison between actual and predicted future choices of various pacemakers. In this 1979 study the dark bars represent the actual application of each pacemaker type based on current availability; note that 68 percent of patients received VVI pacers. The hatched bars are a prediction of how these devices would have been used had they all been readily available; note that >40 percent would have been dual chambered. (Reproduced from Sutton et al: PACE 3:216, 1980, by permission of Futura Publishing Co., Inc.)

"pacemaker syndrome" (Fig. 15–3).[37–39] Patients with intact retrograde (VA) conduction who pace intermittently, such as those with intermittent heart block, carotid sinus hypersensitivity, or episodic sinus pauses, are the most likely to develop such symptoms.

In order to understand pacemaker syndrome and the possibilities for providing patients with an improved pacing mode, it is necessary to briefly review oxygen transport at rest and during exercise. Total oxygen consumption is about 0.25 liters per minute at rest in humans.[36] In an untrained individual this might

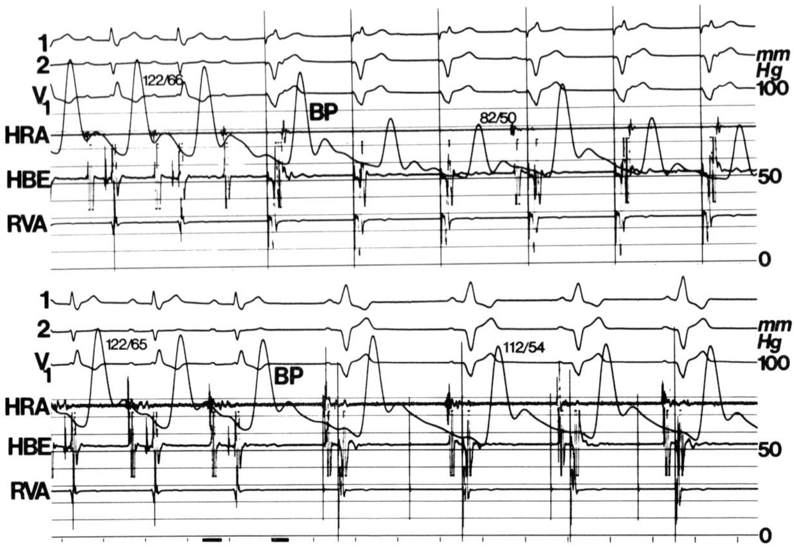

Figure 15–3. Hemodynamic and electrophysiologic parameters in a patient with pacemaker syndrome. The records in both panels are organized as ECG leads 1, 2, and V1; intracardiac electrograms from the high right arium (HRA), His bundle (HBE), and right ventricular apex (RVA), and blood pressure (BP) on a 100 mg Hg scale. In the top panel, following beat 3, carotid sinus pressure produces sinus slowing and AV block and a chronically implanted VVI pacemaker takes over. BP falls to a low of 82/50 and varies tremendously depending upon the random relationship of atrial systole. In the lower panel a change to atrial synchronous pacing completely averts the fall in BP. This patient suffered severe symptoms of pacemaker syndrome, which were completely abolished by change-over to a DDD device.

increase to 3 to 4 liters per minute with heavy work loads. Increased amounts of oxygen are made available to working muscles through three basic mechanisms: (1) an increase in cardiac output, (2) redistribution of blood flow, and (3) an increase in arteriovenous oxygen difference. In a normal individual, the amount of increase in cardiac output is determined by the peripheral oxygen demands and is largely the result of an increase in heart rate rather than stroke volume. In a typically normal untrained athlete, cardiac output may rise from 5 to more than 20 liters per minute.

Although redistribution of blood flow to working muscles may occur during exercise, at rest redistribution of flow and increase in arteriovenous oxygen difference should not be operative. In failing hearts with low resting cardiac output these two compensatory mechanisms may already have come into play. Further, since an already dilated heart may not be capable of mustering an increase in stroke volume during exercise, the ability to increase rate becomes the sole remaining compensatory mechanism. This explains why many patients with ventricular demand pacers become exercise restricted.

Properly timed atrial systole allows (1) maintenance of a reduced filling pressure, thereby facilitating venous return; (2) completion of ventricular filling assisting AV valve closure; and (3) enhancement of ventricular filling, causing further stretching of ventricular muscle fibers to produce a more complete and vigorous contraction.[36] These mechanisms typically augment cardiac output by approximately 20 percent. However, loss of atrial systole in normal patients does not result in a stroke volume decrease of corresponding magnitude because compensatory mechanisms come into play. Mean atrial pressure increases, resulting in a greater driving force, and left ventricular end-diastolic pressure rises, resulting in an increase in muscle fiber length to a suitable preload and more efficient ventricular contraction. On the other hand, patients with stiff, noncompliant ventricles may be devastated by loss of atrial function. In these patients, ventricular filling is restricted and is largely dependent on atrial systolic contribution. With loss of atrial systole and the inability of the ventricle to dilate, cardiac output may fall dramatically. Moreover, mean atrial and left ventricular end-diastolic pressure rise, resulting in pulmonary congestion. In contrast, in patients with dilated compliant ventricles with poor systolic function, as in congestive cardiomyopathies, loss of atrial kick may have little effect, since the degree to which it contributes to ventricular volume is negligible. Pacemaker syndrome is common in patients with normal or noncompliant hearts that pace intermittently because the compensatory mechanisms that do exist do not have time to develop.

As heart rate increases, the role of atrial contraction becomes even more important. During exercise, diastolic filling time is compromised so that the part of filling occurring during atrial contraction increases proportionately. The AV interval is also important and has been said to be optimal between 100 and 200 msec.

During ventricular pacing VA conduction may be absent or intact, with varying retrograde patterns. If the atria contract against closed AV valves, ventricular filling is decreased, leading to a low stroke volume. Mitral regurgitation may occur, and the patient may develop palpitations and symptomatic neck vein pulsations. When VA conduction is 1:1 (as it is in 65 percent of patients with sick sinus syndrome and 30 percent of patients with complete heart block) and all atrial contractions occur against a closed mitral valve, patients frequently feel tired, dizzy, and unable to perform adequate work loads.

In summary, the ability to vary rate during exertion and maintain appropriately timed atrial systole has important hemodynamic consequences that provide a rational basis for dual-chamber pacing.

Technical Considerations

Dual-chamber pacing is not only theoretically sensible; it is also technically achievable. Figure 15–4 shows the impressive survival rate of lithium pulse generators.[1] Second-generation dual-chamber pacers should maintain an equally impressive longevity, especially in combination with newly designed low-threshold leads and appropriate programming. Innovations in lead design and fabrication have made dislocations, perforations, and fractures a rarity. The development of the atrial J lead and the screw-in lead have markedly improved atrial lead survival (Fig. 15–5) and allow low thresholds and acceptable P-wave

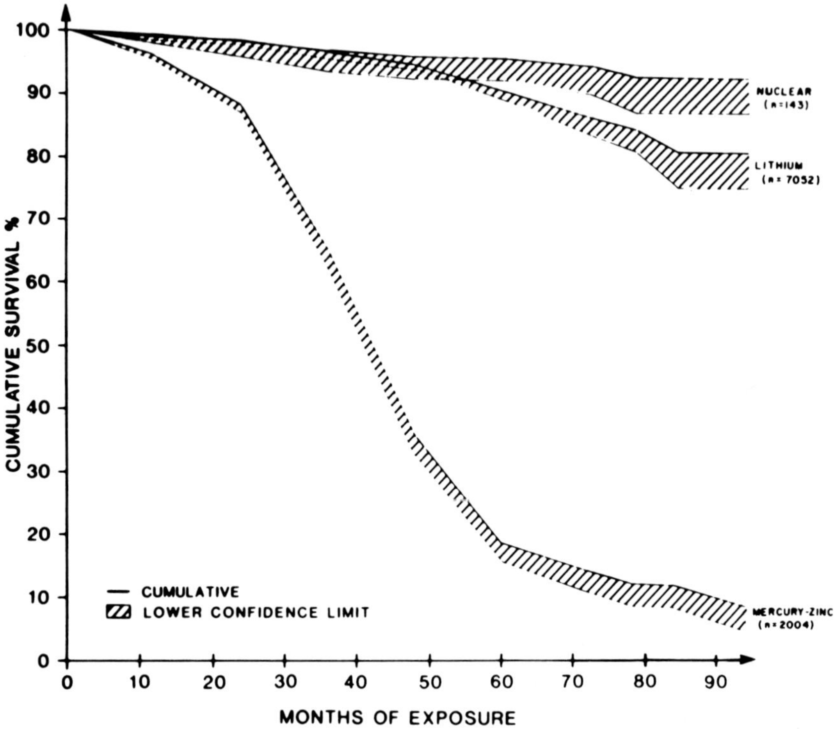

Figure 15–4. Actuarial survival of pulse generators as a function of power source. Note the >80 percent survival of lithium batteries at 90 months compared with the previously used mercury-zinc batteries. (Reproduced from Parsonnet and Bernstein: JACC 1:342, 1983, by permission of Elsevier Science Publishing Co., Inc.)

amplitudes (Fig. 15–6).[1, 40, 41] Finally, multiprogrammability and telemetry of programmed and real-time parameters have added tremendous versatility to all units, decreasing by 15 to 20 percent the need for reoperations (Fig. 15–7).

PACEMAKER CODES

In 1974, in response to the need for a simple means of describing triggered and inhibited pacing systems that had replaced asynchronous units, the Inter-Society Commission on Heart Disease (ICHD) devised a three-letter code for pacing modes.[42] As pulse generators became increasingly more complex, with multiple programming features and antiarrhythmic functions, this code was expanded to five letters (Fig. 15–8), which will be expanded still further in the forthcoming 1982 ICHD report.[43] The usefulness of the code's first three letters for providing a succinct and easily verbalized method of describing pacing modes is unquestioned, as evidenced by its wide acceptance. However, the

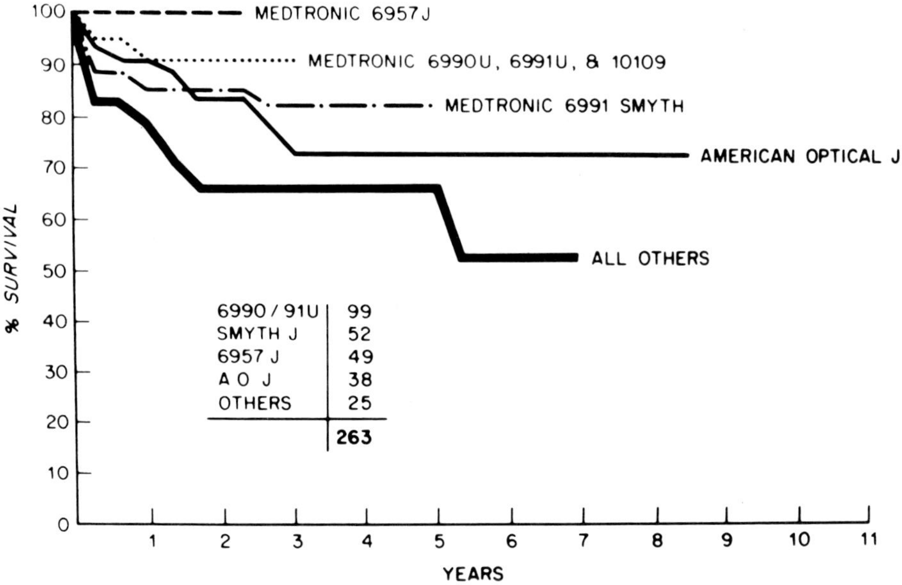

Figure 15–5. Cumulative actuarial survival of atrial leads. The newer leads, such as the Medtronic 6957J and the 6990U, demonstrate excellent performance characteristics. (Reproduced from Parsonnet and Bernstein: JACC 1:342, 1983, by permission of Elsevier Science Publishing Co., Inc.)

CONFIGURATION	FIXATION	STUDY EXPERIENCE					ADDITIONAL EXPERIENCE					
		No.	P-Wave Ampl. (mV)	Threshold (0.5 ms) V	Threshold (0.5 ms) mA	Percent Displacement	Series	No.	P-Wave Ampl. (mV)	Threshold (0.5 ms) V	Threshold (0.5 ms) mA	Percent Displacement
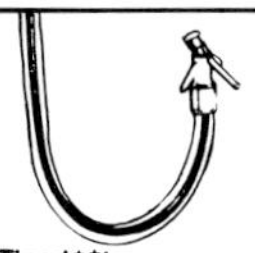 J-Tined**[1]	Passive	6	2.0±1.3	0.8±0.4	2.2±0.9	0	Medtronic	78	3.1±1.6	0.9±.3	2.0±.8	0
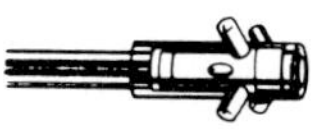 Straight Tined[2]	Passive	1	2.1	0.8	1.2	0	Kruse	14	4.5±1.2	1.7±.7	–	0
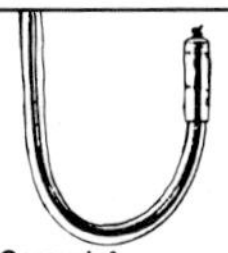 J-Screw-in[3]	Active	9	2.8±1.4	0.5±0.2	0.8±0.3	0	Medtronic	71	2.7±1.2	0.8±.3	1.3±.7	4.2
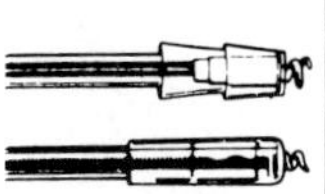 Straight Screw-in[4]	Active	100	3.3±1.8	0.8±0.5	1.3±0.8	1	Perrins	66	3.0±1.4	0.6±.3	1.0±.6	1.5

Figure 15–6. Threshold and amplitude characteristics of various endocardial atrial leads. Note the excellent implant parameters obtained with these leads and the low dislodgement rate. (Reproduced from Sutton et al: Medtronic Bulletin, 1982, by permission of Medtronic, Inc.)

```
PACESETTER SYSTEMS INC.
   Prototype 1.4

DATE:   NOV 16, 1982 10:00 AM

MODEL:  281   SERIAL:       839

PATIENT: ______________________

PHYSICIAN: ____________________________

---------- PROGRAMMED PARAMETERS -----------

MODE ............................ DDD
RATE ............................  70 PPM

VENTRICULAR CHANNEL:
 REFRACTORY ..................... 250 MSEC
 PULSE WIDTH .................... 0.6 MSEC
 PULSE AMPLITUDE ................ 5.0 VOLTS
 SENSITIVITY .................... 2.0 MVOLT

ATRIAL CHANNEL:
 REFRACTORY ..................... 160 MSEC
 PULSE WIDTH .................... 0.6 MSEC
 PULSE AMPLITUDE ................ 5.0 VOLTS
 SENSITIVITY .................... 1.0 MVOLT

AV INTERVAL ..................... 165 MSEC

MAX. TRACK RATE .................  90 PPM

BLANKING PERIOD .................  32 MSEC

MAGNET:  OFF

-------------- MEASURED DATA --------------

PACEMAKER RATE ................. 70.0 PPM

MAGNET RATE .................... 80.0 PPM

CHANNEL MEASUREMENTS:

                   VENTRICLE     ATRIUM
 PULSE VOLTAGE        4.2          4.2     VOLTS
 PULSE CURRENT       16.1         16.1     MAMPS
 PULSE ENERGY          33           34     µJOULES
 PULSE CHARGE           8            9     µCOULOMBS
 LEAD IMPEDANCE ··    236          236     OHMS

BATTERY DATA: ( W.G.8074 - NOM.2.3 AHR )
 IMPEDANCE ......................   1.0 KOHMS
 VOLTAGE ........................  2.68 VOLTS
 CURRENT ........................    43 µAMPS

-------------- TEST RESULTS ---------------

VENTRICULAR R-WAVE AMPLITUDE: 4.0 MVOLTS
      SAFETY MARGIN: 2.0:1

VENTRICULAR CAPTURE THRESHOLD: 3.0 VOLTS
      AT 0.6 MSEC PULSE WIDTH
```

Figure 15–7. Telemetry printout from a Pacesetter's DDD pacemaker. This device allows telemetric monitoring of not only programmed but also real-time parameters, thus improving the ability to diagnose and program around potentially difficult postimplant problems in pacemaker performance.

fourth and fifth letters have not been used frequently, possibly because of some inaccuracies and incompleteness in the presentation of arrhythmia coding and the fact that the fourth letter seems superfluous when referring to complex devices that, by their very nature, must be multiprogrammable.

A complementary code, more suitable for written communication, computer use, and teaching and more specific as to the information imparted, has been devised by Brownlee and colleagues.[44] This code assists in describing dual-chamber devices by placing atrial function in the numerator and ventricular function in the denominator of a ratio format. The symbols P (pace) and S (sense) begin each channel descriptor and are followed by either I (inhibited) or T (triggered) as appropriate. An O indicates no activity in a chamber. A subscript

Position	I	II	III	IV	V
Category	Chamber(s) paced	Chamber(s) sensed	Mode of response(s)	Programmable functions	Special tachyarrhythmia functions
Letters Used	V- Ventricle	V- Ventricle	T- Triggered	P- Programmable (rate and/or output)	B- Bursts
	A- Atrium	A- Atrium	I- Inhibited	M- Multiprogrammable	N- Normal Rate Competition
	D- Double	D- Double	D- Double*		S- Scanning
			O- None		
		O- None	R- Reverse	O- None	E- External
Manufacturer's Designation only	S- Single Chamber	S- Single Chamber	Comma optional here		

*Atrial triggered and ventricular inhibited.

Figure 15–8. Five-position ICHD code. Positions I and II indicate the chambers paced and sensed, respectively. Position III indicates the mode of response, where D means both triggered and inhibited and R means reverse function, i.e., a pacemaker that is silent at slow rates and activated by fast rates. In position IV, P represents simple programmability of 1 or 2 functions while M indicates additional capacity such as the ability to change mode, AV delay, etc. Position V involves antiarrhythmic functions such as scanning or normal rate competition as in a "dual-demand" device (see text under Antitachycardia Pacing: An Overview). (Reproduced from Parsonnet et al: PACE 4:401, 1981, by permission of Futura Publishing Co., Inc.)

is used with I and T to indicate the chamber in which the activity is sensed, causing the pacemaker to inhibit or trigger in response—for example, Iv (inhibited by a sensed ventricular event) or Ta (triggered by a sensed atrial event). An example of the use of this code is shown in Figure 15–9. This coding system currently has no descriptors for antiarrhythmic functions and is limited by the fact that it does not lend itself to verbal communication. As shown in Figure 15–9, pictorial coding is also helpful in describing pacer function and, properly applied, may serve as universal terminology.

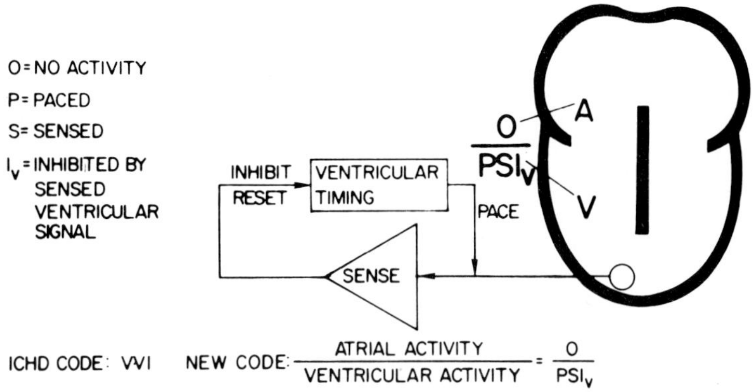

Figure 15–9. "Brownlee code" for a ventricular demand pacemaker. In the ICHD code this pacemaker is a VVI, i.e., it paces and senses in the ventricle and is inhibited. In this new code the numerator shows a 0 to indicate lack of atrial function and the denominator shows a P to indicate pacing, an S to indicate sensing, and an Iv to indicate inhibition by ventricular events. (Reproduced from Brownlee et al: PACE 4:398, 1981, by permission of Futura Publishing Co., Inc.)

None of the current coding systems is perfect, and work on them is still ongoing in several committees. It is likely that the popular three-letter code will remain in use and that specific written and pictorial codes will be further developed for teaching and computer use. In subsequent sections in this chapter, when discussing the function and clinical indications for each device, we will present and explain all three of the codes described above.

PACER FUNCTION AND SELECTION

Atrioventricular Sequential Pacemakers (DVI)

A DVI pacemaker is a system that paces in the atrium and ventricle (D), senses only in the ventricle (V), and the mode of sensing response is inhibited (I) (Fig. 15–10). The AV interval may either be preset by the manufacturer or programmable. There are two basic methods of operation characteristic of current DVI pulse generators. The distinction depends on whether or not ventricular sensing continues during the AV interval. If sensing is continuous during the AV interval (as in the Medtronic bipolar 5992 Byrel) or if the device is unipolar and relies upon a brief "blanking" period to assure that an atrial stimulus is not detected in the ventricular sensing circuit, following which ventricular sensing resumes to the end of the AV interval (as in the Medtronic 5993 SX Byrel), the mode of operation is said to be "noncommitted." If sensing does not occur during the AV interval (as in the Pacesetter's Programmalith AV and the Intermedics Cyberlith IV), the mode of operation is said to be "committed."

Noncommitted DVI pacing systems may pace the atrium and ventricles, the

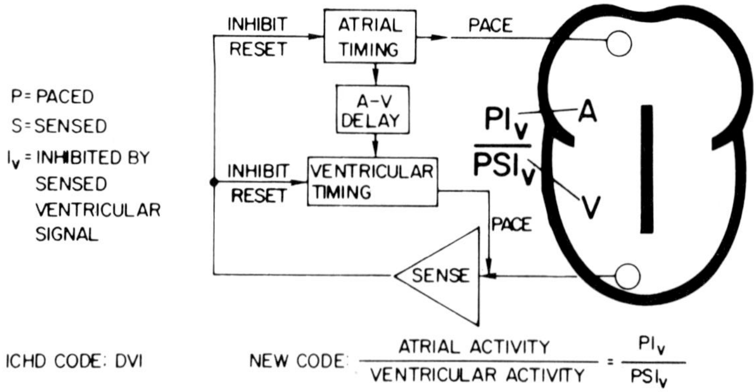

Figure 15–10. "Brownlee code" for an AV sequential pacemaker. The new code and the pictorial code indicate that a DVI pacemaker can pace in both chambers but senses only in the ventricle and that ventricular events inhibit both atrial and ventricular output. Note that atrial events are not sensed. (Reproduced from Brownlee et al: PACE 4:398, 1981, by permission of Futura Publishing Co., Inc.)

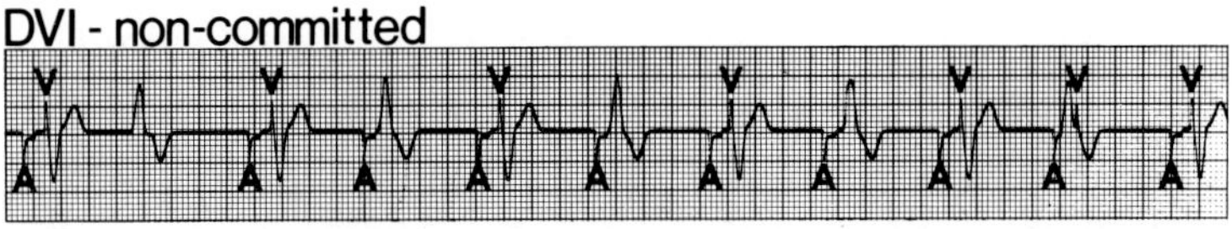

Figure 15–11. "Non-committed" DVI pacing. AV sequential pacing is present on beats 1, 3, 5, 7, 9, and 11. Beat 2 is a PVC that occurs prior to expected atrial output and therefore resets both atrial and ventricular output. Following an atrial spike on beats 4, 6, and 8, late cycle PVCs occur during the AV interval but beyond a brief atrial blanking period; ventricular output is therefore suppressed. On beat 10, a QRS occurs inside the atrial blanking period and a ventricular spike is therefore emitted.

atrium only, or be totally inhibited, depending on where an R wave is detected with respect to the pulse generator's timing cycle (Fig. 15–11). Committed pacing systems must put out a ventricular stimulus once an atrial stimulus is emitted and are more likely to result in fusion and so-called "pseudopseudo fusion" than are noncommitted systems (Fig. 15–12). Since sensing in the atrium does not occur, VA conduction will not result in pacemaker-mediated tachycardia. However, inability to sense in the atrium may result in confusing EKG patterns and in competitive atrial arrhythmias, including atrial fibrillation (see below, Complications of Dual-Chamber Pacemakers).[45]

DVI pacemakers are indicated in sick sinus syndrome associated with AV nodal or His-Purkinje disease or in AV block with accompanying evidence of abnormal sinus node function, where hemodynamic benefit from appropriately timed atrial systole can be shown. This mode of pacing is obviously not indicated in patients with predominant atrial fibrillation. In patients with bradycardia-tachycardia syndrome and paroxysmal atrial fibrillation, on the other hand, in whom episodes of atrial fibrillation may be bradycardia related, DVI pacers may decrease the frequency of episodes. Particular improvement in hemodynamic performance with this mode may be obtained in patients with 1:1 VA conduction during ventricular pacing. Further, DVI pacing may have application to reentrant supraventricular tachyarrhythmias as a termination mode (see below, Antitachycardia Pacing).

Atrial Synchronous Pacemakers (VDD)

In normal operation a VDD pacemaker will sense atrial activity and be triggered, after a programmable AV delay, to pace the ventricle (Fig. 15–13). If

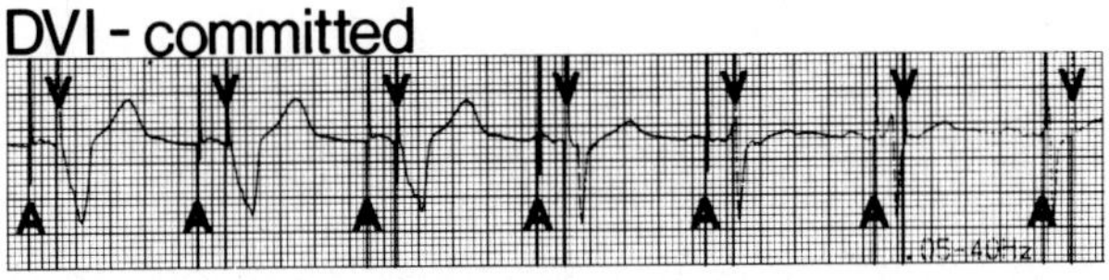

Figure 15–12. "Committed" DVI pacing. AV sequential pacing is present on beats 1, 2, and 3. Following atrial output on subsequent beats a ventricular spike is emitted despite the presence of normally conducted complexes during the AV interval.

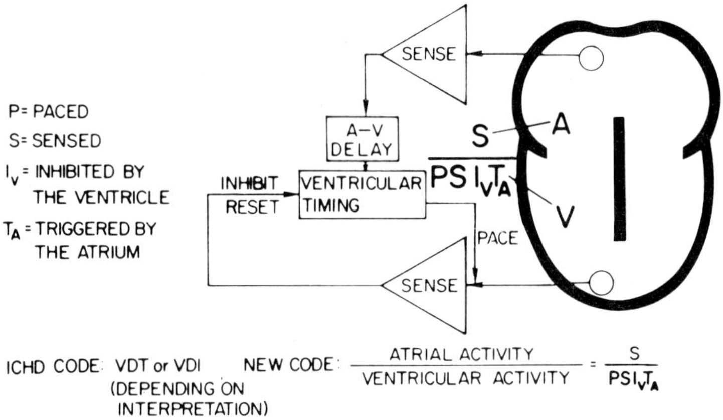

Figure 15–13. "Brownlee code" for an atrial synchronous pacemaker. The ICHD code now designates these devices as VDD. As indicated in the fractional and pictorial codes these pacemakers sense only in the atrium and pace and sense in the ventricle. Ventricular events inhibit ventricular output while atrial events trigger ventricular output. (Reproduced from Brownlee et al: PACE 4:399, 1981, by permission of Futura Publishing Co., Inc.)

the atrial rate falls below a selected base rate, the pacemaker functions as a ventricular demand unit (Fig. 15–14). Sensed ventricular events inhibit ventricular output. This pacing system currently requires both atrial and ventricular leads. However, a recently introduced Cardiac Pacemakers Inc. pacemaker with VDD mode capability employs a single lead, averages atrial rate, and then adjusts the ventricular response up or down in a frequently non-1:1 AV synchronous fashion. This pacemaker has been said to be more forgiving at rate extremes for two reasons. First, at low rates it is still rate responsive as long as a change in atrial rate occurs, even if only from 40 to 50 beats per minute; and second, during atrial arrhythmias, sudden rate swings are avoided since the pacemaker does not maintain 1:1 AV synchrony. The above operation has been called "rate smoothing." Once an upper rate limit of 115 beats per minute has been reached with this device, it gradually decays to its base rate via algorithm control. Standard VDD pacemakers go into a blocking mode, either 2:1 or an artificial form of Wenckebach, once an upper rate limit is exceeded. Within certain limits the upper rate limit characteristics are programmable and vary with each manufacturer.

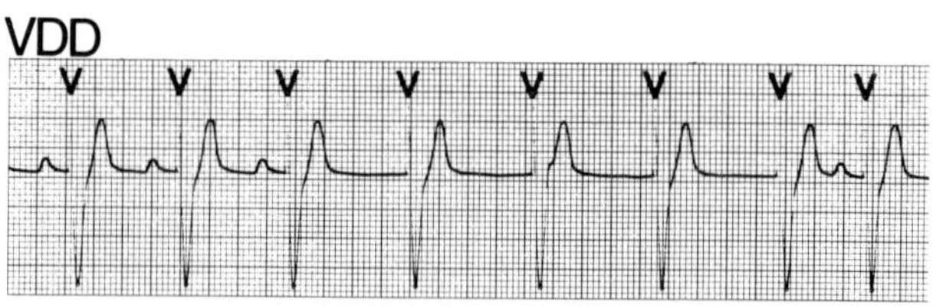

Figure 15–14. VDD pacing. Beats 1, 2, 3, and 8 show typical atrial synchronous pacing with sensed atrial events triggering ventricular output following an appropriate AV delay. When a sinus pause occurs, the pacemaker becomes a ventricular demand device.

Atrial synchronous pacemakers are indicated for patients with complete or intermittent heart block and normal sinus node function in whom the hemodynamic benefit of atrial tracking can be shown. Because these units are rate responsive they offer significant hemodynamic advantages for patients who exercise as compared to DVI pacemakers, which can only pace at a base rate.[9, 11, 15] VDD pacers are contraindicated for patients who develop angina at moderate heart rates and for patients with predominant atrial tachyarrhythmias and sick sinus syndrome. Individuals with only moderate degrees of sinus node dysfunction may, however, be good candidates for the CPI rate-smoothing unit as long as their atrial rates increase somewhat with exercise.

The ability of VDD pacemakers of the standard type to sense atrially may allow reentrant supraventricular tachycardia to occur, in which the pacemaker acts as an artificial bypass tract (see below, Complications of Dual-Chamber Pacemakers).[46–49] In addition, ventricular ectopic beats may be conducted retrogradely to the atrium and trigger a return ventricular beat at a close coupling interval (see below, Complications of Dual-Chamber Pacemakers).[50] These possible undesirable consequences of atrial sensing were not fully appreciated in early models of such devices; newer versions have programmable or automatically extending atrial refractory periods (the time from a ventricular sensed or paced event to the next sensed atrial event), so that in most patients pacemaker-induced arrhythmias can be avoided.

In an attempt to find a method of providing rate-responsive pacing to patients with sinus node dysfunction, some investigators have turned to other indicators of physiologic demand besides the atrium. These devices are not classically VDD in mode, and the exact method of coding for them is not established. Although experiments have been conducted with pH-triggered pacemakers, induction-sensitive pacemakers, temperature-sensitive pacemakers, and respiration frequency-sensitive pacemakers, only units with Po_2 and QT interval sensors have actually been implanted. Po_2 sensors are oxygen-sensitive electrodes implanted in subcutaneous tissue, whereas QT devices measure stimulus-to-T wave interval and adjust rate accordingly. These devices obviously do not provide AV synchrony.

Fully Automatic Pacemakers (DDD)

A DDD pacemaker can sense and pace in both chambers and is either triggered or inhibited or both (Fig. 15–15). In normal operation this unit would sequentially pace both atrium and ventricle with a suitable time delay when natural atrial activity falls below the preset base rate and atrial pacing is not followed by ventricular depolarization. When natural atrial activity exceeds the base rate, the pacemaker switches into an atrial synchronous mode with ventricular pacing following atrial sensing when a natural QRS does not occur within the programmed AV interval (Fig. 15–16). Sensed ventricular events such as premature ventricular beats inhibit both atrial and ventricular output and reset the atrial escape interval. The upper rate characteristics and blocking modes are

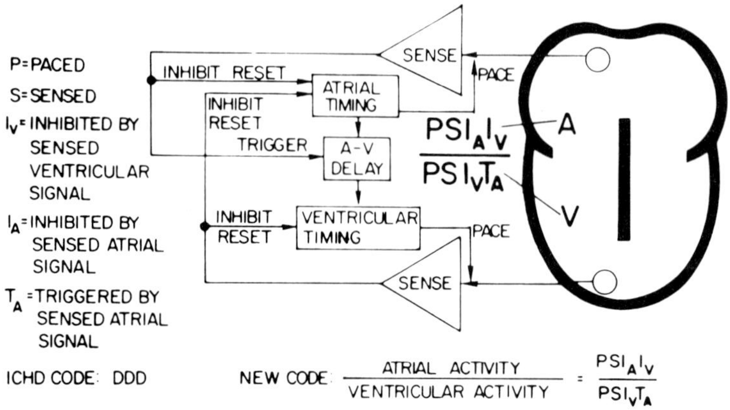

Figure 15–15. "Brownlee code" for fully automatic pacing. In the ICHD code this is a DDD pacemaker. The fractional and pictorial codes show that this device, as programmed, can pace and sense in both chambers; atrial output is inhibited by both sensed atrial and ventricular events, and ventricular output is inhibited by ventricular events and triggered by atrial events. (Reproduced from Brownlee et al: PACE 4:399, 1981, by permission of Futura Publishing Co., Inc.)

similar to the standard VDD systems described above. Most DDD units are noncommitted, employing an atrial blanking period following atrial stimuli to avoid sensing of such events on the ventricular channel.

DDD pacemakers are indicated in patients with AV block and evidence of sick sinus syndrome, AV block with normal sinus node function, and in patients with moderate sick sinus syndrome and AV nodal or His-Purkinje disease who maintain at least some ability to increase atrial rate with exercise. For the most part, VDD pacers will be replaced by DDD units, since the indications for implantation and difficulties of dealing with retrograde atrial sensing are similar and the ability to pace the atrium in DDD pacemakers gives added flexibility to the device.

The major problems in the use of DDD pacemakers are physiologic and are similar to those discussed under VDD pacing. First, DDD pacemakers currently in use cannot distinguish between pathologic and physiologic atrial tachycardias; once the programmed upper rate limit is exceeded, some form of blocking mode takes over. Second, the presence of intact VA conduction allows some patients to develop supraventricular arrhythmias using the pacemaker as one limb of the reentrant circuit (see below, Complications of Dual-Chamber Pacemakers).[46–49]

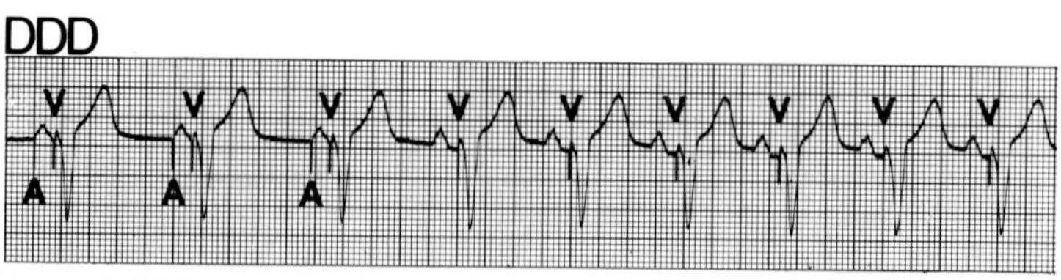

Figure 15–16. DDD pacing. AV sequential pacing is present on beats 1, 2, and 3. As this patient begins exercise the atrial rate increases above the programmed base rate and atrial synchronous pacing begins.

HEMODYNAMIC PROOF OF THE VALUE OF DUAL-CHAMBER PACERS

Having established that dual-chamber pacing is physiologically sensible and mechanically "do-able," one still needs to know if studies are available to *prove* the hemodynamic advantage of such devices over simpler, single-chambered pacemakers in multiple patient series. Such studies have been done; in this section the results will be presented for DVI and VDD/DDD pacing separately.

DVI Pacing

Sutton and colleagues compared atrial or AV sequential pacing to ventricular demand pacing in 24 patients with sick sinus syndrome.[11] The two groups were separated arbitrarily, depending on whether a statistically significant rise in cardiac output was demonstrated. Seventy percent of patients showed a 20 percent increase in cardiac index associated with a 10 percent reduction in pulmonary arterial wedge pressure during atrial or DVI pacing compared to ventricular pacing. In addition, when stroke work index was calculated for all patients and plotted against wedge pressure, atrial or DVI pacing was found to produce a significant elevation of stroke work index and simultaneous fall in wedge pressure in all patients ($p < 0.01$) (Fig. 15–17). Many other similar studies have reported comparable results for DVI pacing in well-trained athletes, in patients with impaired ventricular function, in patients with idiopathic hypertrophic subaortic stenosis or mitral stenosis, and in patients after cardiac surgery.[7, 8, 10, 12–14, 16] It is important to keep in mind that these studies were all performed on patients at rest. Adequate hemodynamic studies comparing DVI to VVI pacing during exercise are not available.

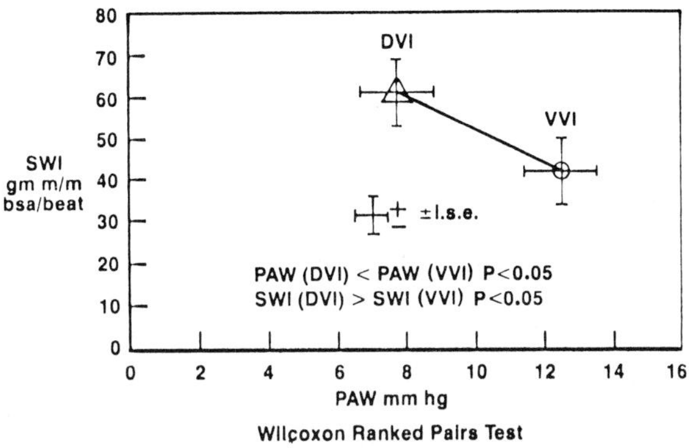

Figure 15–17. Ventricular function in ventricular pacing and atrioventricular pacing at the same heart rate. Note that during DVI pacing, stroke work index (SWI) increases and wedge pressure (PAW) decreases significantly. (Reproduced from Sutton: *In* Current Clinical Applications of Dual-Chamber Pacing, Proceedings of a symposium in Dallas, Texas, p. 92, 1981, by permission of Medtronic Inc.)

Morley and colleagues have established an important role for DVI pacing in patients with carotid sinus hypersensitivity.[17] Twelve patients with persistent symptoms following ventricular demand pacemaker insertion for carotid sinus hypersensitivity and syncope were found to have (1) a significant vasodepressor response, (2) a significant hypotensive response to ventricular pacing ("pacemaker effect"), and (3) a severe hypotensive response to carotid sinus massage with the introduction of ventricular pacing, which reproduced symptoms in all patients. AV sequential pacing eliminated the hypotensive effect of ventricular pacing and was thought to be the treatment of choice for patients with both a cardioinhibitory and vasodepressor component to their carotid hypersensitivity syndrome.

Long-term results of DVI vs. VVI pacing have recently been presented by Stone and colleagues in a large patient population paced for treatment of sick sinus syndrome.[16] Syncope responded well to either pacing mode. Neurologic symptoms were more consistently controlled by DVI pacing (97 percent vs. 52.9 percent $p < 0.000$), as was congestive heart failure, which was eliminated in 89.3 percent of the DVI-treated patients and only 53.6 percent of the VVI-treated patients ($p = 0.003$). Low-output symptoms were alleviated in 80.7 percent of DVI vs. 32.7 per cent of VVI patients, again a highly significant difference ($p < 0.000$). Similar results were found for angina relief with 67.7 percent improvement in DVI patients vs. only 11.5 percent in VVI patients ($p < 0.000$). Sixty-three percent of the DVI population became symptom-free following pacer insertion, compared to 23.9 percent with VVI pacing. Moreover, embolic events appeared to be decreased by DVI pacing, and atrial fibrillation was transient and occurred in only 5.8 percent of DVI patients. No direct hemodynamic investigations were performed in this study, but the degree of symptom relief with DVI vs. VVI pacing is very impressive. These data need to be confirmed by other investigators.

VDD/DDD Pacing

A carefully designed study comparing the hemodynamic benefits of VDD vs. VVI pacing has recently been published by Kruse and colleagues.[9] They evaluated 16 patients with pacemakers that could be programmed to either ventricular-inhibited or atrial synchronous modes, so that each patient served as his own control. Maximal work capacity was determined by bicycle ergometry; Swan-Ganz catheters were used to measure outputs and pressures. There was a mean increase of 24 percent in work capacity with VDD compared with VVI pacing ($p < 0.001$) (Fig. 15–18). During VDD pacing, cardiac output was significantly higher, particularly during exercise, as a result of the capability for heart rate increase and despite a substantial compensatory increase in stroke volume during VVI pacing. Similarly, AV oxygen difference and arterial blood lactate levels were much greater during VVI pacing than during VDD pacing

(Fig. 15–19). Finally, in response to a patient questionnaire, 10 of 15 patients felt that VDD pacing removed their limits on physical exercise (Fig. 15–20). Although similar data have been reported by Karlof, also from Sweden, the results need to be confirmed in other centers with larger patient groups and with substratification data on cardiac diagnosis and baseline function.[15]

In summary, current data strongly support a role for advanced-grade pacemakers. As devices with physiologic sensors other than changing atrial rate and single-lead systems that are not 1:1 AV synchronous but still rate responsive become available, further hemodynamic and long-term follow-up studies will need to be performed so that the patient populations best suited to particular devices can be defined.

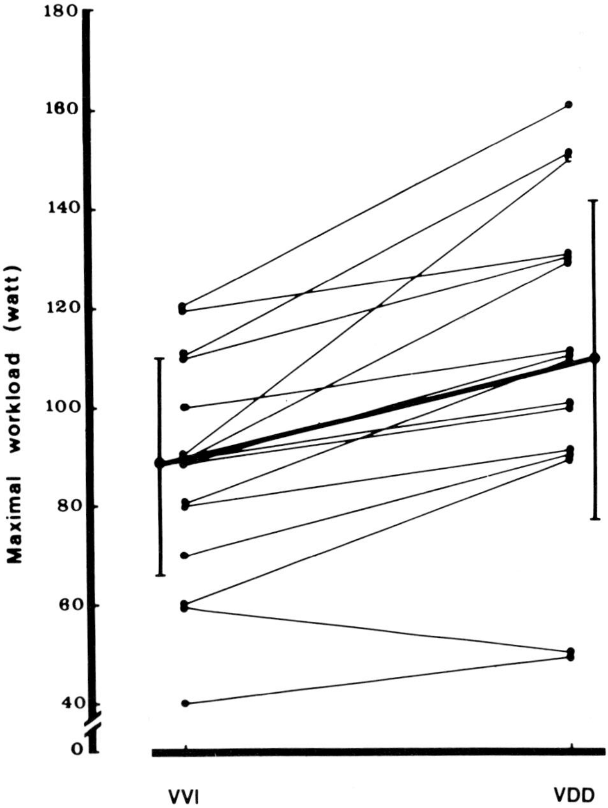

Figure 15–18. Maximal work capacity with ventricular inhibited and atrial synchronous ventricular inhibited pacing. In this study each patient served as his own control. Individual data and the mean ±SD for the group (heavy line) are shown. (Reproduced from Kruse et al: Circulation 65:849, 1982, by permission of the American Heart Association, Inc.)

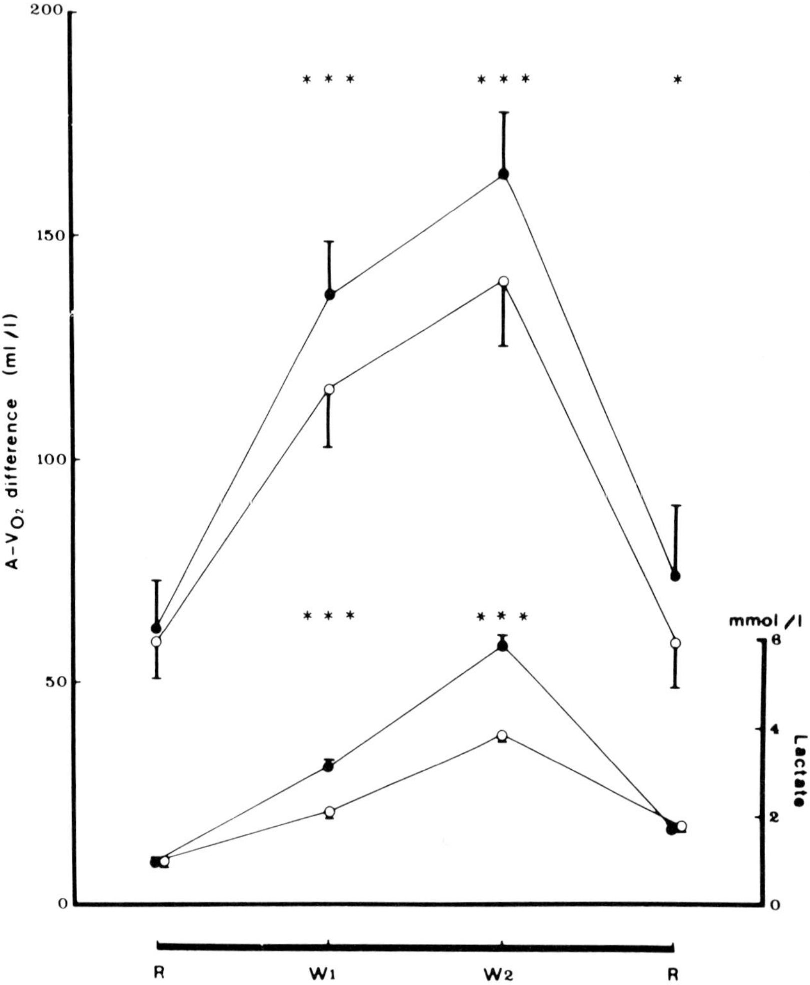

Figure 15–19. Arteriovenous oxygen difference and blood lactate during rest and exercise with ventricular inhibited and atrial synchronous ventricular inhibited pacing. The closed circles represent VVI pacing and the open circles VDD pacing. Note the lower lactate production and AV O_2 difference during VDD pacing. (Reproduced from Kruse et al: Circulation 65:851, 1982, by permission of the American Heart Association, Inc.)

COMPLICATIONS OF DUAL-CHAMBER PACEMAKERS

There is no question that the inherent complexity of dual-chamber devices increases (1) the likelihood of mechanical problems related to the leads and pulse generators, (2) the frequency of confusing EKG patterns during both normal and abnormal operation, and (3) the possibility of pacemaker-induced rhythm disorders. Furthermore, since not all DVI and DDD pacemakers have the same specifications, proper programming and follow-up can be difficult and time-

General Condition on Ventricular Inhibited and Atrial Synchronous Ventricular Inhibited Pacing

Class	General condition	Pacing mode: VVI	Pacing mode: VDD
I	Fine (no physical restriction)	1	11
II	Fair (some physical restriction)	13	5
III	Bad (very restricted)	2	

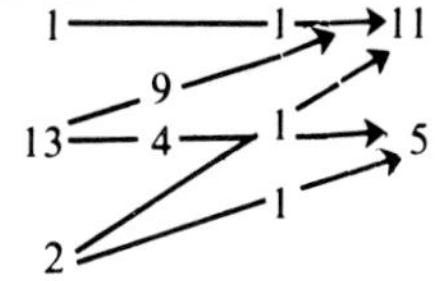

Figure 15–20. Change in symptoms associated with ventricular inhibited and atrial synchronous ventricular inhibited pacing. Note that 11 of the 16 patients felt subjectively improved with changeover to the VDD mode. (Reproduced from Kruse et al: Circulation 65:851, 1982, by permission of the American Heart Association, Inc.)

consuming. Parsonnet has demonstrated, for example, that there are over 42 million potential programming combinations in the Cordis DDD Gemini 415A (Fig. 15–21).[1] Moreover, several programmers have been discovered to have design abnormalities that would allow abnormal sequences to be programmed or lock in rates not intended by the user.

For physicians following patients with dual-chamber devices, the most important problems involve EKG interpretation of function. Therefore, in the

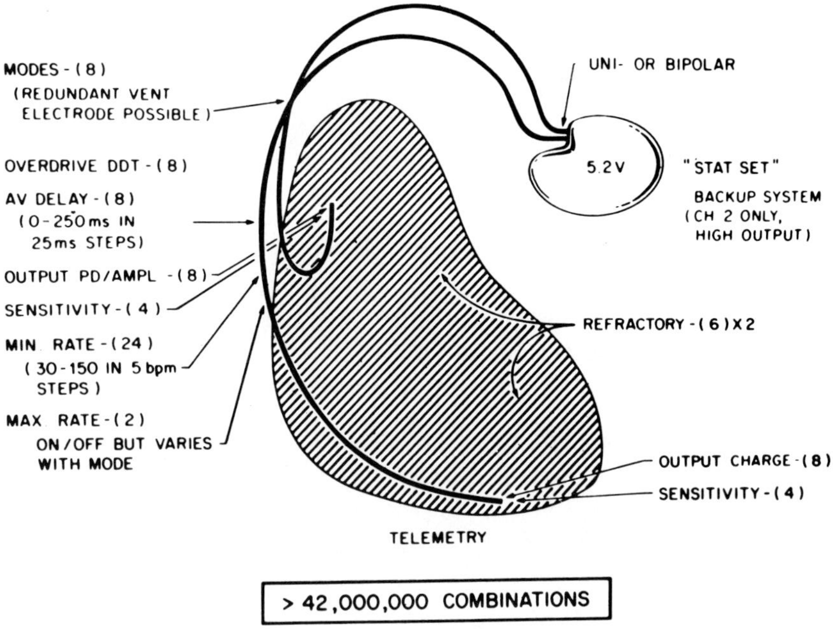

Figure 15–21. Schematic representation of the Cordis Gemini 415A DDD pacemaker. The vast number of potential programming combinations contributes to the complexity of such devices. (Reproduced from Parsonnet and Bernstein: JACC 1:341, 1983, by permission of Elsevier Publishing Co., Inc.)

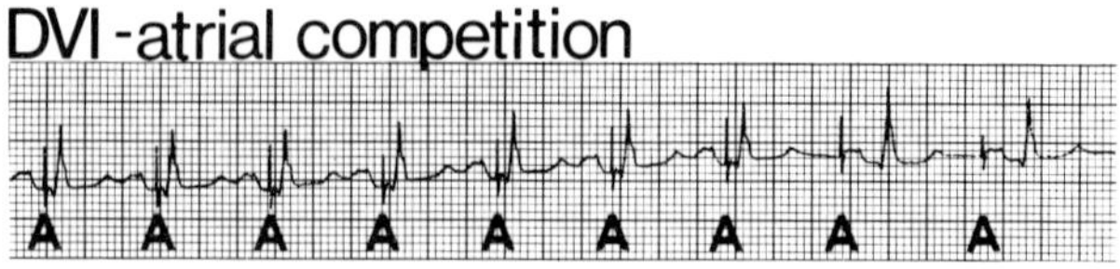

Figure 15–22. Atrial competition during DVI pacing. This pacemaker is programmed to a rate of 80 beats/min or 750 msec and an AV interval of 250 msec. The resultant VA interval is therefore 500 msec. This means that an atrial spike will be emitted 500 msec following a sensed QRS unless another QRS occurs. As a consequence, atrial spikes fall in close relationship to P waves on beats 1 to 7. As the atrial rate slows on beats 8 and 9 atrial capture results. No ventricular spikes are seen because this noncommitted device senses naturally occurring QRS's during the long programmed AV interval of 250 msec.

following section we will concentrate on EKG troubleshooting and the analysis of pacemaker-related arrhythmias.

DVI Mode

One of the most common and least understood manifestations of DVI pacing is atrial competition, a natural consequence of the inability of such devices to sense atrially and the interaction between the VA interval and the patient's intrinsic rate. The VA interval is determined by the pacing rate and AV interval programmed (Fig. 15–22). For example, if the pacing rate is set at 70 beats per minute (857 msec) and the AV interval at 150 msec, the resultant VA interval will be 707 msec. This means that 707 msec after a ventricular sensed or paced event, an atrial spike will be emitted regardless of the patient's own atrial activity, unless a sensed ventricular event occurs. A ventricular spike may or may not be emitted after the atrial spike, depending on whether a committed or noncommitted system is in use. When analyzing EKG strips in patients with DVI pacers, therefore, one must know the rate and AV interval programmed, convert the rate to milliseconds by dividing beats per minute into 60,000, and subtract the AV interval to arrive at the VA interval. By this method, one can determine during periods of atrial competition whether pacer function is normal or abnormal.

Lack of atrial sensing and atrial competition can result in the induction of atrial arrhythmias, especially atrial fibrillation. Furman and Cooper reported that 5 of 31 patients (16 percent) with recently implanted DVI pacemakers developed new-onset atrial fibrillation and suggested that pacemakers with atrial sensing capability are preferable (Fig. 15–23).[45] Other authors have not confirmed this high an incidence of induced atrial fibrillation, but it certainly can occur in this setting and must be considered when selecting an AV sequential pacing mode, especially for patients with a prior history of atrial arrhythmias.

VDD/DDD Modes

The addition of atrial sensing to dual-chamber pacemakers establishes the electrophysiologic milieu necessary for the development of AV reentrant tachy-

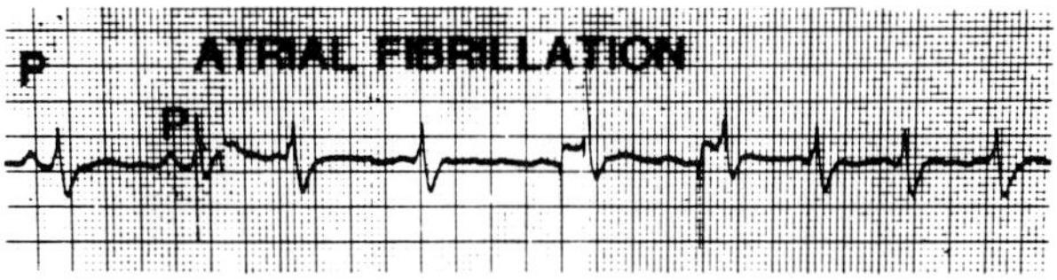

Figure 15–23. Induction of atrial fibrillation by a DVI pacemaker. Lack of atrial sensing, inherent to such devices, results in induction of atrial fibrillation when a pacemaker stimulus falls in the atrial "vulnerable period." (Reproduced from Furman and Cooper: PACE 5:134, 1982, by permission of Futura Publishing Co., Inc.)

cardia, in a manner analogous to the Wolff-Parkinson-White syndrome.[46–49] In pacemaker patients, this arrhythmia has been nicknamed "pacemaker-mediated" or "endless loop" tachycardia.[49] With a dual-chamber system in place there are two antegrade routes to the ventricle (the pacemaker and the AV node and His-Purkinje system) but only one retrograde route to the atrium (the His-Purkinje system and AV node), since no conduction can occur retrogradely through the pacemaker itself. If the retrograde conduction time (VA interval) through the normal conduction system is longer than the atrial refractory period of the pacemaker (the time following ventricular paced or sensed events during which atrial sensing will not occur), pacemaker-mediated supraventricular tachycardia can occur (Fig. 15–24). For example, a premature ventricular beat may be conducted through the His-Purkinje system and AV node retrogradely to the atrium, where activity will be sensed if it occurs outside the atrial refractory period. Following the programmed AV interval, the ventricle is then restimulated via the pacemaker. This activity then again conducts retrogradely, is again sensed in the atrium, and a reentrant circuit is established. Similarly, an atrial premature beat may be blocked antegradely in the AV node or His-Purkinje system so that antegrade conduction must occur over the pacemaker. Activity may then spread retrogradely to the His bundle or AV node, both of which by this time are no longer refractory and can conduct. If the VA interval is long enough and exceeds the atrial refractory period, retrogradely returning atrial activation will be sensed and a reentrant tachycardia may be initiated. These events are shown graphically in Figure 15–25. In some cases even small spontaneous changes in sinus cycle length can produce antegrade AV block and allow a tachycardia to develop.

Many case reports describing pacemaker-mediated tachycardia have appeared in the literature. Pacemakers with short atrial refractory periods are

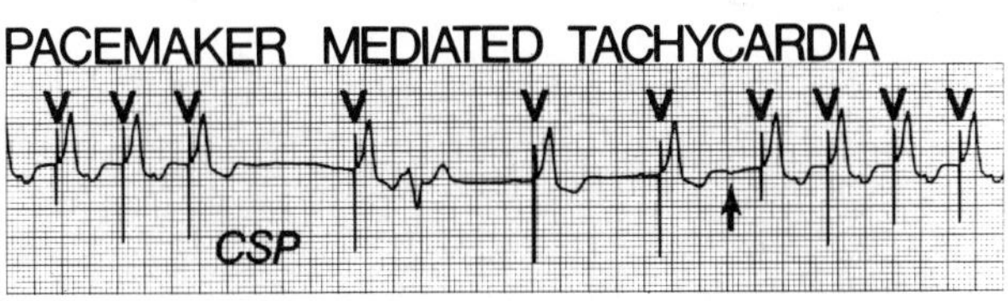

Figure 15–24. Termination and reinitiation of pacemaker-mediated tachycardia. In this patient an episode of pacemaker-mediated tachycardia was readily terminated by carotid sinus pressure (CSP), which produced retrograde AV nodal block. However, the tachycardia was easily reinitiated by a spontaneous APD (marked with an arrow), which blocked antegradely in the AV node and conducted to the ventricle via the pacemaker.

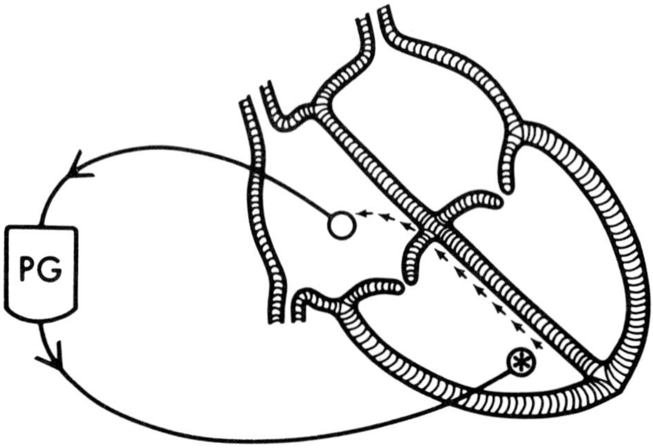

Figure 15–25. Schematic diagram of the mechanism of pacemaker-mediated tachycardia. The open circle denotes sensing; and the circle with the asterisk, sensing and pacing. Each time the ventricle is depolarized by the pacer stimulus, the impulse is retrogradely conducted to the right atrium and detected by the atrial electrode. The pacemaker then triggers the next stimulus into the ventricle and cycle is repeated. (Reproduced from Tolentino et al: PACE 5:258, 1982, by permission of Futura Publishing Co., Inc.)

obviously most prone to the problem. Although the exact frequency with which pacemaker-mediated tachycardia occurs is unknown, Parsonnet and Bernstein state that 50 percent of the Medtronic Versatrax units implanted at Newark Beth Israel Hospital had to be reprogrammed from the DDD to DVI mode to avoid paroxysmal tachycardia.[1] The Versatrax has an atrial refractory period of only 155 msec. Newer DDD pacers employ either a programmable atrial refractory period, which allows selection of an interval appropriate to the patient, or automatic refractory period extension following a premature ventricular contraction (e.g., Versatrax II), which requires no programming yet still allows a long enough refractory period to prevent reentrant arrhythmias in the majority of patients.

Several studies have demonstrated that VA conduction is intact in approximately two-thirds of patients with sinus node dysfunction and 14 to 35 percent of patients with complete heart block.[51–53] This means that 50 percent of all patients receiving VDD/DDD pacemakers may be prone to pacemaker-mediated tachycardia. Hayes and Furman recently reported a series of 53 patients in whom they analyzed VA conduction during incremental pacing.[54] The mean VA conduction time was 235 msec, with a range of 110 to 380 msec. The authors then used this information to select and program specific DDD devices; subsequently no patient developed pacemaker-mediated tachycardia. Despite this report, most investigators have found that measurements made at the time of implantation have little bearing on future conduction patterns because of day-to-day changes in resting vagal tone, heart rate, and other factors. Moreover, since most pacemaker-mediated tachycardia is initiated by ventricular premature beats, further studies need to be performed using the ventricular extrastimulus technique to evaluate VA conduction, before Hayes's findings can be accepted.[53]

It is likely that V to A times will be longer with premature beats than during straight ventricular pacing, because His-Purkinje refractoriness shortens with pacing but not with ventricular premature beats. It is doubtful that conduction studies will generate one number that represents an upper limit of V to A time for all patients. Rather it should be realized that **most** patients have VA times less than 350 msec and that pacemakers that allow the atrial refractory period to be programmable or to extend automatically following premature beats are preferable.

Another consequence of atrial sensing and intact VA conduction is the potential for the development of ventricular arrhythmias. Freedman and colleagues reported such a patient with a Medtronic 2409 ASVIP pacemaker who developed sustained ventricular tachycardia partially mediated by the pacemaker (Fig. 15–26).[50] Ventricular premature beats that are conducted retrogradely may be sensed in the atrium and allow the ventricle to be restimulated, essentially producing a ventricular couplet. In patients with poor ventricular function and coronary artery disease who are prone to life-threatening ventricular arrhythmias, this can allow arrhythmia initiation. The ASVIP had three features designed to prevent such events: (1) ventricular sensing with ventricular-inhibited escape, (2) an atrial refractory period of 170 msec, and (3) a limit on the maximum rate at which ventricular stimuli will follow atrial depolarizations, programmable from 150 to 175 paced beats per minute. Despite this, however, sustained ventricular tachycardia still occurred in the patient presented. Newer DDD pacers with longer and programmable atrial refractory periods will make close coupling intervals less likely and further reduce the potential for ventricular tachycardia induction.

One of the normal features of VDD/DDD pacemakers that is poorly understood and frequently leads to confusing EKGs is called "upper rate behavior." Each VDD/DDD device must include a logic system to respond to atrial arrhythmias, such as atrial flutter, in a non-1:1 pattern to avoid ventricular stimulation at high rates. Figure 15–27 shows the upper rate response of the Medtronic Versatrax, a pseudo form of Wenckebach periodicity. Other units go into a 2:1 block mode once the programmed upper rate limit is exceeded. For an exercising patient (swimming toward the deep end of a pool, for instance) this may be quite dangerous. One must therefore be sure to select for such patients an upper rate limit that is beyond their predicted physical capability.

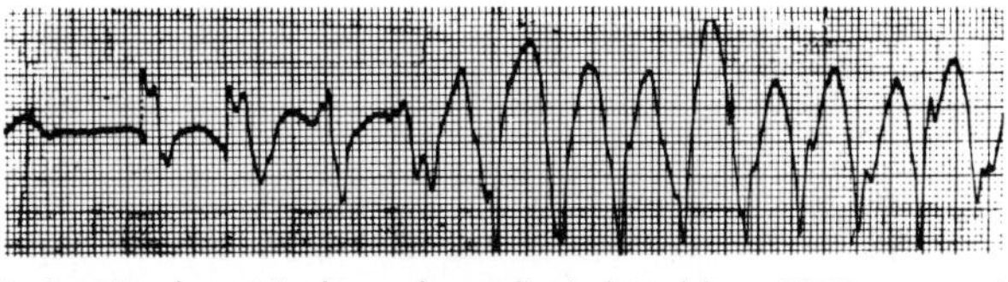

Figure 15–26. Sustained ventricular tachycardia induced by a VDD pacemaker. The first beat is a paced ventricular escape beat. This is followed by an early atrial synchronously paced beat on which the P wave is not well seen. Sustained ventricular tachycardia results. (Reproduced from Freedman et al: PACE 5:492, 1982, by permission of Futura Publishing Co., Inc.)

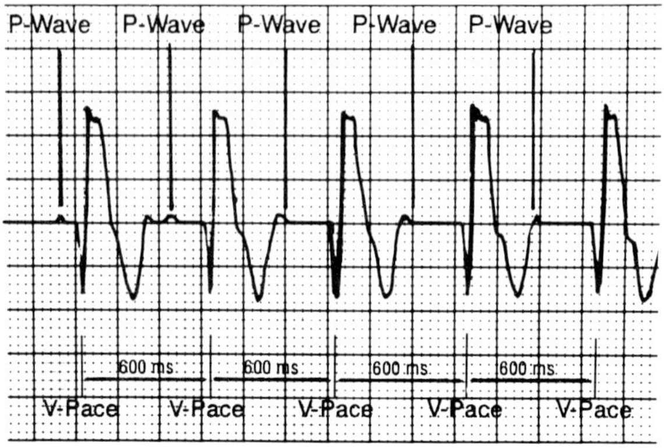

Figure 15–27. Upper rate behavior of the Medtronic Versatrax. The programmed upper rate for this particular individual was 100 beats/min or 600 msec. Once the spontaneous atrial rate exceeded this programmed maximum rate the pacemaker responded with gradual lengthening of the PR interval to maintain the rate at 100 beats/min. (Reproduced from Medtronic ECG Interpretation Guide, p. 58, 1983, by permission of Medtronic, Inc.)

One pacemaker, the Cordis Sequicor, allows the user to choose between a 2:1 block response and a programmable "fallback" response in which the pacer automatically shifts from atrial-synchronized ventricular pacing to the ventricular demand mode. The ventricular rate then gradually decreases until the programmable fallback rate is achieved. Pacing continues at the fallback rate in the VVI mode until the atrial rate falls below the maximum rate by 5 to 10 paced beats per minute. Interestingly enough, however, most patients with implanted Sequicors have eventually been programmed to the 2:1 block mode to avoid induction of pacemaker-mediated tachycardia.

Finally, EKG analysis of pacemaker malfunction is much more difficult with dual-chamber than with single-chamber devices. Figure 15–28 is an example of the confusing patterns that can be produced by units such as the Cordis Gemini 415A DDD pacer, which shows intermittent loss of atrial sensing. Normally the pacemaker senses the atrium and paces the ventricle (beats 1, 2, 4, and 7). When atrial sensing is lost (beats 3, 5, and 6) the pacemaker reverts to the noncommitted DVI mode, since it assumes that P waves are absent. Because the patient retains his own escape rhythm, beats 3 and 5 are partial fusions. On beat 7, only an atrial spike is emitted, since a sensed QRS occurs outside the atrial refractory period.

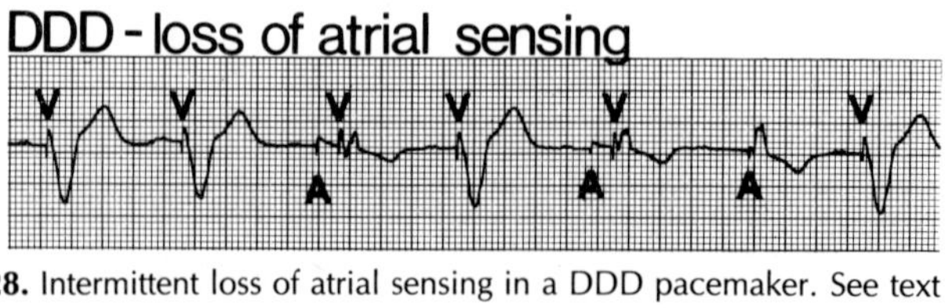

Figure 15–28. Intermittent loss of atrial sensing in a DDD pacemaker. See text for explanation.

CONCLUSIONS

In summary, dual-chamber pacing for bradyarrhythmias makes physiologic sense, is technically achievable, and has proven symptomatic and hemodynamic advantages over single-chamber pacemakers for properly selected patients. It also certainly requires a major physician commitment to understanding the use of such units and the potential for device-related complications.

ANTITACHYCARDIA PACING: AN OVERVIEW

The treatment of recurrent supraventricular and ventricular tachycardia or fibrillation using either conventional or experimental antiarrhythmic drugs remains the preferred approach to therapy but is frequently limited by drug inefficacy, patient intolerance, or noncompliance. Moreover, in patients with ventricular tachyarrhythmias, a single episode of drug failure may result in sudden cardiac death. Surgery remains a second option but requires a specialized facility capable of sophisticated catheter and intraoperative activation mapping and, for many patients, is ruled out because of global pump dysfunction or inaccessible tachycardia circuitry. Therefore, implantable antitachycardia pacemakers have become a viable third option for properly selected subjects.

Invasive electrophysiologic studies using intracardiac recording and stimulation techniques have added greatly to our understanding of the mechanism of human tachyarrhythmias and demonstrated that most supraventricular and ventricular tachycardias may be reliably initiated and terminated.[55, 56] These studies have allowed various pacing modalities to be examined under controlled conditions and have undoubtedly been responsible for the recent advance in pacing therapy for tachyarrhythmias.[21, 25]

As currently conceived, implantable devices may be used to prevent, ameliorate, or terminate tachyarrhythmias.[21, 57] Since most sustained tachyarrhythmias are thought to be reentrant in mechanism and therefore amenable to termination, the greatest attention has been paid to, and in fact the greatest success found in, pacing termination of established arrhythmias. The following factors have been found to affect the ability to terminate reentrant arrhythmias using timed stimuli: (1) the size and site of the tachycardia circuit, (2) the distance between the site of stimulation and the site of the tachycardia circuit, (3) the rate of the tachycardia and the timing of stimulation relative to the tachycardia, (4) the electrophysiologic properties of the tissues between the site of stimulation and the tachycardia circuit, (5) the number of stimuli, and (6) the energy of stimulation.[25, 58]

Coupled with improvements in lead design and pacemaker technology, these concepts have allowed the development of antitachycardia implantable

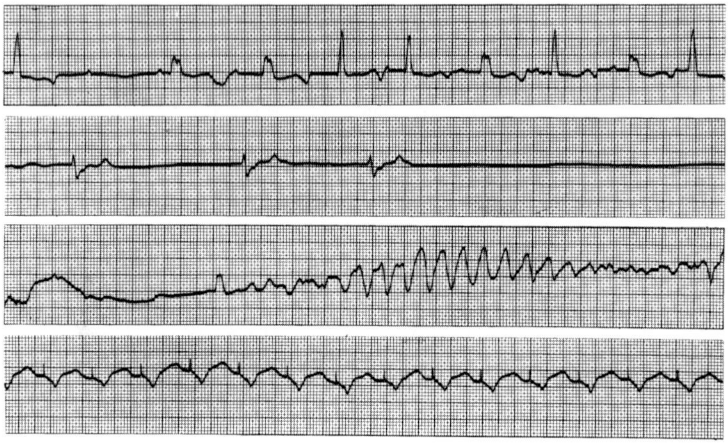

Figure 15–29. Rate support for tachycardia prevention. This patient developed ventricular fibrillation in association with heart block and asystole. Simply maintaining heart rate by pacing prevented arrhythmia reccurrence.

units that provide a definite alternative to antiarrhythmic drugs and surgery. In this section we will examine the various pacing techniques now in use or under investigation, identify available devices and their proper application, and consider current limitations.

Tachycardia Prevention

Rate Support

Patients with bradycardiac rhythms due either to sick sinus syndrome or to high-grade AV block frequently suffer from supraventricular or ventricular tachyarrhythmias or both. In some of these patients tachyarrhythmias can be prevented simply by increasing the heart rate by pacing (Fig. 15–29). Stabilization of heart rate also allows the use of antiarrhythmic agents without fear of further depressing the rate.

Overdrive Suppression

In some patients the number of premature beats may be reduced by pacing at a rate slightly faster than the spontaneous rhythm. However, this form of therapy, even if effective on a temporary basis, is rarely effective chronically, and it is important to realize that there is no direct relationship between the presence of premature beats and the development of sustained tachycardia. Moreover, in patients with ischemic heart disease, pacing may actually result in an increase in arrhythmia.

In patients with the long-QT syndrome, overdrive suppression may be an especially effective temporary therapy, although β-blocking agents remain the basis of chronic treatment (Fig. 15–30). Occasionally, permanent pacing can be effectively applied to such patients but should be undertaken only when temporary pacing has demonstrated long-term reliability and drug therapy is contraindicated.[59]

Dual Site Stimulation

In patients with paroxysmal supraventricular tachycardia, AV pacing may theoretically prevent recurrences of arrhythmia by producing impulse collision in a region of slow conduction, thereby precluding the development of reentrant beats. Studies by Coumel and colleagues, Spurrell and Sowton, Castellanos and colleagues, and Sung and colleagues have demonstrated the efficacy of several programmable pacers (either VAT or DVI in type) set to deliver relatively short AV intervals in preventing arrhythmia recurrences.[23, 33, 60, 61] There are however several major disadvantages to this technique, including (1) the risk that closely coupled ventricular beats may result from atrial premature depolarizations; (2) the possibility that atrial tachycardia may be "tracked," resulting in rapid ventricular rates; and (3) the development of adverse hemodynamics secondary to AV pacing with a short AV delay. Few of these devices have actually ever been implanted.

Tachycardia Amelioration

Continuous Overdrive Pacing

In patients with incessant supraventricular tachycardias, atrial pacing at rates sufficient to produce AV block and a reduction in ventricular rate may

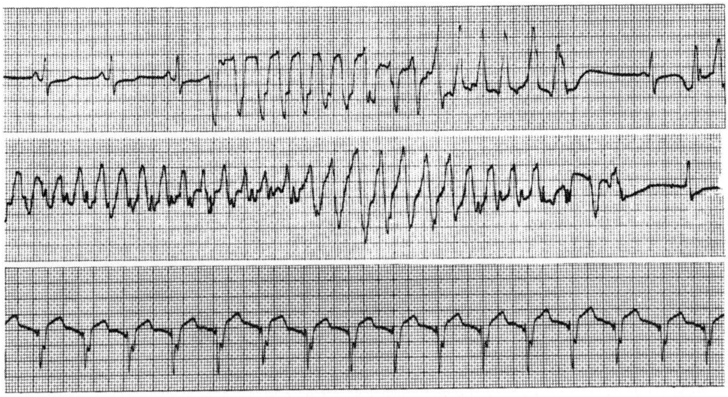

Figure 15–30. Overdrive suppression for long QT syndrome. In this patient, episodes of torsades de pointes occurred in association with familial long QT syndrome. Simple ventricular pacing temporarily prevented recurrence of this arrhythmia until a beta-blocking agent could be started.

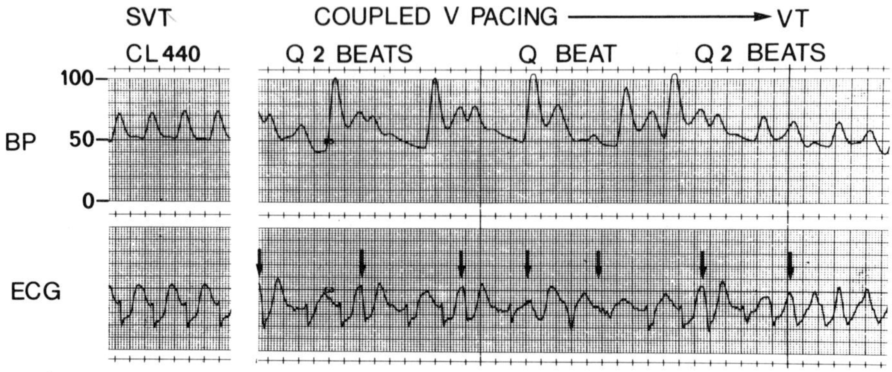

Figure 15–31. Precipitation of ventricular tachycardia during coupled ventricular pacing. This patient had an incessant supraventricular tachycardia with a LBBB/LAD configuration and a systolic blood pressure of 70 that was resistant to conventional therapy. Coupled ventricular pacing was initiated with a favorable hemodynamic response. However, sensing problems developed in the stimulator, resulting in periodic stimulation after every second tachycardia beat, and ventricular tachycardia ensued. (Reproduced from Fisher et al. Am J Cardiol 49:196, 1982, by permission of Technical Publishing Co.)

ameliorate symptoms.[62] Although occasional success has been reported with this technique, for the most part, powerful β-blocking and calcium-blocking antiarrhythmic agents in combination with digitalis have made such an approach unnecessary.

Paired and Coupled Pacing

In paired pacing an initial stimulus (S1) is followed by a second stimulus (S2) in such a way that the S1-S2 interval is shorter than the S2-S1 interval.[21, 63] In coupled pacing, the patient's own depolarization becomes the S1 and the pacing stimulus becomes the S2, which is delivered to the ventricle and critically timed to produce an electrical but no mechanical response. Using this technique the tachycardia continues at an essentially unchanged rate, but mechanical responses are halved (Fig. 15–31). Again this technique has little practical application given newer antiarrhythmic agents, and carries with it the risk of precipitating ventricular tachycardia or fibrillation.

Pacing for Tachycardia Termination

Timed Stimuli

In 1967 Durrer and colleagues established that critically coupled premature beats were capable of terminating supraventricular tachycardia in selected patients with AV bypass tracts.[64] Since then, many studies have demonstrated similar findings for both paroxysmal supraventricular and recurrent sustained ventricular tachycardia. The explanation given for this phenomenon has been penetration of the reentrant circuit by the induced premature beat with creation of a region of refractoriness ahead of the advancing wave front. Block presumably develops in that part of the reentrant circuit with the longest functional refractory period and results in termination of the tachycardia. Ward and colleagues have shown that single extrastimuli are most successful in terminating tachycardias whose circuitry involves the stimulated chamber.[65] Rowlands and colleagues have shown that single extrastimuli and underdrive pacing are generally ineffective in terminating supraventricular tachycardia of the AV nodal reentrant type, presumably because single remote extrastimuli cannot penetrate a small circuit.[66] Further, Wellens and colleagues have demonstrated that unless the reentrant loop is large, as in arrhythmias incorporating an AV bypass tract, multiple extrastimuli are required for termination once the tachycardia rate exceeds 160 beats per minute.[25]

There are many pacing techniques that result in delivery of timed single or multiple extrastimuli. Slow competitive or underdrive pacing is the simplest form and may be readily accomplished by placement of a magnet over an AAI or VVI pacemaker, thereby converting it to the asynchronous AOO or VOO mode (Fig. 15–32). For patients who do not require bradycardia support, this form of pacing may also be accomplished by implantation of a radio-frequency pacemaker set to a slow rate. In this device the power supply is a simple 9-volt battery that is incorporated into the handheld transmitter (see below, Available Devices). Underdrive pacing (as well as many other pacing modes) can also be performed using experimental devices like the Cordis Omni-Orthocor, which functions as a demand pacer that can be converted to the triggered mode using a magnet that is incorporated into an overdriver. The overdriver is a software programmable

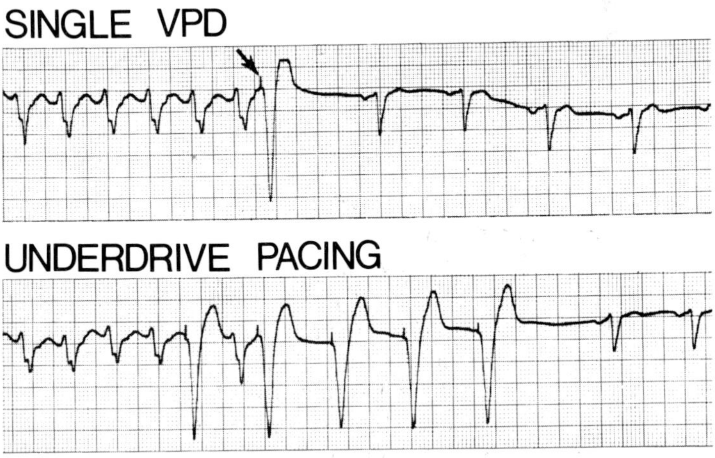

Figure 15–32. Termination of ventricular tachycardia by underdrive pacing. In this patient, during electrophysiologic testing, single ventricular extrastimuli were able to reproducibly terminate ventricular tachycardia. Therefore, a VVI pacemaker was implanted and activated by the patient using a magnet to the VOO mode during clinical episodes of sustained tachycardia. Successful termination of the arrhythmia was readily achieved when a single capture occurred at the appropriate coupling interval.

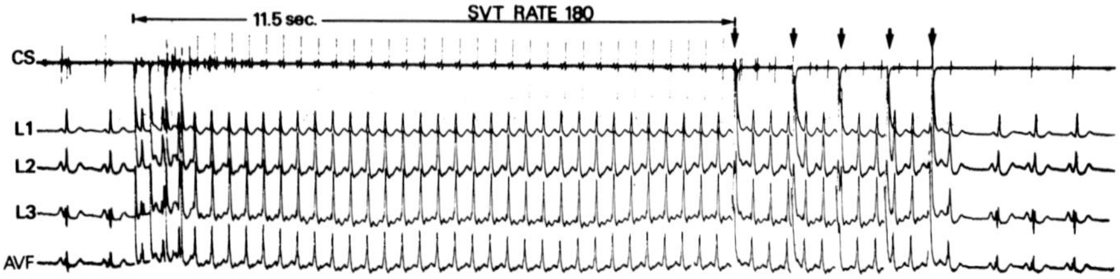

Figure 15–33. Termination of supraventricular tachycardia by an "upside-down demand" underdrive pacemaker. Surface ECG leads are displayed along with a coronary sinus (CS) electrogram. The tachycardia is initiated on the left with programmed extrastimuli. After a tachycardia confirmation period of 11.5 seconds the device paces into the arrhythmia at an average rate of 70 beats/min. Pacing continues until termination of the SVT which in this case occurred after 5 complexes. (Reproduced from Fisher et al: Am J Cardiol 49:197, 1982, by permission of Technical Publishing Co.)

stimulator that delivers a prescribed pacing sequence once activated by the patient or physician (see below, Available Devices).

Automatic versions of underdrive pacemakers include dual demand and reverse mode or "upside-down" demand pacers. A dual demand pacemaker operates as a standard demand device to prevent bradycardia. During tachycardia, this unit is automatically activated to pace at the same rate as the demand rate until the tachycardia terminates. Upside-down pacemakers respond automatically to tachycardia with slow competitive pacing but have no bradycardiac function (Fig. 15–33). It should be emphasized that all devices for underdrive pacing are applicable only to patients whose tachyarrhythmias can be demonstrated to be consistently terminated by single ventricular extrastimuli during electrophysiologic study and who can tolerate their tachycardias without hemodynamic embarrassment.

Recently devices have become available that can deliver single or multiple extrastimuli at specified coupling intervals during tachycardia. The Cordis Omni-Orthocor is one such system that can deliver as many as three extrastimuli using the patient-activated stimulator discussed above. In this system the coupling intervals do not change automatically but can be readily altered using the computer program. The Medtronic Interactive Tachycardia Terminating System is a similar system conceptually but can also scan the cardiac cycle with extrastimuli (see below, Available Devices). In this device changes in the program must be made at the factory. Spurrell and colleagues have recently designed an implantable extrastimulus pacemaker capable of automatically detecting tachycardia and scanning the cardiac cycle with as many as two independently adjustable extrastimuli (see Available Devices) (Fig. 15–34).[31] Finally, Fisher and colleagues and Spurrell and Sowton have described systems that deliver a short train of extremely rapid stimuli at coupling intervals of 2 to 40 msec, timed to begin during the refractory period and calculated to have a duration resulting in a single capture.[67, 68] However, inherent in this system is the risk of the development of unwanted new arrhythmias. It is of course essential that electrophysiologic testing that demonstrates reliable termination of the tachyarrhythmias

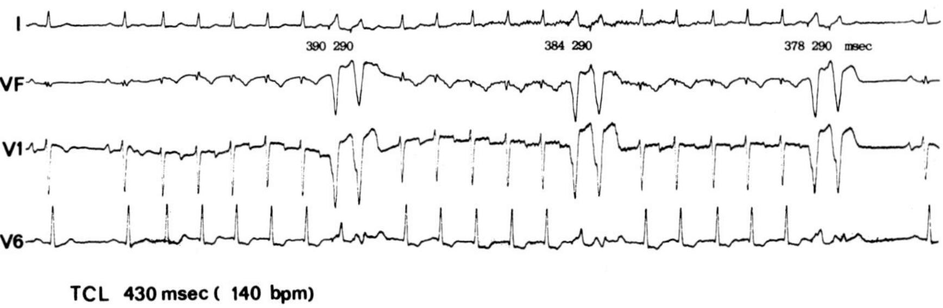

Figure 15–34. Termination of supraventricular tachycardia by double scanning extrastimuli. A spontaneous episode of tachycardia occurs after the second sinus beat. The arrhythmia is terminated by two ventricular premature beats with a coupling interval of 378 and 290 msec, respectively. (Reproduced from Spurrell et al: Am J Cardiol 49:757, 1982, by permission of Technical Publishing Co.)

under study by premature extrastimuli be performed prior to placement of any of these pacemakers.

Overdrive Pacing

This technique consists of pacing at a rate above the tachycardia rate and can be successful when single or double extrastimuli are not (Fig. 15–35). It is assumed that shortening of the refractory period at the site of stimulation induced by the rapid paced rate enables shorter coupling intervals to reach and potentially invade and terminate the reentrant circuit.

The most commonly employed form of overdrive pacing is simple burst pacing in which multiple stimuli are delivered at a fixed stimulus-to-stimulus interval. Bursts may be coupled to the tachycardia or asynchronous and may vary in rate and number of stimuli. On a temporary basis, burst pacing is an excellent technique for acute termination of atrial flutter, especially in patients with lung disease in whom anesthesia poses a risk and in patients who are just recovering from cardiac surgery.[69] On a permanent basis, radio-frequency pacers have been the most frequently used devices for delivery of asynchronous, manually activated bursts.[22, 32, 34, 35] Newer implantable pacemakers have now

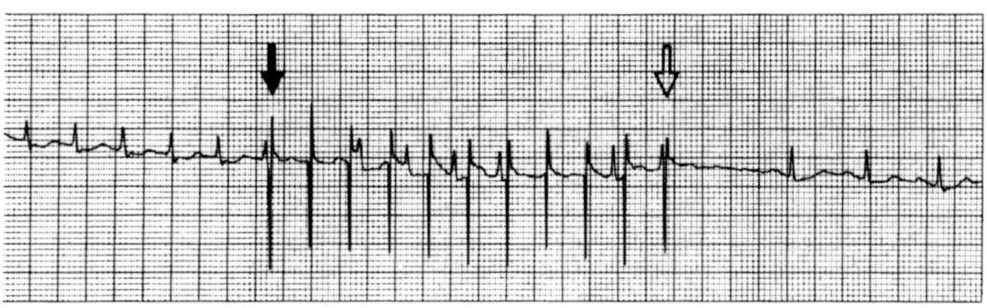

Figure 15–35. Termination of supraventricular tachycardia by "burst" pacing. Re-entrant supraventricular tachycardia is present at the beginning of the strip. An asynchronous burst of 11 stimuli at a rate of 200/min successfully terminates the arrhythmia.

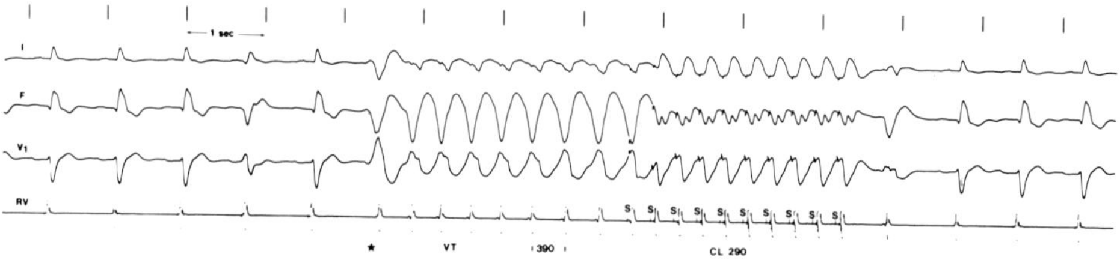

Figure 15–36. Termination of ventricular tachycardia by automatic burst pacing using the Intermedics Cybertach. Surface ECG leads and a right ventricular electrogram are displayed. Ventricular tachycardia with a cycle length of 390 msec (155 bpm) is initiated by a premature ventricular beat. When the R wave following the eighth short interval is sensed, the pacemaker begins pacing at a cycle length of 295 msecs (206 bpm). With cessation of pacing sinus rhythm is restored. (Reproduced from Griffen et al: PACE 4:584, by permission of Futura Publishing Co., Inc.)

become available that can deliver bursts automatically (see below, Available Devices) (Fig. 15–36). Ramp or autodecremental pacing is another form of overdrive pacing, but in this technique the stimulus-to-stimulus intervals vary continuously in a systematic fashion, either up or down.

The principal hazard of bursts of rapid pacing is in the application of this technique to ventricular arrhythmias, where one risks acceleration of the tachycardia or induction of ventricular fibrillation (Fig. 15–37). Fisher described these complications in 4 percent of attempts to terminate arrhythmias with bursts.[21] More importantly, however, such episodes occurred at least once in 43 percent of these patients. Although in this series accleration could be avoided by changing the rate or duration of the terminating burst or by altering the patients' antiarrhythmic drug regimen, most investigators continue to be concerned about the risks of implantable burst pacemakers as a primary chronic therapy.

Cardioversion and Defibrillation

The concept of terminating ventricular fibrillation using an intrathoracic lead system has been extensively evaluated by Mirowski.[29] The current system, the automatic implantable defibrillator (AID), relies on a sensing circuit that

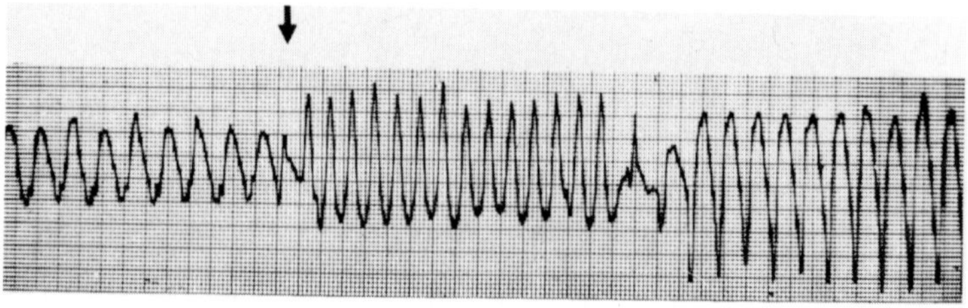

Figure 15–37. Acceleration of ventricular tachycardia by burst pacing. Ventricular tachycardia is present at the beginning of the strip. A burst is initiated via a patient-activated hand held device which usually readily terminates the tachycardia. In this instance the arrhythmia is accelerated and results in hemodynamic collapse.

recognizes the absence of isoelectric potential segments and delivers a 25-joule truncated exponential pulse within 15 to 25 seconds of arrhythmia onset (see below, Available Devices) (Fig. 15–38). In 1981 Mirowski reported on 16 patients who had this device implanted.[29] Twenty-five episodes of tachyarrhythmia were documented in the hospital after implantation; 8 occurred spontaneously, and 17 were induced using programmed extrastimuli. All spontaneous arrhythmias and 14 of the 17 induced arrhythmias were correctly identified and converted to normal sinus rhythm. However, in 3 patients spurious discharges have occurred during sinus rhythm, and occasional failure of the device to recycle has also been observed. Mirowski reports that further device refinements have eliminated such problems.

The patient population appropriate to the use of the AID remains to be defined. Certainly it should **not** be implanted in every patient at high risk for sudden cardiac death, as some have suggested. Mirowski's own requirements currently are that patients must have survived at least two cardiac arrests unassociated with myocardial infarction, and ventricular fibrillation must have been documented at least once.[29] In addition, extensive antiarrhythmic drug therapy must have been attempted and failed.

Zipes and colleagues have recently investigated the feasibility of transvenous cardioversion.[26] In an initial series of canine experiments, they used a specially designed transvenous lead and an external cardioverter capable of delivering a truncated exponential waveform 6 msec in duration at 9 different energy levels ranging from 0.0005 to 2.5 joules. In 14 dogs, 3 to 8 days following an acute infarction, 627 episodes of ventricular tachycardia were evaluated. Eighty-three

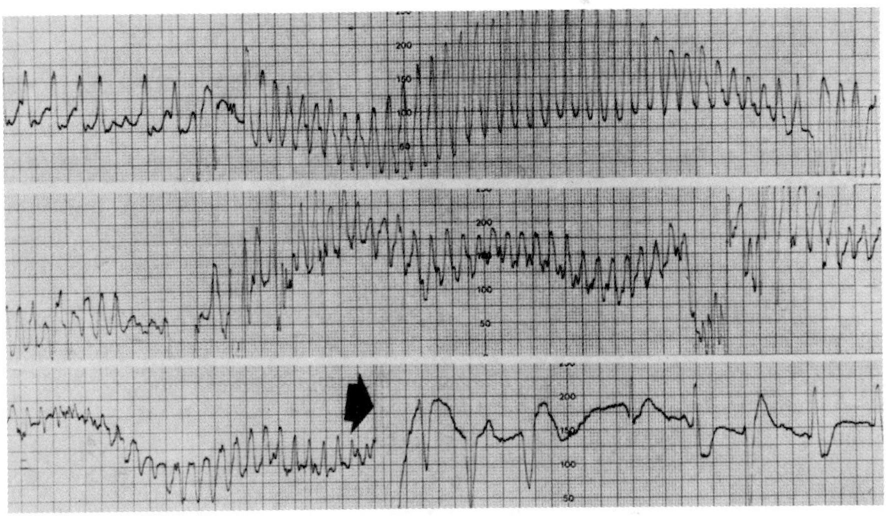

Figure 15–38. Restoration of sinus rhythm by the automatic implantable defibrillator (AID). Ventricular flutter-fibrillation was initiated in this patient by 2 spontaneous ventricular premature beats during atrial fibrillation. The arrhythmia was automatically terminated by a single 25-joule discharge 23 seconds later (arrow). (Reproduced from Mirowski et al: Am Heart J 102:267, 1981, by permission of C. V. Mosby Co.)

percent of the tachycardias having cycle lengths ≥200 msec could be terminated by shocks of 1 joule or less delivered in the first 80 percent of the QRS. Atrial arrhythmias and repetitive ventricular responses were precipitated uncommonly. Faster tachycardias with cycle lengths <200 msec required higher energies, and in 2 cases ventricular fibrillation was induced by shocks of low energy early in the QRS.

Further studies using the same Medtronic 6880 transvenous lead system and a modified Medtronic external cardioverter with 12 energy settings (0.0075 to 2.0 joules) have been performed with human subjects. Zipes and colleagues reported 7 patients with remote infarctions, in 5 of whom the technique was effective with thresholds of between 0.025 and 2.0 joules.[26] Forty-seven of 50 (94 percent) episodes of ventricular tachycardia were terminated, 1 was accelerated, and 2 did not respond prior to hemodynamic compromise.

Direct comparisons between pacing modalities and transvenous cardioversion, using the patient as his own control, are not available as yet. However, most investigators have found that tachycardias with slower rates respond to both techniques and that when cardioversion is effective, pacing is **usually** also effective, as illustrated in Figure 15–39. In faster tachycardias, when pacing is ineffective the cardioverter also tends to be ineffective at tolerable energy settings.

Zipes has found that energies of <0.5 joules are appreciated by the patient as a giant hiccup or a moderate blow to the chest, whereas higher energies

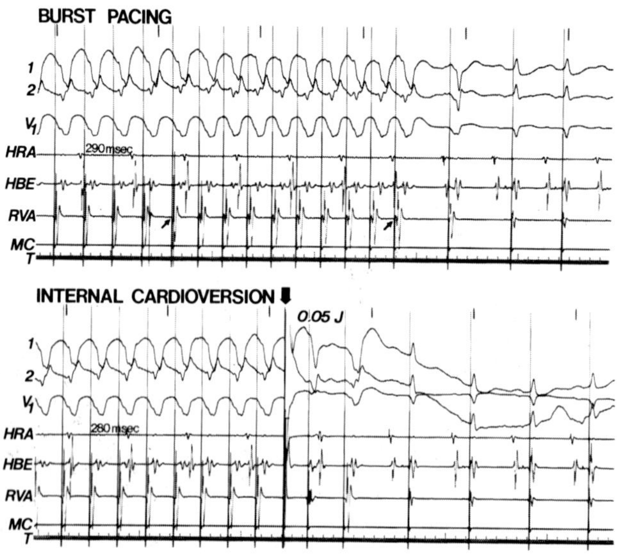

Figure 15–39. Termination of ventricular tachycardia by internal cardioversion. In both panels records are organized as ECG leads 1, 2, and V1 and intracardiac recordings from the high right atrium (HRA), His bundle (HBE), right ventricular apex (RVA), a marker channel (MC), and time lines (TL). Induced ventricular tachycardia is terminated by burst pacing in the upper panel and by a 0.05-joule shock in the lower panel, which the patient described as a slight blow to the chest.

produce greater discomfort. Standard pacing stimulation is generally entirely painless. On the other hand, transvenous cardioversion does not appear to carry the same risks of tachycardia acceleration as does burst pacing and is clearly applicable to patients in whom pacing modalities are ineffective.

Defibrillation and cardioversion techniques require considerably more exploration. The first two implants of the Medtronic Cardioverter have only recently taken place. Indications for the use of such devices remain to be completely developed, and current devices are still undergoing mechanical refinements.

Criteria for Selection of an Antitachycardia Device

With a variety of implantable pacing systems to choose from, as well as several other available therapeutic choices in addition to pacing, it is important that criteria be developed for choosing or rejecting pacing as a chronic therapy. At present, such selection criteria are primarily relevant to tachycardia termination systems.

In our own current decision-making processes, pacemaker therapy is usually considered in the following instances: (1) only after the patient has demonstrated lack of responsiveness to both conventional and experimental medications, as judged by electrophysiologic testing and clinical observation. (However, if the patient has infrequent tachycardia episodes, has demonstrated efficacy with pacing, and prefers not to take antiarrhythmic agents, an implantable device may be used. This applies especially to young patients with paroxysmal supraventricular tachycardia who may have a lifelong requirement for expensive and potentially toxic antiarrhythmic drugs); (2) only if the patient refuses surgery, has a tachyarrhythmia not amenable to surgery, or if the risk of surgery appears greater than the risk of arrhythmia acceleration or failure of termination by a pacing device; and (3) only if the proposed pacing system has been proven efficacious by electrophysiologic testing. This means that the tachycardia must be terminated successfully 50 to 100 times, spread out over several days, either without drugs or on the proposed drug regimen that will be used in conjunction with the pacing system. If a pacemaker is still considered appropriate for a patient in whom occasional failure or termination or acceleration is noted, then a manually activated device used only by a physician would be selected.

Fisher and colleagues have indicated that **manually** activated antitachycardia pacemakers are appropriate for patients whose tachycardias fall into the following categories: (1) non–life-threatening, (2) hemodynamically stable enough to permit the patient time to get to the hospital or activate the device personally, (3) easily recognized by the patient, (4) of varying rates or morphologies that require repeated manipulation of parameters, or (5) are occasionally accelerated by pacing.[21] **Automatic** devices are considered for the following patients: (1) those in whom severe symptoms could develop before a manual unit could be activated, (2) those who are unaware of the tachycardia for long periods of time, (3) those who are physically or mentally incapable of using a manually activated system, or (4) those who prefer automatic activation for psychosocial reasons.[21]

We consider using an implantable defibrillator only in the following patients: (1) those who have had at least one cardiac arrest, (2) those who have reproducibly inducible polymorphic ventricular tachycardia or ventricular fibrillation in the electrophysiology laboratory unresponsive to antiarrhythmic drug testing and inappropriate for standard pacing systems, and (3) those who are not surgical candidates. An implantable cardioverter is relevant to patients with stable recurrent sustained ventricular tachycardia who are (1) unresponsive to drug therapy, (2) poor surgical candidates, (3) have demonstrated inefficacy or acceleration with standard pacing modes, and (4) can tolerate cardioversion without anesthesia. For both of these units the physician must also repeatedly demonstrate device efficacy prior to implantation.

Available Devices

Once having decided that a patient is a candidate for an antitachycardia device, the physician choosing this therapy must be aware of the specific types of devices that can be accessed for implantation. Specific data on currently available (although in many cases still experimental) antitachycardia pacing systems will be presented in the sections that follow.

Medtronic (Model 5998) Radio-Frequency Pacemaker

This device is the most frequently used manually activated burst pacemaker. It is a radio-frequency-coupled stimulator system consisting of an external transmitter and an implantable receiver designed for use with a bipolar myocardial lead system. The transmitter operates on a simple 9-volt battery that can be changed easily. When activated, the transmitter generates a pulse-modulated radio-frequency carrier signal that is coupled (transmitted) to the implanted receiver via the antenna loop located within the transmitter module that is held over the receiver site. The implanted receiver demodulates and filters the transmitted energy and delivers the resultant stimulation pulses to the lead system. The stimulation rate is adjustable from 50 to 400 pulses per minute and is selected simply by turning a screw in the back of the transmitter. The major advantages of this system are its simplicity, the small size of the implanted receiver, and its wide range of selectable pacing rates.

Intermedics Cyberlith

This pacemaker is designed for automatic tachycardia detection and burst pacing termination. It is a multiprogrammable, bipolar, lithium-powered unit that also functions as a standard inhibited pacemaker. The tachycardia terminating response may be inhibited noninvasively. Other programmable features include 2 basic pacing rates (60 and 80 pulses per minute), 15 pulse durations

(0.15 to 2.29 msec), and 7 input sensitivity levels (0.6 to 2.8 mv). The automatic tachycardia terminating features are also programmable. Twenty-eight combinations of burst rate and duration are available, ranging from 180 to 1440 pulses per minute for 0.33 to 5.3 seconds. The presence of an arrhythmia is determined by rate, and this feature is also programmable. Input signals with a rate greater than 350 per minute are rejected as noise, no tachycardia terminating response is delivered, and asychronous pacing is initiated. Magnetization converts the Cyberlith to an asynchronous mode without tachycardia terminating capability.

If a tachyarrhythmia occurs, the event is stored, and on subsequent telemetry a large-amplitude artifact indicates that the pacemaker has sensed a tachycardia since the last programming.

Cordis Omni-Orthocor

This system consists of the Omni-Orthocor 234A implantable pacemaker and external overdriver. The 234A is a lithium-powered unipolar pacemaker with programmable rates (50 to 120 pulses per minute) and current outputs (2 to 9 ma). The refractory period is 350 msec at all programmed rates but shortens to 175 msec in the presence of a magnet, which allows synchronization with external pulses up to a rate of 350 pulses per minute. The overdriver is software computer programmable via the Orthocor Proscriber to (1) deliver up to three timed extrastimuli, (2) burst pace at selectable intervals (160 to 400 msec) and number of pulses (1 to 20), (3) ramp pace with selectable initial and final intervals and rate, and (4) burst pace and give up to three extrastimuli. The overdriver incorporates a magnet that places the pacer in a triggered mode. In the extrastimulus program the overdriver senses the output pulses of the pacemaker and, following depression of the activation button, delivers the preselected therapy. In all other modes, depression of the activation button allows the selected pulse train to be delivered immediately without coupling to intrinsic activity.

The exciting feature of this manually activated pacemaker is its extreme versatility, offering multiple antitachycardia mode selections and allowing an individual patient's pacing needs to be altered with ease should electrophysiologic conditions change.

Teletronics (Model 4151) Pasar

This device is designed for automatic scanning of as many as two extrastimuli. It is a bipolar lithium-powered pacemaker that is fully programmable. A tachycardia is detected when four consecutive cycles are seen by the device at a rate faster than a programmed trigger rate. After the fourth cycle, an extrastimulus is emitted with a preset coupling interval from the preceding sensed intracardiac potential. The first coupling interval can be programmed to 12 different settings between 200 and 390 msec. If tachycardia continues, a further extrastimulus occurs after every four cycles with the coupling interval reduced by 6 msec. This continues for 15 decrements if the tachycardia does not terminate, thereby resulting in scanning 90 msec of the cardiac cycle. If the tachycardia still has not terminated, then the pacemaker recycles and repeats the scan. If two extrastimuli are required for termination, an additional stimulus can be introduced, although with a fixed interstimulus coupling interval (16 choices between 125 and 310 msec).

When one or more appropriately timed premature beats terminates the tachycardia, stimulation stops and the extrastimulus sequence resulting in termination is retained in the pacemaker's memory. At the next onset of tachycardia this sequence is used first.

The pacemaker has three available pulse widths and two available sensitivity settings. There are two trigger rates between 130 and 225 as well as a low trigger rate of 40 to allow testing of the device during sinus rhythm. The Pasar can be deactivated at any time, either by the application of a magnet over the site of implantation or by application of a small personal pocket programmer that emits coded magnetic pulses.

Medtronic Interactive Tachycardia Terminating System

This manually activated system consists of the three following components: (1) an implantable demand pulse generator (nonprogrammable with a base pacing rate of 50 beats per minute) with a magnetically enabled short refractory period and the ability to transmit radio-frequency impulses synchronous with each cardiac cycle and trigger from external radio-frequency signals transmitted from a patient activator; (2) an external control unit (patient activator), which receives impulses from the implanted pacemaker and responds, if tachycardia detection criteria are met, by transmitting radio-frequency signals to activate a previously prescribed tachycardia termination pacing sequence; and (3) a prescription formulator that is an external stimulator used to test potential termination sequences and derive the appropriate pacing technique to be built into the activator. This stimulator can be used at the time of invasive electrophysiologic studies or noninvasively via the implanted pulse generator.

The formulator has the capacity to (1) burst asynchronously or burst and give extrastimuli; (2) deliver up to three independently variable extrastimuli; (3) scan up to three extrastimuli; (4) sequentially add up to three extrastimuli should a single extrastimulus fail to terminate a tachycardia; (5) sequentially scan and add extrastimuli; and (6) adapt to rate changes in the tachycardia by delivering extrastimuli based on a percentage of the cycle length.

There are two sensitivities, and pulse width is adjustable from 0.25 to 2.0 msec in increments of 0.25 msec. Having derived a prescription for an individual patient's tachycardia, the activator is programmed to this sequence at the factory. Changes in the program must also be made at the factory. This system has an amazingly wide range of potential pacing programs for patients who are candidates for manually activated antitachycardia pacemakers and requires extensive understanding of the formulator.

Medrad Automatic Implantable Defibrillator (AID)

This device is similar in size and shape to early pacemakers and weighs 250 g. The defibrillating electrodes are constructed from titanium and silicone rubber. One electrode, designed for placement in the superior vena cava near the right atrial junction, is located on the distal end of an intravascular catheter. The second electrode, in the form of a cup or of a flexible rectangular patch, is placed extrapericardially over the cardiac apex. The device is powered by lithium batteries with low internal impedance and high-energy density to provide the capability of delivering approximately 100 discharges.

Ventricular fibrillation is identified by a probability density function for electrical activity, which detects the absence of isoelectric potential segments characteristic of nonsinusoidal rhythms. The device then delivers a truncated exponential pulse of 25 joules within 15 to 25 seconds of arrhythmia onset. The pulse duration varies from 3 to 8 msec as a function of interelectrode resistance. The AID can recycle as many as three times if the previous discharge is ineffective, with the strength of the third and fourth pulse increased to 30 joules. Following the fourth discharge, approximately 35 seconds of nonfibrillating rhythm are required to reset the counter and allow another series of shocks.

Noninvasive testing of the AID can be accomplished using an external analyzer. Magnet placement over the device initiates the capacitor-charging cycle with the charge delivered into a built-in test-load resistor rather than to the patient. Increases in the capacitor-charging time denote battery depletion, whereas failure to initiate the charging cycle indicates abnormal operation. Continuous application of the magnet over the pulse generator disables the device and can deplete the batteries if necessary.

The AID, while continuing to undergo further refinements, represents an impressive scientific and technological achievement with great potential application to patients surviving cardiac arrest.

Medtronic Internal Cardioverter

This system consists of a specially designed lead (the Model 6882), the SP 6000 programmer, and the Model 7210 pulse generator. The 7210 is designed to detect and treat ventricular tachycardia by delivering low-energy ($\leq$2 joules) cardioversion pulses in synchrony with intrinsic ventricular depolarization. When the device is not treating ventricular tachycardia, it operates in a VVI pacing mode. It may be programmed to operate only in VVI mode or in VVI mode in conjunction with an automatic cardioversion modality. When not in an automatic mode, a cardioversion sequence may still be programmed into the pacemaker but can only be activated on a temporary manual basis using the programmer.

Three VVI pacing parameters and four cardioversion parameters may be independently programmed. Basic pacing rate is programmable from 30 to 100 in steps of 5 paced beats per minute, pulse width is programmable from 0.05 to 1.6 msec in increments of 0.1 msec, and sensitivity can be set at either 1.5 or 3.0 mv. Cardioversion parameters include an interval change threshold (off or

25 to 200 msec in 25-msec increments), a tachycardia trigger interval (205 to 545 msec in 10-msec increments, a number of intervals to trigger (2 to 32 in increments of 1), and a cardioversion pulse energy (0.6, 0.2, 0.5, 1.0, 1.8, and 2.0 joules).

Automatic detection of ventricular tachycardia is accomplished by selecting one of two programmable methods. Method one identifies ventricular tachycardia when the R-R interval is less than the programmed value (tachycardia trigger interval) for a programmed number of consecutive intervals (number of intervals to trigger). Method two adds the additional criteria of a sudden decrease in the R-R interval as compared to the previous interval (interval change threshold) to avoid detection and treatment of sinus tachycardia in patients with relatively slow ventricular tachycardia.

The pulse generator has two independent power sources: one lithium-iodine cell powers the unit's electronic circuits for timing, sensing, and so forth, and two lithium-thionyl chloride cells provide power to the capacitors for pacing and cardioversion. Once a tachycardia is detected, the capacitor charges (over 1 to 10 seconds depending on selected energy) and enters a sensing period, awaiting a suitably timed R wave to which it can synchronize the delivery of the cardioversion pulse. The preselected energy is delivered 7.8 msec after the R wave is sensed. The device will attempt up to three cardioversions at programmed parameters and then two further attempts at 2 joules. Following this fifth attempt the Cardioverter is disabled until such time as one paced or sensed interval is of longer duration than the programmed tachycardia trigger interval.

This unit also has full telemetry and several temporary modes, including underdrive and overdrive pacing, delivery of timed extrastimuli, and manual cardioversion. Application of a magnet converts the 7210 to the VVI mode with automatic cardioversion modality off.

Like the AID, the Cardioverter is an impressive technological achievement still in its early stages of testing. The breadth of its clinical application remains to be determined.

CONCLUSIONS

This chapter has attempted to review in detail the current status of both antibradycardia and antitachycardia pacemaking. It should be emphasized that this is a rapidly evolving field, and it is likely that many new devices not even mentioned here will be available within the next several years. Nevertheless, it is necessary to begin to grasp current technology since advanced-grade pacemakers are destined to occupy an increasingly important position in modern cardiologic practice.

REFERENCES

1. Parsonnet V, and Bernstein AD: Cardiac pacing in the 1980s: Treatment and techniques in transition. J Am Coll Cardiol 1:339, 1983.
2. Goldman BS, and Parsonnet V: World survey on cardiac pacing. *In* Meere C (ed): Proceedings of the VI World Symposium on Cardiac Pacing. Montreal, PACE 2(5):W1–W17, 1979.
3. Gordon PL, Calfee RV, and Baker RG: Multiprogrammable pacemaker technology. *In* Barold SS, and Mugila J (eds): The Third Decade of Cardiac Pacing. New York, Futura, 1982, p. 137.
4. Gold RD: The state of the art in pacemaker technology. Proceedings of the AAMI technology assessment conference. Cardiac monitoring in a complex patient care environment. December 1–2, 1981, Arlington, Virginia. Association for the Advancement of Medical Instrumentation, 1981, p. 51.
5. Bilitch M, Hauser RG, Goldman BS, et al: Performance of cardiac pacemaker pulse generators. PACE 5:628, 1982.
6. Neumann G, Funke H, Kirchhoff PG, and Schaede A: Clinical experience with the universal DDD pacemaker. *In* Barold SS, and Mugila J (eds): The Third Decade of Cardiac Pacing. New York, Futura, 1982, pp. 225–248.
7. Shemin RJ, Scott WC, Kastl DG, and Morrow AG: Hemodynamic effects of various modes of cardiac pacing after operation for idiopathic hypertrophic subaortic stenosis. Ann Thorac Surg 27:137, 1979.
8. Hartzler GO, Maloney JD, Curtis JJ, and Barnhorst DA: Hemodynamic benefits of atrioventricular sequential pacing after cardiac surgery. Am J Cardiol 40:232, 1977.
9. Kruse I, Arnman K, Conradson TB, and Ryden L: A comparison of the acute and long-term hemodynamic effects of ventricular inhibited and atrial synchronous ventricular inhibited pacing. Circulation 65:846, 1982.
10. Reiter MJ, and Hindman MC: Hemodynamic effects of acute atrioventricular sequential pacing in patients with left ventricular dysfunction. Am J Cardiol 49:687, 1982.
11. Sutton R, Perrins J, and Citron P: Physiologic cardiac pacing. PACE 3:207, 1980.
12. Leinbach RC, Chamberlain DA, Kastor JA, et al: A comparison of the hemodynamic effects of ventricular and sequential AV pacing in patients with heart block. Am Heart J 78:502, 1969.
13. Sutton R, and Citron P: Electrophysiologic and hemodynamic basis for application of new pacemaker technology in sick sinus syndrome and atrioventricular block. Br Heart J 41:600, 1979.
14. Yashar JJ, Kitzel DL, Arif M, et al: Atrioventricular sequential pacemakers: Indications, complications, and long-term follow-up. Ann Thorac Surg 29:91, 1980.
15. Karlof I: Hemodynamic effect of atrial triggered versus fixed rate pacing at rest and during exercise in complete heart block. Acta Med Scand 197:195, 1975.
16. Stone J, Bhakta RD, and Lutgen J: Dual-chamber sequential pacing management of sinus node dysfunction: Advantages over single-chamber pacing. Am Heart J 104:1319, 1982.
17. Morley CA, Perrins EJ, Grant P, et al: Carotid sinus syncope treated by pacing: Analysis of persistent symptoms and role of atrioventricular sequential pacing. Br Heart J 47:411, 1982.
18. Griffin JC, Mason JW, and Calfee RV: Clinical use of an implantable automatic tachycardia-terminating pacemaker. Am Heart J 100:1093, 1980.
19. Greene HL, Gross BW, Preston TA, et al: Termination of ventricular tachycardia by programmed extrastimuli from an externally activated permanent pacemaker. PACE 5:434, 1982.
20. Griffin JC, Mason JW, Ross DL, and Calfee RV: The treatment of ventricular tachycardia using an automatic tachycardia terminating pacemaker. PACE 4:582, 1981.
21. Fisher JD, Kim SG, Furman S, and Matos JA: Role of implantable pacemakers in control of recurrent ventricular tachycardia. Am J Cardiol 49:194, 1982.
22. Peters RW, Shafton F, Frank S, et al: Radiofrequency-triggered pacemakers: Uses and limitations. Ann Intern Med 88:17, 1978.
23. Castellanos A, Waxman HL, Moleiro F, et al: Preliminary studies with an implantable multimodal AV pacemaker for reciprocating atrioventricular tachycardias. PACE 3:257, 1980.
24. Ward DE, Camm AJ, Gainsborough J, and Spurrell RAJ: Autodecremental pacing—A microprocessor-based modality for the termination of paroxysmal tachycardia. PACE 3:178, 1980.

25. Wellens HJJ, Bar FW, Gorgels AP, and Muncharaz JF: Electrical management of arrhythmias with emphasis on the tachycardias. Am J Cardiol 41:1025, 1978.
26. Zipes DP, Jackman WM, Heger JJ, et al: Clinical transvenous cardioversion of recurrent life-threatening ventricular tachyarrhythmias: Low-energy synchronized cardioversion of ventricular tachycardia and termination of ventricular fibrillation in patients using a catheter electrode. Am Heart J 103:789, 1982.
27. Fisher JD, Matos JA, and Kim SG: The sparking joules of internal cardiac stimulation: Cardioversion, defibrillation, and ablation. Am Heart J 104:177, 1982.
28. Arbel ER, Cohen HC, Langendorf R, and Glick G: Successful treatment of drug-resistant atrial tachycardia and intractable congestive heart failure with permanent coupled atrial pacing. Am J Cardiol 41:336, 1978.
29. Mirowski M, Reid PR, Watkins L, et al: Clinical treatment of life-threatening ventricular tachyarrhythmias with the automatic implantable defibrillator. Am Heart J 102:265, 1981.
30. Wiener I: Pacing techniques in the treatment of tachycardias. Ann Intern Med 93:326, 1980.
31. Spurrell RAJ, Nathan AW, Bexton RS, et al: Implantable automatic scanning pacemaker for termination of supraventricular tachycardia. Am J Cardiol 49:753, 1982.
32. Solti F, Szabo Z, Czako E, et al: Refractory supraventricular reentry tachycardia treated by radiofrequency atrial pacemaker. PACE 5:275, 1982.
33. Sung RJ, Styperek JL, and Castellanos A: Complete abolition of the reentrant supraventricular tachycardia zone using a new modality of cardiac pacing with simultaneous atrioventricular stimulation. Am J Cardiol 45:72, 1980.
34. Ruskin JN, Garan H, Poulin F, and Harthorne JW: Permanent radiofrequency ventricular pacing for management of drug-resistant ventricular tachycardia. Am J Cardiol 46:317, 1980.
35. Hartzler GO, Holmes DR, and Osborn WJ: Patient-activated transvenous cardiac stimulation for the treatment of supraventricular and ventricular tachycardia. Am J Cardiol 47:903, 1981.
36. Ryden L: Physiologic pacing—Pacemaker selection. *In* Sutton R (ed): Proceedings of a Mini-symposium—Physiologic Pacing. Florence, Medtronom, 13, 1981, pp. 16–19.
37. Haas JM, and Strait GB: Pacemaker-induced cardiovascular failure: Hemodynamic and angiographic observations. Am J Cardiol 33:295, 1974.
38. Johnson AD, Laiken SL, and Engler RL: Hemodynamic compromise associated with ventriculo-atrial conduction following transvenous pacemaker placement. Am J Med 65:75, 1978.
39. Werres R, Parsonnet V, Gilbert L, and Zucker IR: Symptomatic unilateral cannon "A" waves in a patient with a ventricular pacemaker. Chest 73:539, 1978.
40. Perrins EJ, Sutton R, Kalebic B, et al: Modern atrial and ventricular leads for permanent cardiac pacing. Br Heart J 46:196, 1981.
41. Smyth NPD, Citron P, Keshishian JM, et al: Permanent pervenous atrial sensing and pacing with a new J-shaped lead. J Thorac Cardiovasc Surg 72:565, 1976.
42. Parsonnet V, Furman S, and Smyth NPD: Implantable cardiac pacemakers: Status report and resource guideline. Am J Cardiol 34:487, 1974.
43. Parsonnet V, Furman S, and Smyth NPD: A revised code for pacemaker identification. PACE 4:400, 1981.
44. Brownlee RR, Shimmel JB, and DelMarco CJ: A new code for pacemaker operating modes. PACE 4:396, 1981.
45. Furman S, and Cooper JA: Atrial fibrillation during AV sequential pacing. PACE 5:133, 1982.
46. Tolentins AO, Javier RP, Byrd C, and Samer P: Pacer-induced tachycardia associated with an atrial synchronous ventricular inhibited (ASVIP) pulse generator. PACE 5:251, 1982.
47. Bathen J, Gundersen T, and Forfang K: Tachycardias related to atrial synchronous ventricular pacing. PACE 5:471, 1982.
48. DenDulk K, Lindemans FW, Bar FW, and Wellens HJJ: Pacemaker-related tachycardia. PACE 5:476, 1982.
49. Furman S, and Fisher JD: Endless loop tachycardia in an AV universal (DDD) pacemaker. PACE 5:486, 1982.
50. Freedman RA, Rothman MT, and Mason JW: Recurrent ventricular tachycardia induced by an atrial synchronous ventricular inhibited-pacemaker. PACE 5:490, 1982.
51. Levy S, Corbelli JL, Labrunie P, et al: Retrograde (ventriculo-atrial) conduction. PACE 6:364, 1983.
52. Akhtar M: Retrograde conduction in man. PACE 4:548, 1981.
53. Mahmud R, Lehmann M, Denker S, et al: Atrioventricular sequential pacing: Differential effect on retrograde conduction related to level of impulse collision. Circulation 68:23, 1983.

54. Hayes DL, and Furman S: Atrio-ventricular and ventriculo-atrial conduction times in patients undergoing pacemaker implant. PACE 6:38, 1983.
55. Wellens HJJ, Schuilenberg RM, and Darrer D: Electrical stimulation of the heart in patients with ventricular tachycardia. Circulation 46:216, 1972.
56. Josephson ME, Horowitz LN, Farshidi A, and Kastor JA: Recurrent sustained ventricular tachycardia: I. Mechanisms. Circulation 57:431, 1978.
57. Camm J, and Ward D: Management of tachycardia: General principles. *In* Pacing for Tachycardia Control. Colorado, Telectronics, 1983, pp. 13–23.
58. Camm J, and Ward D: Electrophysiological methods. *In* Pacing for Tachycardia Control. Colorado, Teletronics, 1983, pp. 25–41.
59. Segni ED, David D, Katzenstein M, et al: Permanent overdrive pacing for the suppression of recurrent ventricular tachycardia in a newborn with long QT syndrome. J Electrocardiol 13:189, 1980.
60. Coumel P, Cabrol C, Fabiato A, et al: Tachycardie permanente par rhythme reciproque. Arch Mal Coeur 60:1830, 1967.
61. Spurrell RAJ, and Sowton E: Pacing techniques in the management of supraventricular tachycardias. Part 2. J Electrocardiol 9:89, 1976.
62. Preston TA, Haynes RE, Gavin WA, and Hessel EA: Permanent rapid atrial pacing to control supraventricular tachycardia. PACE 2:331, 1979.
63. Langendorf R, and Pick A: Observations on the clinical use of paired electrical stimulation of the heart. Bull NY Acad Med 41:535, 1965.
64. Durrer D, Schoo L, Schuilenberg RM, and Wellens HJJ: The role of premature beats in the initiation and termination of supraventricular tachycardia in the Wolff-Parkinson-White syndrome. Circulation 36:644, 1967.
65. Ward DE, Camm AJ, and Spurrell RAJ: The response of regular reentrant supraventricular tachycardia to right heart stimulation. PACE 2:586, 1979.
66. Rowlands E, Curry PVL, and Krikler DM: The assessment of underdrive pacing in the early termination of reentrant atrioventricular tachycardia. *In* Meere C (ed): Proceedings of the VI World Symposium on Cardiac Pacing. Montreal, PACE 2(5):A22, 1979.
67. Spurrell RAJ, and Sowton E: Pacing techniques in the management of supraventricular tachycardia. J Electrocardiol 8:287, 1975.
68. Fisher JD, Kim SG, and Ostrow E: Ultra-rapid single capture train stimulation for termination of ventricular tachycardia (abstract). Clin Res 29:191A, 1981.
69. Waldo AL, MacLean WAH, Karp RB, et al: Entrainment and interruption of atrial flutter with atrial pacing: Studies in man following open-heart surgery. Circulation 56:737, 1977.

Appendix I

Commentary: Clinical Perspectives in Cardiac Pacing

JOEL MORGANROTH, M.D.

The data in this book clearly indicate that the last decade has brought evolutionary change to the field of cardiac pacing. The earliest application of external electrical stimuli applied to the chest in 1952 has now evolved to include the currently available multiprogrammable dual-chamber pacemaker with provisions for transcutaneous programming, physiologic adaptations, and potential control of various arrhythmias. As in other areas of technological advance in medicine, determination of appropriate indications and adequate cost-benefit analysis unfortunately follow rather than parallel the developing advances. Thus questions of suitable clinical priorities are now being raised.

Several developments in the 1970s allowed for this emergence of dual-chamber multiprogrammable pacemakers. Advances in lithium battery technology with improved lead and connector systems and ease of implantation without thoracotomy have led to rapid acceptance of these devices. Electrode malfunction is now uncommon, and multiprogrammability allows for adaptable electrophysiologic changes, solving many problems that in the past would have required a surgical approach. With the development of easy implantation methods and the relatively trouble-free performance of pacemaker units, the safety of this new technology is becoming unquestioned. Emerging problems involving the complexities of programmer maintenance and analysis of electrocardiographic patterns to achieve proper pacemaker functioning will be solved through experience. What is now more important is whether such devices are efficacious. As in the case of other biomedical devices, the evaluation of efficacy is often based on the patient's assessment of clinical response rather than more definitive objective criteria. With ill-defined indications for pacing and the concern for medical cost in these times of escalating health care expenditures, the definition of efficacy is an important issue.

Recent investigation into the frequency of pacemaker implantation in the United States has raised claims that many pacemakers are implanted without proper justification. This suspicion has arisen not only from retrospective analyses of patient charts but also from results of published reports after removal of pacemakers and changing utilization patterns after institution of peer review and quality assurance. This issue has been heightened by recent reports in the national press of unethical marketing practices in the pacemaker industry. As in many other areas of cardiology practice, standardization of nomenclature and indications for cardiac pacing, and proper quality control and follow-up has yet to be achieved. Even simple guidelines for the routine follow-up of new pacemakers have become less certain. It is hoped that advancing technology will allow the basic follow-up information to be stored for access by transtelephonic computer commands.

The vexing questions regarding the appropriate application of clinical electrophysiology studies for selecting a suitable cardiac pacemaker and methods of determining more precise indications for cardiac pacing, as well as the details and complications of the various methods of implantation, are all addressed in this book. Even if there were a clear consensus concerning such matters, some controversy would still exist. Methods to evaluate outpatient cardiac status with high-cost technology (ultrasonography, radionuclide scintigraphy, computerized x-ray tomography, and the emerging use of nuclear magnetic resonance) and invasive in-hospital clinical electrophysiologic testing can add large costs to the assessment of potential pacemaker patients if applied indiscriminately. Decisions regarding the extent of testing performed on patients before pacemaker implantation will have a major impact on the general health care cost.

It is the challenge to cardiology in the 1980s to derive more precise algorithms for the management of the patient's medical needs and the cost-benefit analysis. Hospital administrators will become more vocal and intrude more upon the physician's previously unchallenged domain in this regard, since hospital reimbursement will no longer be based on actual expenditures but on the efficiency of medical care for a particular diagnosis. Thus physicians will have to justify their choice of diagnostic and therapeutic modalities rather than, as in the past, abnegating concern with cost issues. The incentives to determine precise indications and requirements in pacemaking must evolve soon. This book details the data to help in this process, but as yet a consensus has not been reached on the ideal algorithms regarding the various aspects of cardiac pacing. Hopefully this information will serve as a springboard for careful experiments in clinical decision making, to help solve these dilemmas in the near future.

Appendix II

Atlas of Pacemaker Generators and Leads

BIOTRONIK

6024 S.W. Jean Road, B-4, P.O. Box 1988
Lake Oswego, Oregon 97034
503-635-3594

INTRODUCTION

Biotronik was founded in 1963 in Berlin, West Germany, by Professor Max Schaldach, a physicist, and Otto Franke, an electrical engineer. Since the first successful implant in 1964, Biotronik has been a world leader in pacemaker and lead technology. The company's headquarters are located in West Berlin, with other offices in the United States, England, Switzerland, France, Canada, and Austria.

PULSE GENERATORS

Throughout Biotronik's history, its pulse generators have become progressively smaller, more versatile, and more dependable, with longer service life. Most presently available units are multiprogrammable, with a choice of rates, pulse amplitudes, pulse widths, and sensitivities. Currently available models include the following:

Diplos 03 ("double beat"). The Diplos is a unipolar, multiprogrammable pulse generator designed for AV sequential (DDD) pacing but is also programmable to the VVI (R-wave inhibited) mode. Its 400-msec atrial refractory period reduces the possibility of retrograde conduction. Expected lifetime is 52 months at factory-programmed parameters. The Diplos 04 is suitable for all indications for pacing, including the following:

1. Mobitz second-degree AV block
2. Complete AV block
3. Intermittent AV block

4. Multifascicular block
5. Sinus bradycardia
6. Sick sinus syndrome
7. Tachyarrhythmias
8. Congestive heart failure
9. Syncope/dizziness

The Diplos 03 is contraindicated in patients with atrial flutter or fibrillation. It is especially effective in patients with marginal cardiac status who may benefit from the atrial contribution to cardiac output.

Kalos 03 ("beautiful"). A unipolar or bipolar, multiprogrammable VVI pacemaker, the Kalos is 8.8 mm thin and weighs 49 g. Expected lifetime is 95 months at factory-programmed parameters. It is indicated for the treatment of the following conditions:

1. AV block, either third-degree or second-degree, especially if symptomatic
2. Sinus node dysfunction, such as sick sinus syndrome or carotid sinus syndrome
3. Tachyarrhythmias refractory to drug treatment and terminable by pacing
4. Atrial fibrillation or flutter with slow ventricular response

Eikos 04 ("natural"). A unipolar, multiprogrammable AAI (P-wave inhibited) pacemaker, Eikos 04 has higher sensitivity settings but shape, weight, and other specifications are identical to the Kalos. Atrial pacing is indicated in symptomatic bradycardias with normal AV conduction and provides the benefit of the atrial contribution to cardiac output.

Leukos 03 ("bright"). This device is either unipolar or bipolar, VVI, and identical to Kalos but nonprogrammable. Factory specifications are as follows:

1. Basic rate: 72 paced beats per minute (ppm)
2. Pulse amplitude: 4.8 V
3. Pulse width: 0.5 msec
4. Sensitivity: 3.2 mv
5. Refractory period: 300 msec
6. Expected lifetime: 95 months

Archos 05 ("roots"). This is a unipolar, AAI pacemaker identical to Eikos but nonprogrammable.

Neos 01 ("new"). This unipolar or bipolar, multiprogrammable VVI or AAI pacemaker became available in the summer of 1983. Its size (57 × 41 × 8.8 mm) and weight (37 g) make it one of the smallest and lightest pacemakers available. Clinically relevant parameters are programmable over a wide range. The telemetry feature provides program content.

Diplos 04 ("double beat"). This pacemaker, which will be available in the fall of 1984, is the second generation of dual-chamber models. It is a unipolar, multiprogrammable pulse generator with 10 available modes: DDD, DOO, DVI, VVI, VOO, VDD, VAT, AAI, AOO, and DAT. It offers a programmable atrial refractory period and committed or uncommitted ventricular response, as well as hysteresis. The telemetry feature provides program content and state of battery.

Pacemaker Characteristics

Pacemaker	Classification	Parameters	Salient Features
Diplos 03 ("double beat")	DDD, DOO, VVI, VOO (multiprogrammable)	Mode, rate, pulse width, sensitivity, AV delay, pulse amplitude	Projected market availablility spring 1984 Unipolar configuration 400-msec atrial refractory period reduces possibility of retrograde conduction

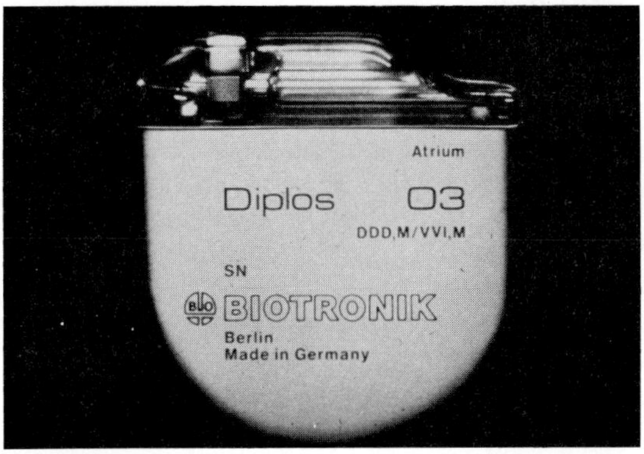

Pacemaker	Classification	Parameters	Salient Features
Kalos 03 ("beautiful")	VVI, VOO (multiprogrammable)	Rate, pulse amplitude, pulse width, sensitivity, hysteresis	Unipolar or bipolar configuration Only 8.8 mm thick, lightweight (49 g)

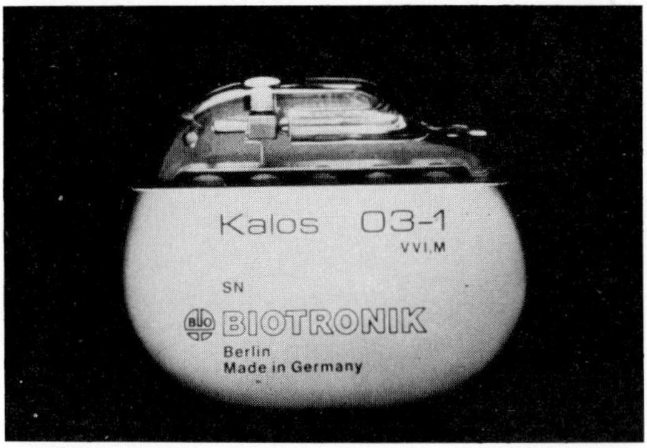

Table continued on following page

Pacemaker Characteristics *Continued*

Pacemaker	Classification	Parameters	Salient Features
Leukos 03 ("bright")	VVI (nonprogrammable)	Basic rate: 72 ppm Pulse amplitude: 4.8 V Pulse width: 0.5 msec Sensitivity: 3.2 mv Refractory: 300 msec	Unipolar or bipolar configuration Identical to Kalos in size and shape but nonprogrammable

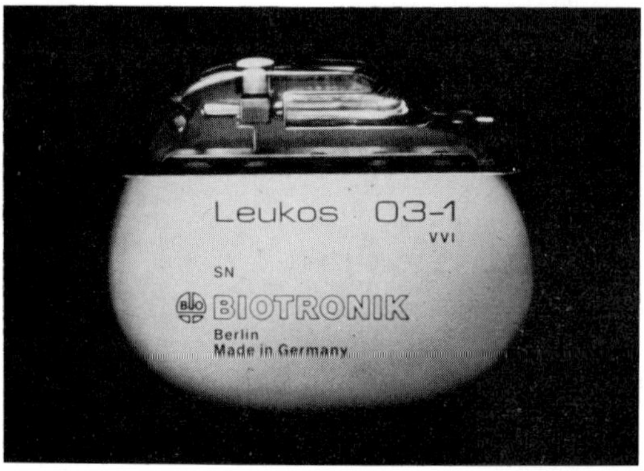

Pacemaker	Classification	Parameters	Salient Features
Eikos 04 ("natural")	AAI, AOO (multiprogrammable)	Rate, pulse amplitude, pulse width, sensitivity, hysteresis	Unipolar Has identical shape, size, and weight to Kalos, but higher sensitivity settings make it suitable for atrial pacing
Archos 05 ("roots")	AAI (nonprogrammable)	Basic rate: 72 ppm Pulse amplitude: 4.8 V Pulse width: 0.5 msec Sensitivity: 0.8 mv Refractory: 400 msec	Unipolar Identical to Eikos but nonprogrammable

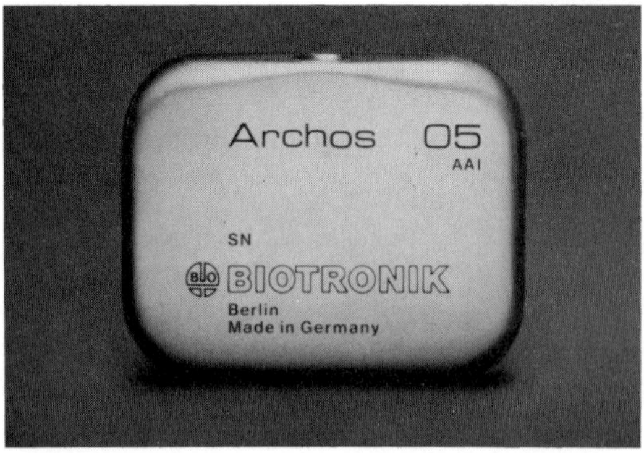

Pacemaker Characteristics *Continued*

Pacemaker	Classification	Parameters	Salient Features
Diplos 04 ("double beat") 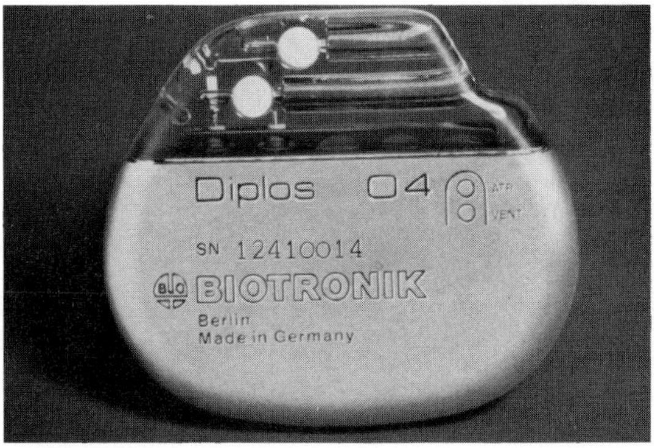 	DDD, DOO, DVI, VVI, VOO, VDD, VAT, AAI, AOO (multiprogrammable)	Mode, rate, atrial pulse width, ventricle pulse width, atrium sensitivity, ventricle sensitivity, AV delay, AV delay fallback, atrium amplitude, ventricle amplitude, atrium refractory, ventricle refractory, upper tracking rates, ventricle output, Wenckebach, hysteresis	Programmable atrial refractory period to reduce possibility of retrograde conduction Telemetry feature provides program content, state of battery Ventricular output either committed or uncommitted Unipolar configuration Projected availability for clinical validation fall 1984
Neos 01 ("new") 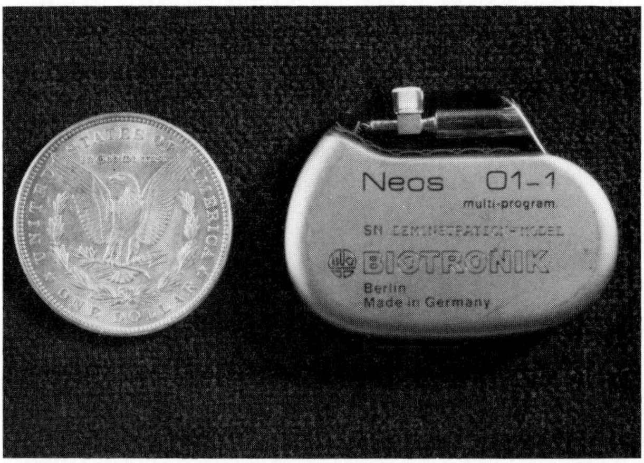 	VVI, VOO, AAI, AOO (multiprogrammable)	Rate, pulse, amplitude, pulse width, sensitivity, refractory, hysteresis	Available since July 1983 Smallest, thinnest pacemaker available (57 × 41 × 8.8 mm) Lightweight (37 g) Suitable for either atrial or ventricular pacing Telemetry feature provides program content, battery Output voltage remains at constant amplitude throughout life of pacemaker. This feature minimizes possibility of exit block

LEADS

The leads that conduct impulses from the implanted pulse generator to the heart are a significant part of pacemaker technology. Biotronik is continually working to improve its leads; this is exemplified by the development of its new, thinner, 5 French Silastic leads that have been available since the fall of 1983. Also, the FH, YC, and N leads are available in high performance silicone with a lead body diameter of only 1.5 mm. Biotronik offers a wide range of leads for both active and passive fixation.

Lead Characteristics

Lead	Description	Salient Features
K-10 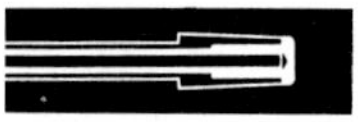	Passive fixation Unipolar, transvenous	Flange tip
N 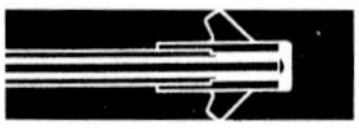	Passive fixation Unipolar, transvenous	Four rubbber tines
I-3 ("Irnich") 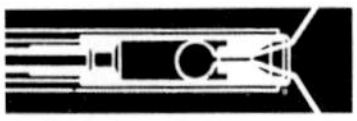	Active fixation Unipolar, transvenous	Retractable metal prongs Indicated for patients at high risk for lead displacement, such as those with dilated right ventricles
FH ("fishhook") 	Active fixation Unipolar, transvenous	Opposed hooks fixed to endocardium by rotation of lead. Designed for atrial use
Y 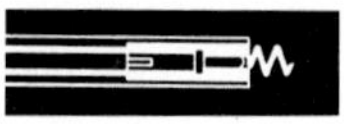	Active fixation Unipolar, transvenous	Retractable screw-in tip, fixed to endocardium by rotation of lead
YR 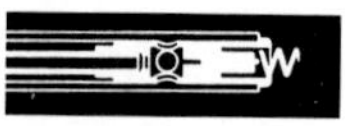	Active fixation Unipolar, transvenous	Retractable screw-in tip, fixed to endocardium by ejection of tip
YC 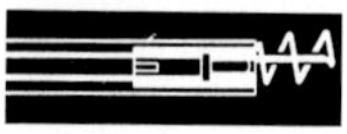	Active fixation	Screw-in coil tip, fixed to endocardium by rotation of lead

CARDIAC PACEMAKERS, INC.

4100 North Hamline Avenue
P.O. Box 43079
St. Paul, Minnesota 55164
612-631-3000

INTRODUCTION

In December, 1978, CPI became a part of Eli Lilly and Company. Founded in 1876, Lilly has both contributed to and benefited from scientific discoveries, and CPI continues to benefit from the 108-year Lilly tradition, which is based on respect for individual needs and achievement.

CPI, a subsidiary of Eli Lilly and Company, Indianapolis, Indiana, manufactures heart pacemakers, insulin infusion devices, and related products. The company distributes its products worldwide with international headquarters in St. Paul, Minnesota and European headquarters in Heerlen, The Netherlands.

CPI was founded in February, 1972, by four men who were certain they could produce a longer life with a more reliable cardiac pacemaker. Since 1959, mercury zinc power sources, with a longevity of only one to two years, had been used in pacemakers. Anthony Adducci, James Baustert, Arthur Schwalm, and Manuel Villafana felt that a lithium power source was the answer. In the fall of 1971, Villafana talked with Wilson Greatbatch regarding his experiments with lithium. Greatbatch, a well-known and respected authority on batteries, had also helped design the first implantable pacemaker in the United States, using mercury zinc cells, which at the time were the most accepted power source for pacemakers. The company recorded its first human implant on November 29, 1972, when a MAXILITH bipolar asynchronous pulse generator was implanted by Dr. H. David Friedberg and Dr. John Burroughs in Milwaukee, Wisconsin. The MAXILITH family was CPI's first generation of pacemakers. Numerous pacemaker types have followed, all powered by lithium batteries.

Pacemaker Characteristics

Pacemaker	Classification	Parameters	Salient Features
CPI Ultra I Model 0531 (unipolar) Model 0631 (bipolar)	VVI, AAI, VOO, AOO	Pacing rate, pulse width, sensitivity, hysteresis, pulse amplitude, refractory period, mode	Memory, telemetry, intracardiac electrogram capabilities, event counters Administrative benefits: storage of pacemaker and patient data in pacemaker using CPI Model 2030 hand-held programmer Diagnostic benefits: verifies pacemaker function using 2030 programmer Intracardiac electrogram capabilities with 2030 programmer and any conventional EKG recorder

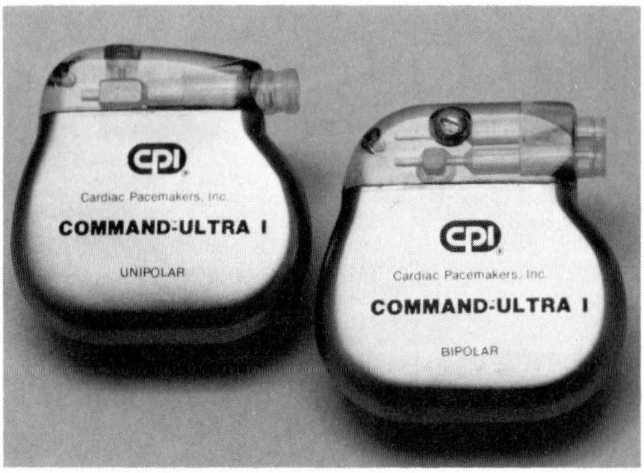

Pacemaker	Classification	Parameters	Salient Features
CPI Ultra II Model 0910	VDD, VAT, VVI, VOO	Pacing rate, pulse width, atrial sensitivity, ventricular sensitivity, pulse amplitude, ventricular and atrial refractory periods, AV delay, upper rate limit, mode	Memory, telemetry, intracardiac electrogram capabilities, event counters Administrative benefits: storage of pacemaker and patient data in pacemaker using CPI Model 2030 hand-held programmer Diagnostic benefits: verifies pacemaker function using 2030 programmer Intracardiac electrogram capabilities with 2030 programmer and any conventional EKG recorder

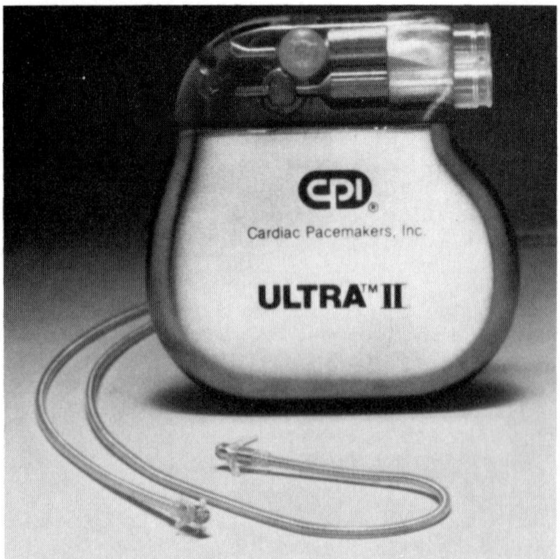

Pacemaker Characteristics *Continued*

Pacemaker	Classification	Parameters	Salient Features
CPI Delta 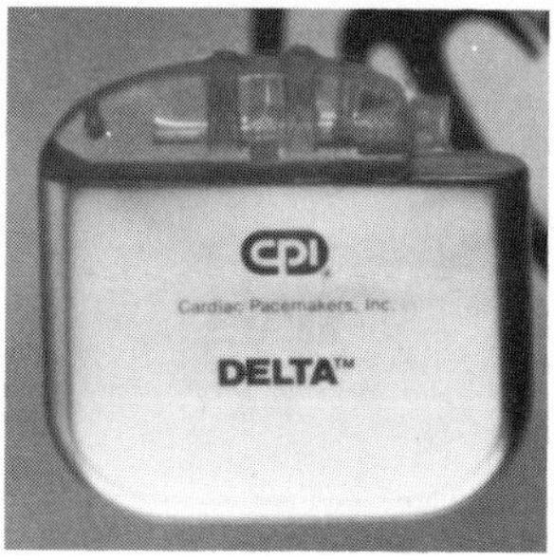	DDD, VDD, DVI, DOO, AAI, AAT, AOO, VVI, VVT, VOO, VAT	Base rate, upper rate limit, hysteresis rate, ventricular pulse width, atrial pulse width, ventricular/atrial pulse amplitude, ventricular sensitivity, atrial sensitivity, AV delay, refractory (paced and sensed), rate smoothing, programmable fallback, magnetic rate, unipolar/bipolar, mode, stat 1 mode, stat 2 mode	Delta began IDE clinical investigation in the USA in December, 1983 Programmable unipolar/bipolar Unique combination of features designed for arrhythmia control Uses the CPI 2040 desk-top programmer with program module and telemetry wand
CPI P5 Model 0530 (unipolar) Model 0630 (bipolar) 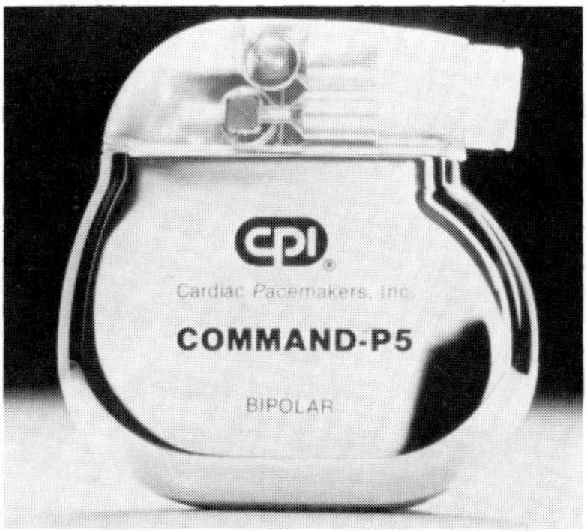	VVI, AAI, VOO, AOO	Sensitivity, refractory period, pacing rate, pacing energy, mode	Verification system for either office or telephone monitoring Lightweight (57 and 59 g) Atrial or ventricular pacing capabilities Demand or asynchronous mode Uses CPI Model 2010 programmer
CPI MICROTHIN P2 Model 0523 (unipolar) Model 0623 (bipolar) 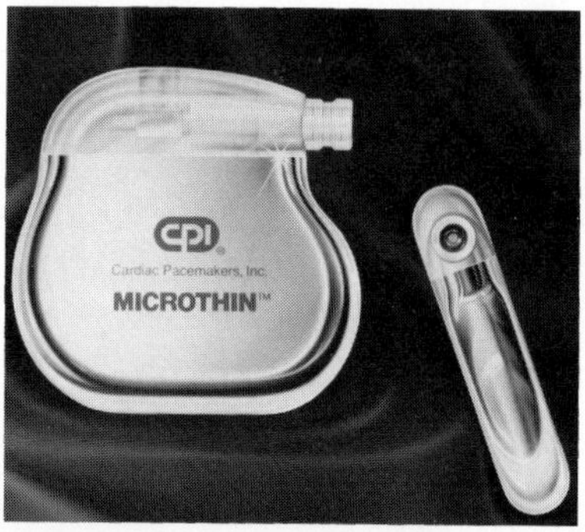	VVI	Pacing rate, pulse width	Thin and lightweight (52 and 54 g) Pacing rate can be changed nonsurgically with CPI Model 2000 or 2001 programmer Verification system for either office or telephone monitoring

Table continued on following page

Pacemaker Characteristics *Continued*

Pacemaker	Classification	Parameters	Salient Features
NP Model 0525 (unipolar) Model 0625 (bipolar)	VVI		Demand pacemaker Thin and lightweight (48 and 49 g) Titanium case

Lead Characteristics

Lead	Description	Salient Features
Thin ventricular endocardial Model 4150 (unipolar) Model 4250 (bipolar)	Tined, porous tip ventricular lead	Ventricular pacing lead 59 cm Silicone-coated material Porous tip for optimum sensing Four tines for easier placement and greater stability Thin for ease of vein entry to reduce patient trauma and postoperative complications Compatible with CPI pulse generators

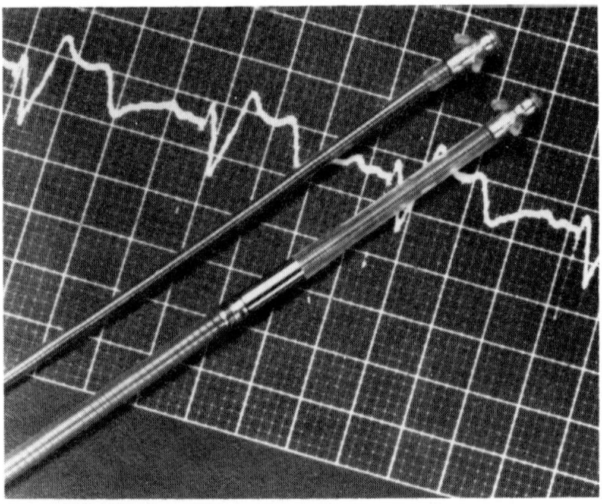

Lead	Description	Salient Features
Thin atrial J endocardial Model 4157 (unipolar) Model 4257 (bipolar)	Tined, porous tip atrial J lead	Atrial pacing lead 59 cm Silicone coated Porous tip Four tines J-shaped for ease of placement in atrium Compatible with CPI pulse generators

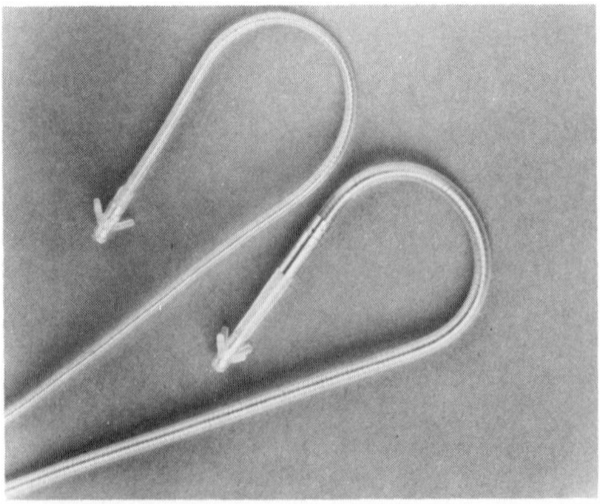

CARDIO-PACE MEDICAL

1120 Red Fox Road
Saint Paul, Minnesota 55112
612-483-6787

INTRODUCTION

Cardio-Pace Medical, Inc. was founded in 1981 to develop a pacing system that would incorporate the latest technology in a straightforward, simple, programmable device that could be brought to the health care system at a price substantially lower than that of comparable units. The Durapulse Models P-101 and P-102 are the result. The company's devices were subject to an Investigational Device Exemption protocol and were granted FDA market release in December, 1982. The following quote from a paper by Dr. John Strobeck expresses this young company's early history: "The Durapulse pacemakers mark the beginning of a much-needed, cost-conscious era of pacemaker therapy in which implanting physicians must choose for their patients a pacemaker capable of providing clinically relevant pacemaker function and state-of-the-art pacer electronics, at the lowest possible cost."*

PULSE GENERATORS

The Durapulse Model P-101 (unipolar) and Model P-102 (bipolar) represent the company's initial market entry vehicles. They incorporate a Wilson Greatbatch, Ltd. lithium-iodine battery and highly reliable circuitry in a hermetically sealed, physiologically shaped titanium housing. The Durapulse pulse generators use universal connector dimensions and accept most currently produced pacing leads. Cardio-Pace Medical believes that rate programmability is the single most clinically significant and most frequently used programmable function. Thus Durapulse pulse generators are engineered with a versatile rate-programmable range of 30 to 120 ppm in single-beat increments. Both models are also programmable for mode (asyncronous or demand) and refractory period (305 msec or 410 msec). The devices are radio-frequency programmed and incorporate a patented loop antenna that eliminates the position-sensitive interface problems of programmer and pulse generator associated with other systems.

---

*Strobeck JE: Pacemaker therapy. Cardiovascular Reviews and Reports 4(6), June 1983.

Pacemaker Characteristics

Pacemaker	Classification	Parameters	Salient Features
Durapulse pulse generator Model P_1O_1 (unipolar) Model P_1O_2 (bipolar)	VOO, VVI (programmable)	Rate, refractory period, mode (asynchronous or demand)	Unipolar or bipolar configuration Cost effective Lightweight (45 g unipolar, 49 g bipolar) Projected life 7–10 years

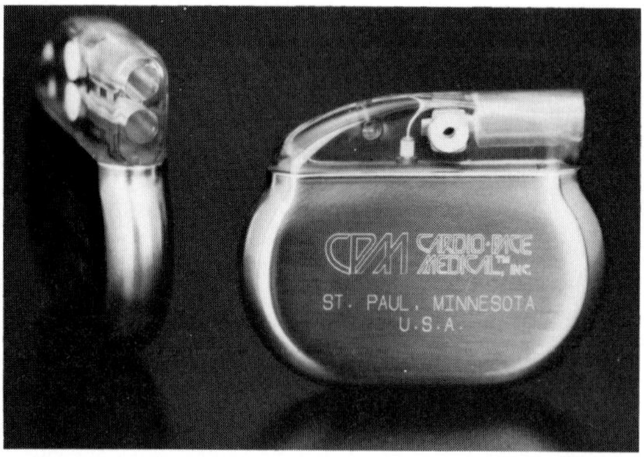

LEADS

Cardio-Pace Medical purchases selected leads under a private label arrangement and markets these leads under the Duraflex trade name.

COOK PACEMAKER CORPORATION

P.O. Box 529
Leechburg, Pennsylvania 15656
412-845-8621

INTRODUCTION

The name Cook has been associated with the medical business for almost 20 years. Cook Group Companies employ over 1000 people worldwide in more than 13 companies. The pioneer company, Cook Incorporated, began in 1963 through the efforts of Bill Cook. Today this company enjoys a fine reputation for its contribution to the development of catheters. The other companies manufacture related medical products such as introducers, surgical needles, and pharmaceuticals.

In a similar fashion, Cook Pacemaker Corporation (CPC)* was founded on March 27, 1981. CPC purchased a 38,000-square-foot ultramodern building located on 37 acres near Pittsburgh, Pennsylvania. The building has three "clean" rooms and the latest equipment, such as the programmable laser welder. During its first year, CPC introduced a multiprogrammable pacemaker with full telemetry complemented by a series of pacemaker leads. This unit, referred to as Model 325T, received an excellent reception in the marketplace because of its round shape and unique telemetry features. This unit has been implanted for more than 2 years without any reports of failures or adverse effects. In addition to producing Model 325T, CPC is currently involved in designing and manufacturing a complete series of atrial ventricular pacemakers to treat a wide range of cardiac arrhythmias. All of the technical and administrative staff have had extensive pacemaker experience.

PULSE GENERATORS

The Cook current product line consists of four "family" groups of pulse generators. The cost-effective pacing series consists of Models 315, 316, and 325D. Models 315 and 316 are thin, lightweight, rate-programmable pulse generators. Model 325D offers programmable rate, refractory period, pulse width, output, sensitivity, and mode.

*CPC is a wholly owned subsidiary of Cook Group, Inc.

The long-life programmable/telemetry series includes Models 325T and 326T. These generators offer more than 10 years of life expectancy with full programming and telemetry capability.

The new Models 327T and 328T have recently been introduced as the VENTRIflex Series. These units offer full programming and telemetry capabilities in a thin, lightweight case.

Model 400 is the first pulse generator of the AVflex Series. This generator is presently under clinical investigation. It offers the physician a simple, easy-to-use dual-chamber pacing system. The rate, AV delay, refractory periods, pulse width, output, and sensitivity are programmable with the same programmer used for all CPC products.

Pacemaker Characteristics

Pacemaker	Classification	Parameter	Features
Model 315 (unipolar) Model 316 (bipolar)	VVI	Rate programmable	Cost effective Thin (9 × 54.9 mm) Lightweight Market availability in 1984

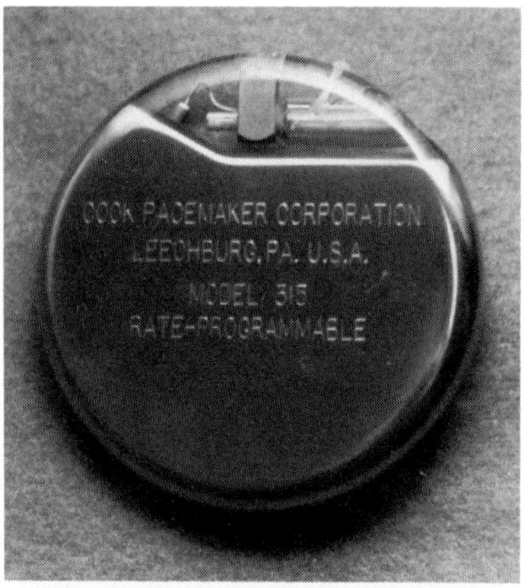

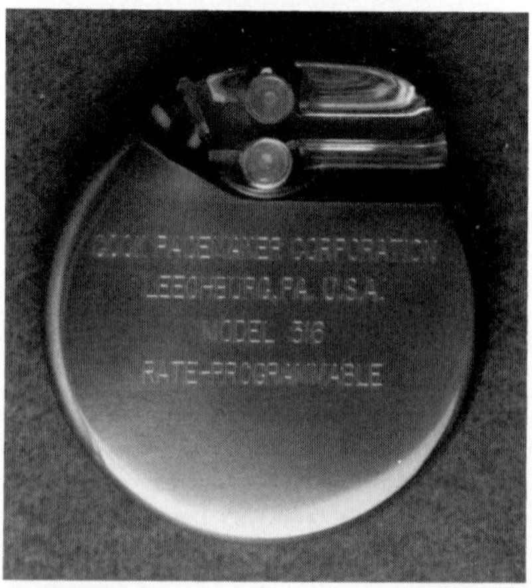

Pacemaker Characteristics *Continued*

Pacemaker	Classification	Parameter	Features
Model 325D (unipolar)	VVI, VOO	Programmable rate, refractory period, pulse width, mode, output, sensitivity	Fully programmable Long life Cost effective
Model 325T (unipolar) Model 326T (bipolar)	VVI, VOO	Programmable with telemetry, rate, refractory period, pulse width, mode, output, sensitivity	Fully programmable with telemetry Long life ERT indicator Unique "audio" confirmation of programming or magnet placement

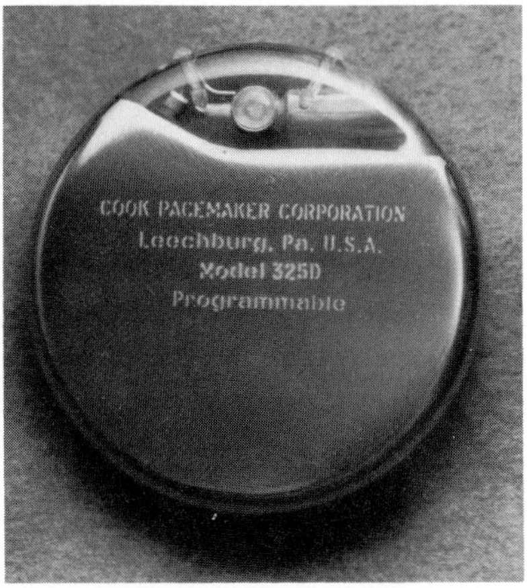

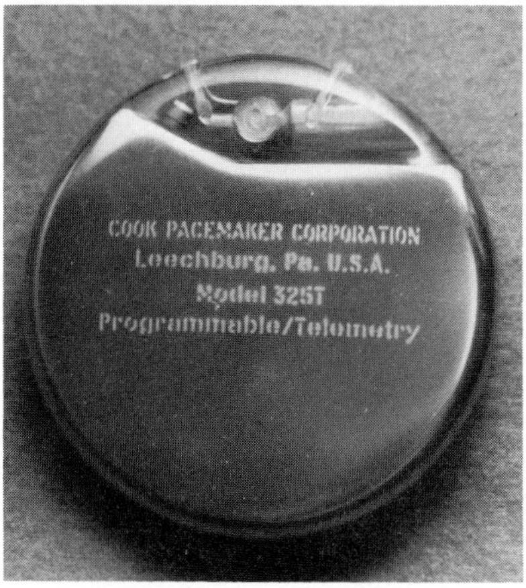

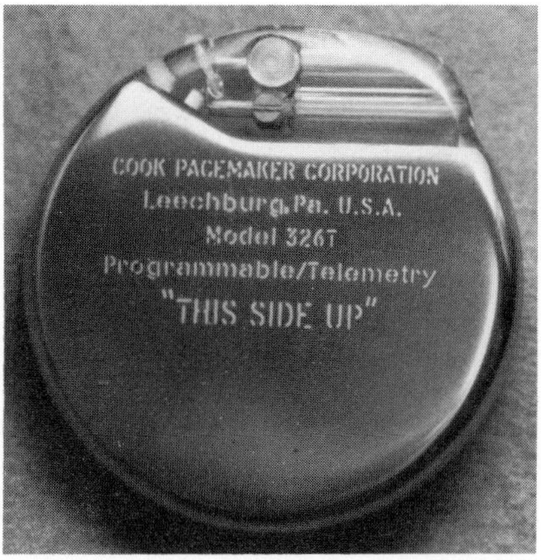

Table continued on following page

Pacemaker Characteristics *Continued*

Pacemaker	Classification	Parameter	Features
VENTRIflex Model 327T (unipolar) Model 328T (bipolar) Model 329T (bipolar in-line)	VVI, VOO	Programmable with telemetry, rate, refractory period, pulse width, output, sensitivity, mode	Thin Fully programmable with telemetry ERT indicator Unique "audio" confirmation of programming or magnet placement Model 329T available in 1984

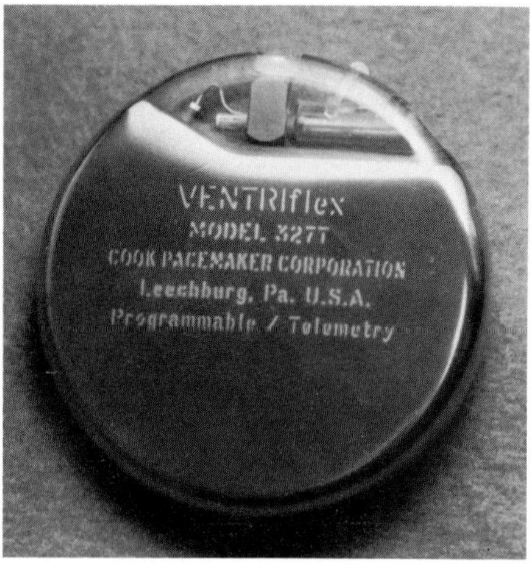

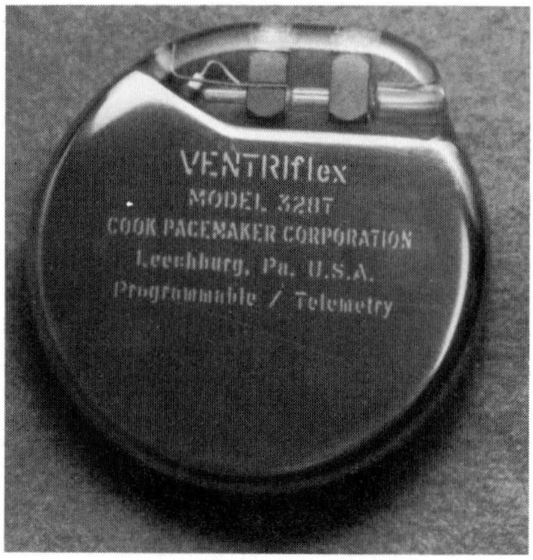

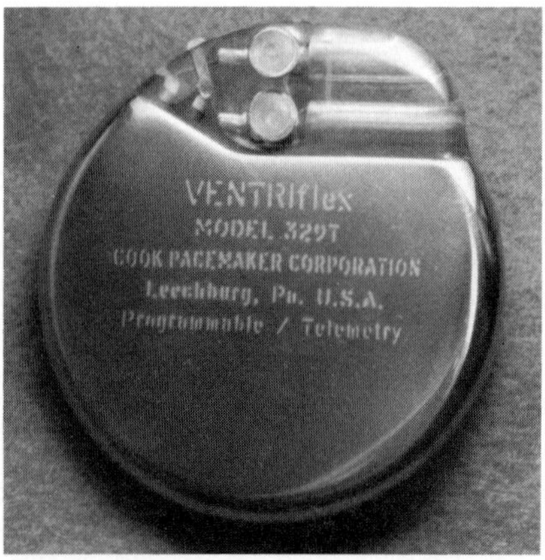

Pacemaker Characteristics *Continued*

Pacemaker	Classification	Parameter	Features
AVflex	DDD, DVI, VVI	Programmable rate, pulse width, sensitivity, AV delay, refractory periods, mode	Long life Programmable Long atrial refractory periods Easy-to-use programmer Noncommitted ventricular stimulation in DDD and DVI modes Under clinical investigation

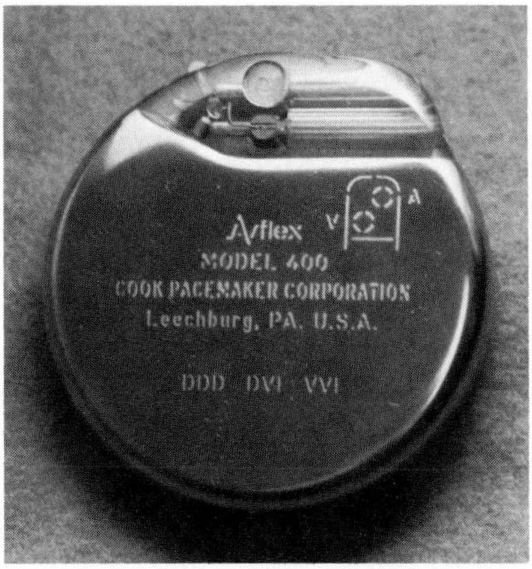

Lead Characteristics

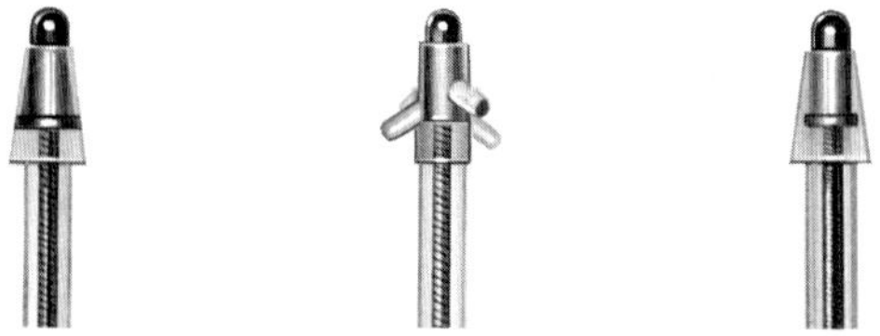

	Model A	Model C	Model B
	Unipolar wedge	Unipolar tined	Bipolar wedge
Catalog number	203–04	206–07	204–05
Length	60 cm	60 cm	60 cm
Conductor material	MP35N-trifilar	MP35N-trifilar	MP35N-trifilar
Insulator material	Silicone rubber	Silicone rubber	Silicone rubber
Electrode material	Platinum iridium	Platinum iridium	Platinum iridium
Electrode surface area	12.5 mm^2	12.5 mm^2	12.5 mm^2
Anode surface area			44 mm^2
Body diameter	2.54 mm (7.7 French)	2.54 mm (7.7 French)	3.17 mm (9.6 French)
Maximum diameter of wedge	3.68 mm		3.68 mm
Diameter with tines released		6.09 mm	
Diameter with tines folded		4.85 mm	
Resistance	58 ohms	58 ohms	56 ohms
			58 ohms
Cook introducer size	11 French	12 French	11 French
Proximal end body diameter	6.2 mm	6.2 mm	5.3 mm

Lead Characteristics *Continued*

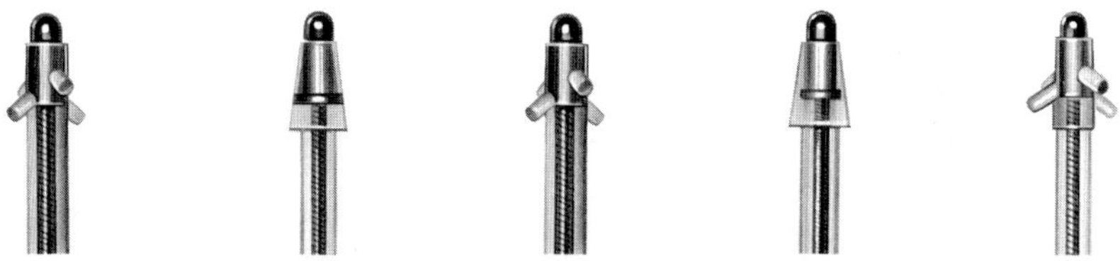

Model D	Model F (01)	Model E (01)	Model F (02)	Model E (02)
Bipolar tined	Unipolar wedge	Unipolar tined	Unipolar wedge	Unipolar tined
207–08	215–16 (01)	214–15 (01)	215–16 (02)	214–15 (02)
60 cm	60 cm	60 cm	60 cm	60 cm
MP35N-trifilar	MP35N-trifilar	MP35N-trifilar	MP35N-trifilar	MP35N-trifilar
Silicone rubber		High-performance medical grade silicone rubber		
Platinum iridium	Platinum iridium	Platinum iridium	Platinum iridium	Platinum iridium
12.5 mm^2	12.5 mm^2	12.5 mm^2	12.5 mm^2	12.5 mm^2
44 mm^2				
3.17 mm (9.6 French)	1.5 mm (4.5 French)	1.5 mm (4.5 French)	1.5 mm (4.5 French)	1.5 mm (4.5 French)
	3.3 mm		3.3 mm	
6.52 mm		6.09 mm		6.09 mm
5.23 mm		4.85 mm		4.85 mm
56 ohms	46 ohms	46 ohms	46 ohms	46 ohms
58 ohms				
12 French	10 French	12 French	10 French	12 French
5.3	5.3 mm	5.3 mm	6.2 mm	6.2 mm

CORATOMIC, INC.

300 Indian Springs Road
P.O. Box 434
Indiana, Pennsylvania 15701
412-349-1811

INTRODUCTION

Coratomic, Inc. manufactures a wide variety of implantable cardiac pacemakers and pacing electrodes. Pacer designs include both multiprogrammable and conventional, lithium-powered and isotopic-powered, and unipolar and bipolar models.

All Coratomic pacemakers feature an ovoid shape to reduce the possibilities of necrosis and erosion through sensitive skin. This gently contoured design, which has set the industry standard, provides a natural fit in the implant site for long-term patient comfort and safety. In addition all Coratomic pacemakers are manufactured with a "velvet grain" external finish for increased conductive surface area.

The programmers used with Coratomic multiprogrammable pacemakers are lightweight in construction, permitting convenient single-hand operation. They feature simplified control knob and switch functions with easy-to-read digital readouts.

MULTIPROGRAMMABLE PACEMAKERS

Model VX5-105. This is a five-function, multiprogrammable, lithium-powered, unipolar design for VVI/VOO operating modes. Programmable parameters include the following:

1. Thirty-two rate selections from 31 ppm to 119 ppm
2. Eight pulse-width selections from 0.15 msec to 1.20 msec
3. Eight sensitivity selections from 1.0 mv to 7.5 mv, plus "off"
4. Two amplitude selections of 2.5 V and 4.6 V (peak voltage)
5. Two refractory-period selections of 305 msec (paced)/250 msec (sensed) or 430 msec (paced)/380 msec (sensed)

The VX5-105 offers real-time telemetry and is designed into a 9-mm-thick case. This unit has a calculated longevity, at nominal settings, of 8 years at 100 percent pacing and 12 years at 50 percent pacing.

Model VX5-205. This is the bipolar version of Model VX5-105. All characteristics are similar, except that Model VX5-205 is 5 mm more in height and weighs 4 g more. Calculated longevity is identical to that of Model VX5-105.

Model VX5-305. This is a low-profile bipolar version of Model VX5-105. The pacer head accepts an in-line, bipolar, coaxial lead. This pacer is 5 mm less in height than the standard VX5-205 bipolar lead. Electrical characteristics are identical.

Ovalife C-101-P. This is a three-function, multiprogrammable, isotopic-powered, unipolar design for VVI/VOO operating modes. Programmable parameters include the following:

1. Thirteen rate selections from 38 ppm to 120 ppm
2. Four sensitivity selections from 1.5 mv to 5.0 mv, plus fixed rate
3. Two pulse amplitude selections of 4 ma and 10 ma

The C-101-P, with its isotopic power source, is one of the most cost-effective pacemakers available in today's marketplace. This unit has a calculated longevity of more than 40 years.

CONVENTIONAL PACEMAKERS

Ovalith-920. This unit is a nonprogrammable, lithium powered, unipolar design for VVI operating modes. It is designed for long-term pacing application when programmability is not required. The Ovalith-920 is supplied in a 12-mm-thick case and has a calculated longevity of 10 years at 100 percent pacing and 15 years at 50 percent pacing.

Ovalith-920BP. This is the bipolar version of the Ovalith-920. Characteristics are similar, except the Ovalith-920BP is 3 mm more in height and 2 g heavier. The calculated longevity of this unit is 8 years at 100 percent pacing and 12 years at 50 percent pacing.

Pacemaker Characteristics

Pacemaker	Characteristics	Parameters	Salient Features
Model VX5-105	VVI-M or VOO (multiprogrammable)	Rate, pulse width, pulse amplitude, sensitivity, refractory period	Lithium powered Unipolar Telemetry 9 mm thick, 45 g Uses hand-held programmer with easy-to-read LED readouts Popular ovoid shape

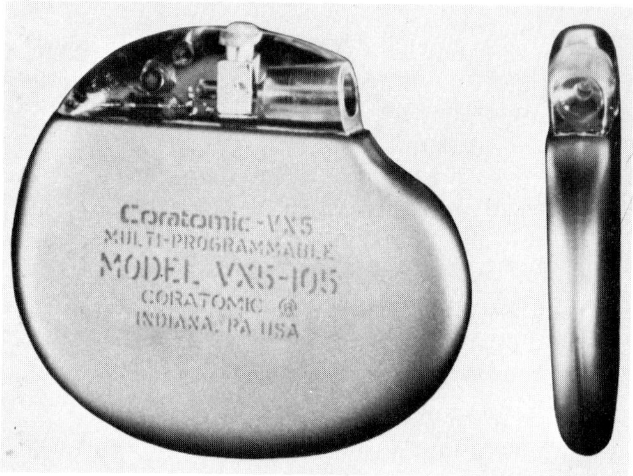

Pacemaker	Characteristics	Parameters	Salient Features
Model VX5-205	VVI-M or VOO (multiprogrammable)	Rate, pulse width, pulse amplitude, sensitivity, refractory period	Bipolar Same features as VX5-105 but accepts a bipolar bifurcated lead Popular ovoid shape
Model VX5-305	VVI-M or VOO (multiprogrammable)	Rate, pulse width, pulse amplitude, sensitivity, refractory period	Low-profile bipolar Same features as VX5-105 but accepts an in-line, coaxial, bipolar lead Popular ovoid shape
Ovalife C-101-P	VVI-M or VOO (multiprogrammable)	Rate, pulse current, and sensitivity	Nuclear powered Unipolar >40 Years projected life Hand-held programmer Only nuclear-powered multiprogrammable pacer available in the industry Popular ovoid shape

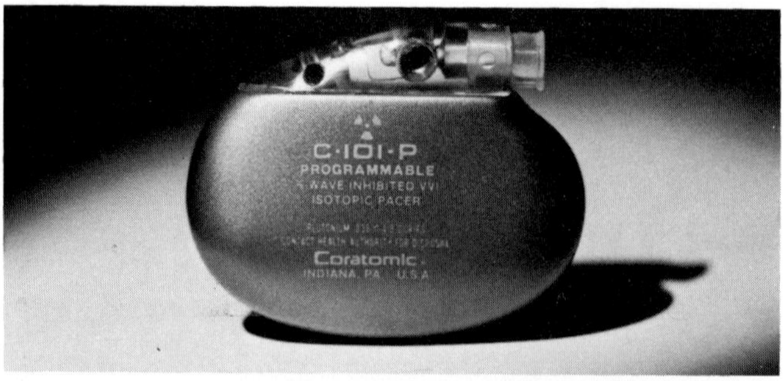

Pacemaker Characteristics *Continued*

Pacemaker	Characteristics	Parameters	Salient Features
Ovalith-920	VVI (nonprogrammable)	Basic rate: 72 ppm Pulse amplitude: 5.3 V Pulse width: 0.5 msec Sensitivity: 2.1 mv Refractory period: 300 msec	Lithium powered Unipolar 11 mm thick, 43 g Popular ovoid shape
Ovalith-920BP 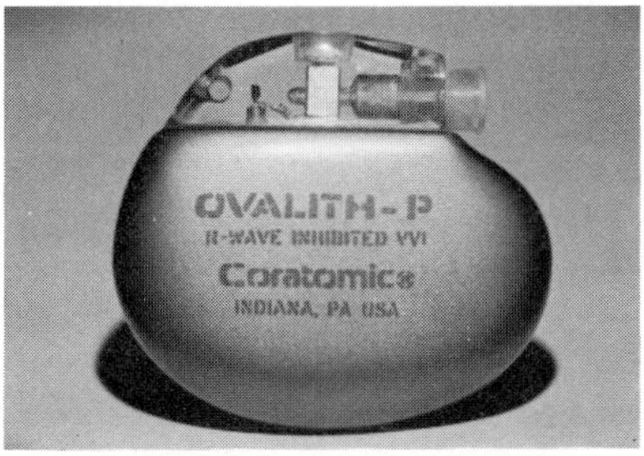	VVI (nonprogrammable)	Basic rate: 72 ppm Pulse amplitude: 5.3 V Pulse width: 0.5 msec Sensitivity: 2.1 mv Refractory period: 300 msec	Bipolar Same features as Ovalith-920, except pacer head is designed to accept a bifurcated lead Popular ovoid shape

PACING ELECTRODES

Coratomic pacing leads with model number and system type are shown below.

SINGLE FLANGE FIXATION PROFILE WITH RING TIP 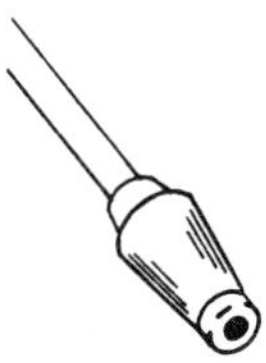			CROWN FLANGE FIXATION PROFILE WITH RING TIP 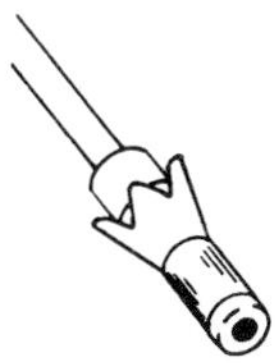		
L-110	L-111	L-112	L-120	L-121	L-122
UNIPOLAR	BIFURCATED BIPOLAR	IN-LINE BIPOLAR	UNIPOLAR	BIFURCATED BIPOLAR	IN-LINE BIPOLAR

RETRACTABLE SCREW-IN FIXATION PROFILE WITH HELIX TIP 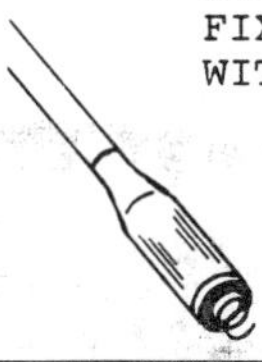			TINED FIXATION PROFILE WITH RING TIP 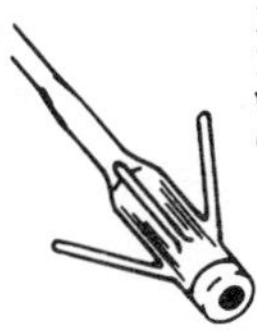		TINED FIXATION PROFILE WITH RING TIP 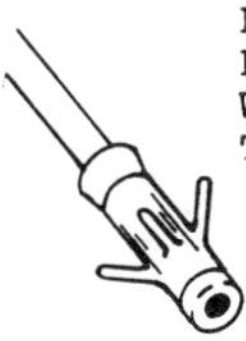	
L-130	L-131	L-132	L-150	L-151	L-160	L-161
UNIPOLAR	BIFURCATED BIPOLAR	IN-LINE BIPOLAR	UNIPOLAR	BIFURCATED BIPOLAR	UNIPOLAR	BIFURCATED BIPOLAR

CORDIS CORPORATION

P.O. Box 025700
Miami, Florida 33102-5700
305-551-2000

INTRODUCTION

Cordis Corporation, a leader in the manufacture of advanced cardiac pacing systems, developed noninvasively programmable cardiac pacers and introduced them to the medical community. Cordis was the first manufacturer to develop a pacer with atrial sensing. Cordis has had more than 20 years of clinical experience, which been applied to the design of sophisticated pacing systems that employ atrial sensing to maintain AV synchrony and greatly improve a patient's physiologic status. Cordis was the first to offer an approved, fully automatic DDD pacer, Sequicor, which was followed by the introduction of their most advanced physiologic pacer—Gemini.

PULSE GENERATORS

All Cordis pacers have been designed as constant-current systems to guarantee that a consistent charge is delivered with each pacer pulse.

The lithium-cupric sulfide batteries used in Cordis pacers lead the industry in performance ratings. These batteries are used because of their easy-to-detect, dual-plateau, end-of-life indicators; the low internal impedance of lithium-cupric sulfide chemistry yields end-of-life characteristics that are more highly predictable than those provided by other currently available chemistries.

The circuitry and batteries of Cordis pacers are sealed in biocompatible titanium cases that are anatomically scaled for minimal pocket bulge. Radiopaque code letters provide rapid x-ray identification of each implanted unit.

All Cordis pacers discussed herein have an exclusive patient safety system, an independent pacing circuit that protects patients in case of random component malfunction.

Cordis pacers are easy to telemeter and program using the hand-held Programmer III. Through Programmer III, nominal pacing parameters can be attained instantaneously, using Stat Set programming.

Pacemaker Characteristics

Pacemaker	Classification	Programmable Parameters	Salient Features
Gemini θ (Theta) Model 415A 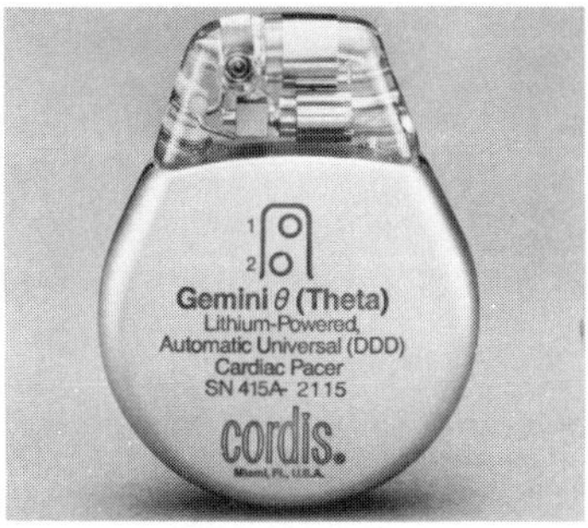	Automatic, universal pacer: DDD, DVI, DDT/I, DDT, VDD, VVI, AAI, and VVT (multiprogrammable, dual-chamber)	Mode, rate, atrial pulse duration/output current, ventricular pulse duration/output current, atrial sensitivity, ventricular sensitivity, atrial refractory period, ventricular refractory period, AV delay, unipolar/bipolar polarity	The ultimate state-of-the-art physiologic pacer Full 10-year predicted service life (at 70 ppm, 0.6 msec/6 ma) Telemetry Programmable unipolar/bipolar pacing configuration is available in certain modes for noninvasive control of exit block, myopotentials, and EMI and helps adapt the pacing system to meet the patient's evolving pacing requirements Automatic block atrial tachycardia response High-output currents of up to 12 ma are available for overcoming exit block Microcomputer-controlled Quartz-crystal oscillator provides an accurate timing base for the microcomputer
Gemini III Model 418A 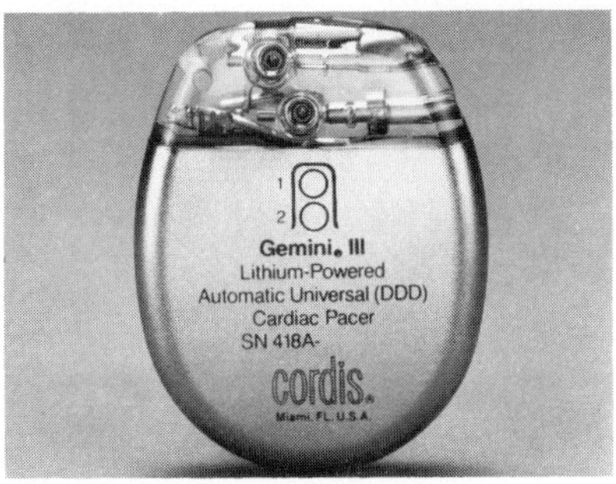	Automatic, universal pacer: DDD, DVI, DDT/I, DDT, VDD, VVI, AAI, and VVT (multiprogrammable, dual-chamber)	Mode, rate, atrial pulse duration/output current, ventricular pulse duration/output current, atrial sensitivity, ventricular sensitivity, atrial refractory period, ventricular refractory period, AV delay, unipolar/bipolar polarity	A lightweight (42 g) compact (10 mm thick) pacing system 5-year predicted service life (at 70 ppm, 0.6 ms/6 ma) Telemetry Programmable unipolar/bipolar pacing configuration Universal 3.2-mm connector

Table continued on following page

Pacemaker Characteristics *Continued*

Pacemaker	Classification	Programmable Parameters	Salient Features
Sequicor II θ (Theta) Model 233F 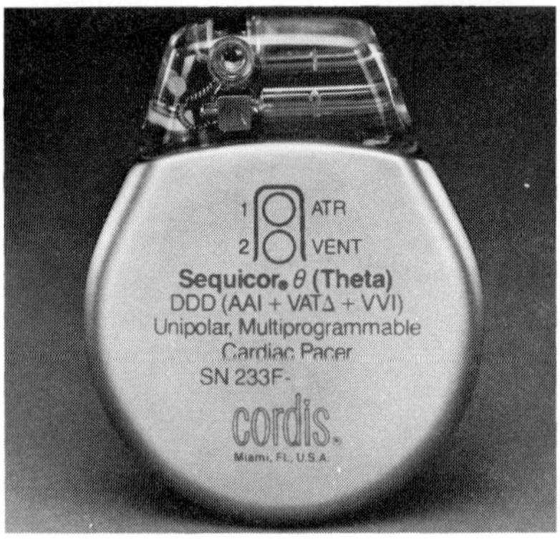	DDD, DVI, VDD, VVI, DAD, VAT, DOO, VOO (multiprogrammable, dual-chamber)	Mode, rate, atrial pulse duration/output current, ventricular pulse duration/output current, atrial sensitivity, ventricular sensitivity, atrial refractory period, ventricular refractory period, AV delay	Fully automatic DDD mode allows pacer to spontaneously and appropriately adapt to meet the patient's needs Telemetry for simplified programming and monitoring Long service life (approximately 10 years at 70 ppm, 0.6 msec/6 ma) Independently programmable atrial refractory periods of up to 500 msec provide retrograde conduction control Automatic block atrial tachycardia response High-output currents up to 12 ma are available for overcoming exit block Quartz-crystal oscillator precisely regulates timing functions Microprocessor-based circuitry Unipolar pacing configuration
Sequicor III Model 233G 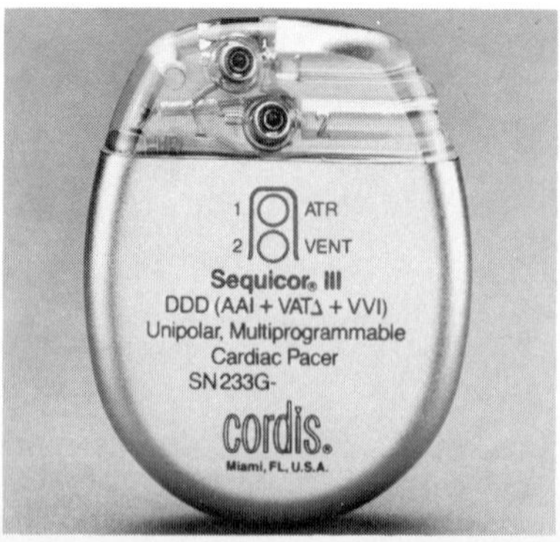	DDD, DVI, VDD, VVI, DAD, VAT, DOO, VOO (multiprogrammable, dual-chamber)	Mode, rate, atrial pulse duration/output current, ventricular pulse duration/output current, atrial refractory period, ventricular refractory period, atrial sensitivity, ventricular sensitivity, AV delay	All of the same features as Sequicor II Unipolar pacing configuration Extremely light DDD pacer (43 g) Thin, 10-mm profile for unchanged cosmetic appearance 5.9-Year predicted service life (at 70 ppm, 0.6 msec/6 ma)

Pacemaker Characteristics *Continued*

Pacemaker	Classification	Programmable Parameters	Salient Features
Multicor II Models 402A, 402B, and 402C	VVI, VVT, VOO, VVIΔ (hysteresis) AAI, AAT, AOO (multiprogrammable, single-chamber)	Mode, rate, unipolar/bipolar polarity, pulse duration/output current, sensitivity (VVI, VVT, AAI, AAT), sensitivity (VVIΔ), refractory period, hysteresis delay	A highly programmable single-channel pacer Easy-to-use linear bipolar connector Telemetry Hysteresis Unique unipolar/bipolar pacing configuration allows the physician to overcome most sensing problems noninvasively to respond to the patient's ever-changing needs Microcomputer-controlled electronics Small, γ-size (57 × 48 × 10 mm) 42 g light Suitable for either atrial or ventricular pacing 6.4-Year predicted service life (at 70 ppm, 0.6 msec/6 ma) Multicor II, Model 402C has a small (4.75-mm) bifurcated connector

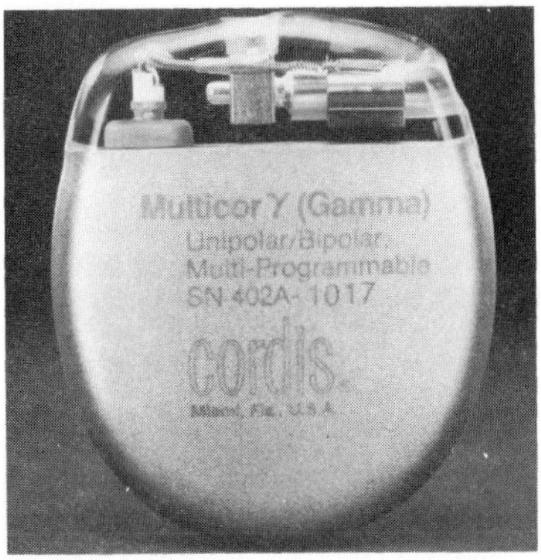

Pacemaker	Classification	Programmable Parameters	Salient Features
Multicor γ (Gamma) Model 337A	VVI, VVT, VOO (multiprogrammable, single-chamber)	Mode, rate, output current, sensitivity	Adjustable atrial refractory periods up to 520 msec Unipolar pacing configuration 8.7-Year predicted service life (at 70 ppm, medium current drain setting)

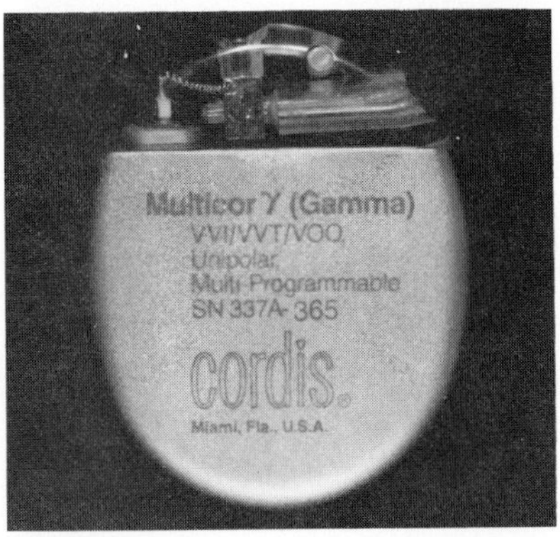

FUTURE CORDIS PACING SYSTEMS

Planned pacers will more closely approximate and restore the patient's natural heart function. A variety of relevant diagnostic functions will be incorporated into these future pacers.

CORDIS ENCOR PERMANENT CARDIAC PACING LEADS

Encor leads can be used with all Cordis pacers, as well as the pacers of other manufacturers. These leads consist of a multifilar cobalt/nickel alloy coil conductor inside Cordis's specially formulated thin polyurethane insulation. This construction provides superior flex strength with only half the body diameter of standard leads.

Encor leads have a porous-surfaced electrode, which encourages and permits tissue ingrowth for improved electrode attachment, lower chronic thresholds, reduced trauma, and lower current of injury. A variety of active and passive fixation devices are available to choose from.

Many Encor leads are now available with a universal (3.2-mm) connector, and for increased flexibility an up-sizing adapter and an up-sizing sleeve are supplied to enlarge the connector size to 4.75 mm or 6.00 mm, respectively. The unique, integral, triple-barrier Peerless seal on the connector helps prevent body fluids from entering the pacer neck.

Lead Characteristics

Lead	Description	Salient Features
Encor unipolar pervenous J atrial leads	Passive fixation, unipolar, transvenous	Silicone elastomer tines anchor electrode within appendage Lengths available are 45, 48, and 52 cm

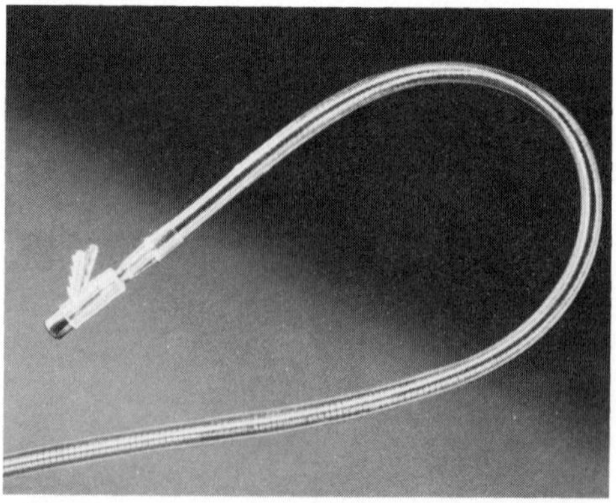

Lead Characteristics *Continued*

Lead	Description	Salient Features
Encor linear bipolar pervenous J atrial leads	Passive fixation, bipolar, transvenous	Through use of linear connector, size of overall pacing system is reduced Proximal band is located 25 mm from electrode Silicone elastomer tines anchor electrode within appendage Lengths available are 45 and 52 cm
Encor unipolar pervenous ventricular leads	Passive fixation, unipolar, transvenous	Fins or tines at the distal tip help to anchor the electrode in the trabeculae Lengths of 52, 58, and 62 cm are available

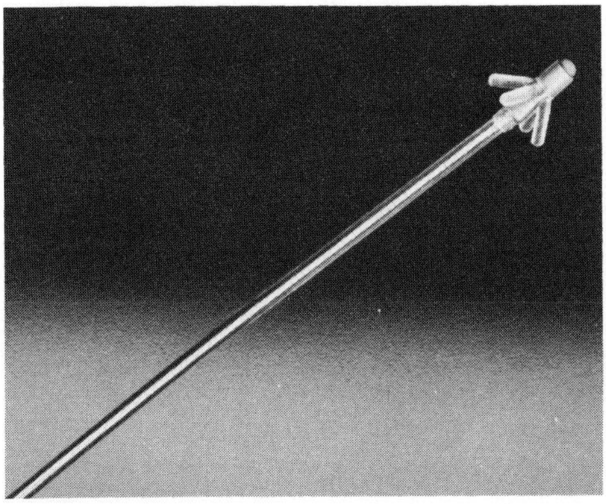

Lead	Description	Salient Features
Encor bipolar pervenous ventricular leads	Passive fixation, bipolar, transvenous	Available in either linear or bifurcated configurations Silicone elastomer tines or fins aid in reducing dislodgment (tines only on bifurcated models) Lengths of 52 and 62 cm are available
Encor pervenous active-fixation lead	Active fixation, unipolar, transvenous, atrial or ventricular	Porous-surfaced ring electrode is electrically isolated Nonconducting stainless steel active-fixation coil is not a part of the electrode and therefore allows better sensing thresholds to be attained Coil is completely retractable Positional stability of electrode is assured, especially in patients with smooth-walled ventricles, hypertrophied hearts, or nonexistent atrial appendages

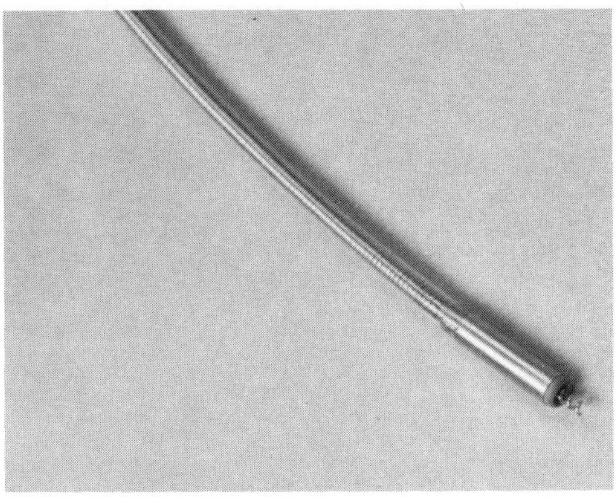

Table continued on following page

Lead Characteristics *Continued*

Lead	Description	Salient Features
Encor epicardial lead with porous-surfaced electrode	Unipolar, epicardial, atrial or ventricular	These are the only epicardial leads available with a porous-surfaced electrode Small size ideal for use with pediatric as well as adult patients Myocardial stab for stability not necessary For increased versatility of application, the soft silicone elastomer pad readily conforms to the contour of the atrium or ventricle Available with removable temporary extension wire

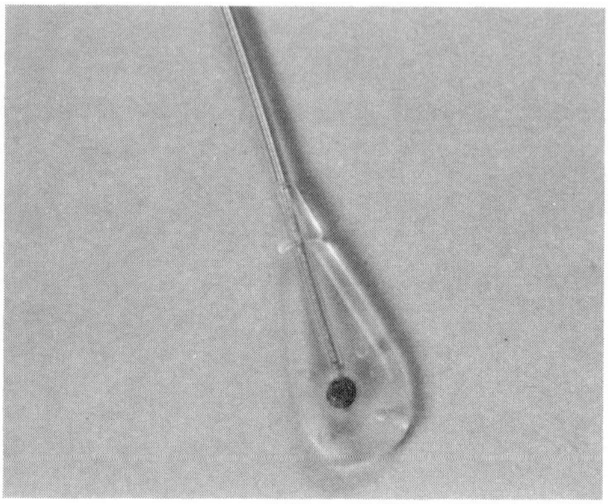

ELA MEDICAL

3740 Williston Road
Minnetonka, Minnesota 55343
612-935-2033

INTRODUCTION

ELA Medical, a pacemaker manufacturer with a long-established reputation for quality and reliability, has been manufacturing and marketing cardiac pacemakers in Europe since 1964 and in the United States since June, 1979.

During its many years of manufacturing and marketing medical devices, ELA has pioneered several technological advances in the field of cardiac pacing. For example, ELA was the first pacemaker manufacturer to incorporate the lithium iodine battery in a demand pulse generator. It was among the leading manufacturers to hermetically seal its pulse generator in titanium. Most recently, it was the first pacemaker company to incorporate microprocessor based circuitry into its multiprogrammable pulse generator, Multilith. The company is presently in the process of developing a fully automated dual chamber pacing system.

PULSE GENERATORS

ELA Medical has a long-established reputation for reliability and quality. Their pulse generators have had the longest projected lives among comparable pacemakers because of their very low current drain circuitry and very high capacity lithium-iodine batteries.

Multilith Models 1140 and 2140. These unipolar and bipolar multiprogrammable pacemakers are programmable to the asynchronous (VVO), R-wave inhibited (VVI), or R-wave triggered modes. Because these units have programmable sensitivity, they also can be used in the atrium. Their projected lifetime is 14 years at nominal* pacing values.

These units can be programmed to high output (7.5 V) for high-threshold patients or for loss-of-pacing situations. The ability to measure thresholds noninvasively enables the physician to tailor the pacemaker's output to the individual's chronic threshold. This feature optimizes both the patient's safety from loss of capture and the pulse generator's longevity.

*Nominal (100 percent pacing, 70 ppm, 5.0 V, 510-ohm load).

Pacemaker Characteristics

Pacemaker	Classification	Parameters	Features
Multilith Model 1140 (unipolar) Model 2140 (bipolar)	VVI, VVT, VOO, AAI, AAT, AOO (multiprogrammable)	Mode, rate, sensitivity, pulse amplitude, refractory period	High-output capability Noninvasive threshold ability Two-way telemetry printer Small hand-held programmer

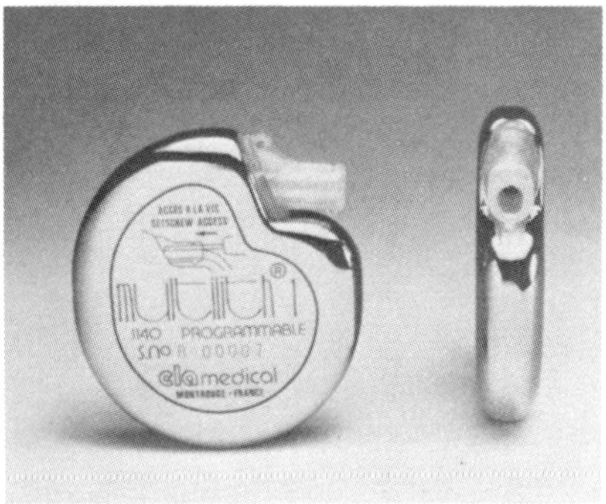

Pacemaker	Classification	Parameters	Features
Multilith Model 1141 (unipolar) Model 2141 (bipolar)	VVI, VVT, VOO, AAI, AAT, AOO (multiprogrammable)	Rate, sensitivity, pulse amplitude, mode, refractory period	High-output capability Noninvasive threshold ability Small hand-held programmer

Multilith Models 1141 and 2141. These units are similar to the Multilith described above, except that they do not have two-way telemetry, which makes them less expensive. The units can be programmed noninvasively but cannot be interrogated.

Unilith Models 7540 and 7542. These are nonprogrammable VVI pulse generators. They, as well as the Multiliths, have a very physiologic shape and unique, single-access connector system.

Multilith II (bipolar and unipolar). These units will be available in 1984 and are the same as the Multilith models 1140 and 2140, except that they will be smaller in size and will have an 8- to 9-year projected lifetime at nominal* values.

Physiolith. This DDD pacemaker will become available in 1984 in both unipolar and bipolar configurations. It will have programmable modes, rates, and AV delays. It will also have programmable amplitudes, pulse widths, and sensitivities and threshold tests in both chambers. This unit is fully automatic and provides intracardiac data from both chambers. It was designed to make EKG interpretation easy and accurate as well as to provide Holter and other diagnostic data to the physician.

*Nominal (100 percent pacing, 70 ppm, 5.0 V, 510-ohm load).

Pacemaker Characteristics *Continued*

Pacemaker	Classification	Parameters	Features
Unilith Model 7540 (unipolar) Model 7542 (bipolar)	 VVI VVI (nonprogrammable)		Small, physiologic shape Pure titanium housing Unique single-access connector
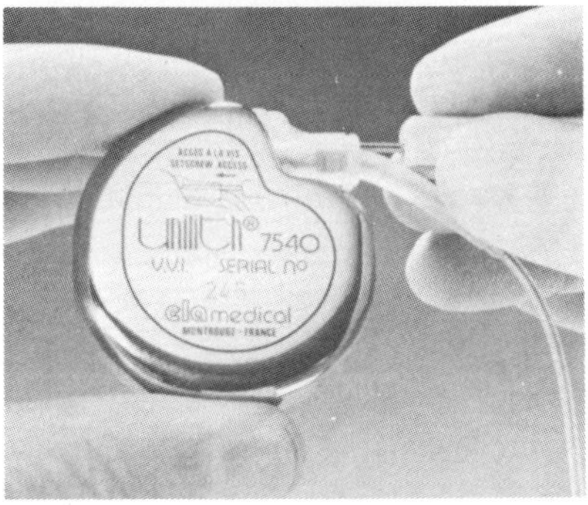			
Physiolith	(See Stimulation mode)	Rate, mode, AV delay, amplitude, pulse width, sensitivity	Currently undergoing clinical evaluation Optimizes AV synchrony and avoids pacemaker-mediated tachycardia Provides accurate intracardiac data from both chambers
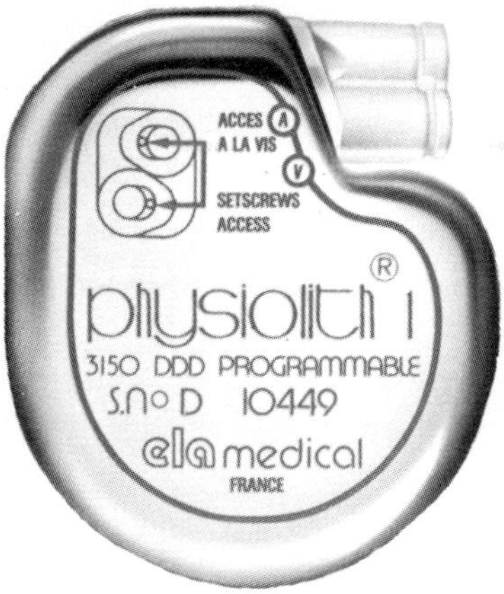			

LEADS

ELA Medical leads are spiral-tined endocardial leads. The tine configuration is unique and is designed to minimize dislodgement and make introduction through a 9-French introducer feasible and easy. ELA leads use a trifilar conducting coil and a high-performance silicone elastomer as an insulating material.

PMAF. This unipolar transvenous leads has an 8 mm^2 electrode surface area made from platinum iridium. The body diameter is 2.3 mm. The small surface area and tine configuration make it very popular. This lead has a standard 1.6-mm terminal pin.

PBAF. This bipolar transvenous lead is similar to the PMAF, except that the body diameter is slightly larger and the conductor is coaxial, permitting both a proximal ring and distal tip electrodes for bipolar pacing. This lead has two standard 1.6-mm terminal pins.

PMCF. This new unipolar transvenous lead is identical to the PMAF lead, except that the electrode material is made of vitreous carbon. The carbon electrode material lowers chronic stimulation thresholds and improves sensing over the standard platinum iridium–tipped electrodes. It will be available in 1984.

Lead Characteristics

Lead	Description	Features
PMA 860	Spiral-tined endocardial lead, unipolar	8 mm^2 surface area 4 spiral tines Fits through 9-French introducer
PBA 860	Spiral-tined endocardial lead, bipolar	8 mm^2 surface area 4 spiral tines Fits through 9-French introducer
PMC 860	Spiral-tined endocardial lead, unipolar	8 mm^2 surface area 4 spiral tines Fits through 9-French introducer Low chronic threshold Better sensing ability

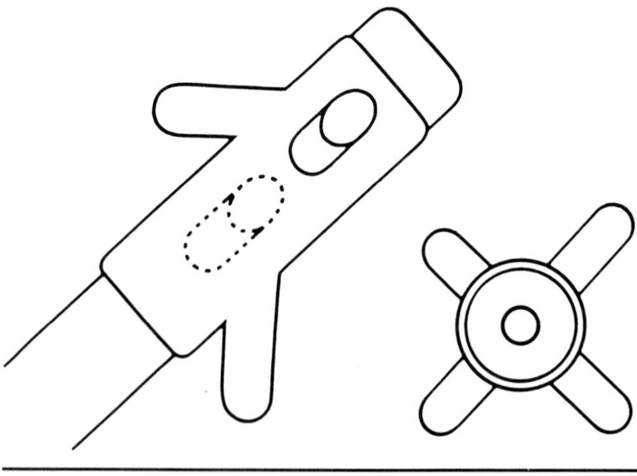

INTERMEDICS, INC.

P.O. Box 617
Freeport, Texas 77541
409-233-8611

INTRODUCTION

Intermedics, Inc., founded in 1973, became the world's second largest manufacturer of cardiac pacing systems in 1979 and is presently one of the world's fastest growing, diversified health care companies.

Through innovative product development, Intermedics has consistently maintained the leading edge in pacing technology. A broad range of cardiac pulse generators, both nonprogrammable and multiprogrammable single- and dual-chamber devices, as well as a large selection of pacing leads, is presently available from Intermedics.

PULSE GENERATORS

The leading Intermedics multiprogrammable pulse generator models include the following:

Avius Model 263–01. This unit is a dual unipolar, multiprogrammable, AV sequential pulse generator. Designed primarily for dual-chamber (DVI) pacing therapy, Avius can also be programmed for DOO or VVI modes of operation. It offers 15 programmable rates, 15 pulse widths, and 7 sensitivity selections. Avius's telemetry provides battery voltage, pace/sense event markers, and positive programming confirmation. Avius's dimensions are 6.0 × 4.7 × 1.1 cm. It weighs 68 g and is powered by a 3.0 ampere hour lithium-iodine cell.

Cosmos Model 283–01. This cardiac pulse generator is a multimodal, multiprogrammable device intended primarily for DDD pacing applications. The extensive programmability of Cosmos, however, makes it a very versatile device for use in the majority of pacing applications, both single- and dual-chamber.

Key features of the Model 283–01 include a total of 12 single- and dual-chamber operating modes; wide ranges of programmable rates, atrial and ventricular refractory periods, ventricular blanking periods, sensitivity levels, output amplitudes, and pulse widths; superior pacemaker-mediated tachycardia controls including a programmable atrial refractory period, a programmable automatic atrial refractory extension after premature ventricular events, and an automatic tachycardia termination algorithm; Wenckebach, gradual fallback, and multiple ratio block upper-rate responses; and extensive telemetry capabilities. Cosmos telemetry capabilities include the following:

1. Inquire data—currently programmed operating parameters
2. Telemetry data—real-time (measured) operating characteristics, battery condition, and lead system parameters; transtelephonic capabilities for transmitting and receiving data
3. Diagnostic data—a cumulative record of pace and sense events stored in the pulse generator's memory registers

An Intermedics Rx 2000 Model 522–06 programmer is used to program the Cosmos and to interrogate the pulse generator's telemetry functions. Close attention to human engineering factors in the design of the Rx 2000 has resulted in a "user-friendly" device that minimizes programming complexity. Data are displayed on the programmer's video display screen, and a permanent record of all data is available via an integral thermal printer.

The 283–01 is a dual unipolar device that accepts unipolar pacing leads with standard 5-mm (diameter) connectors. To prevent possible stimulation of muscles adjacent to the implant site, a conformal polymer coating covers the titanium case of the generator, except for an area that forms an indifferent electrode. Cosmos's dimensions are 6.0 × 7.7 × 1.1 cm. It weighs 65 g and is powered by a 3.0-ampere hour lithium-iodine cell.

Cosmos Bipolar Model 284–02. This pulse generator, which has features identical to the 283–01 but compatible with Intermedics' In-line bipolar pacing leads, is also undergoing clinical evaluation. Projected market availability of Model 284–02 is mid-1984.

Quantum Models 253–19 (unipolar), 254–18 (bipolar), and 254–20 (in-line bipolar). These pulse generators are 8-mm thick multiprogrammable single-chamber (VVI) pacemakers with digital real-time measured telemetry. Multiprogrammability allows the physician to tailor these pulse generators to each patient's specific needs. The Quantum series may be programmed to any of 15 rates, 15 pulse widths, 7 sensitivities, 3 modes, and 3 pulse amplitudes.

The Quantum system (pulse generator, Model 522–03 programmer, 540–02 decoder, 542–02 printer, and 535–03 transmitter) measures and telemeters its programmed values as well as its actual operating parameters with digital real-time telemetry. It may telemeter these measurements to a programmer or a hand-held decoder. The portable hand-held decoder will receive telemetry by either direct patient contact or remotely via transtelephonic transmission. A permanent record of the telemetry is available through the use of the Model 542–02 printer. The Quantum programmer is "user-friendly" in its simplicity. All programmable functions are held in separate displays through all the programming steps. After programming, a confirmation signal is received as visual proof that the pulse generator has accepted its new program. The Quantum series pulse generators also include redundant circuitry (a back-up pacer) to ensure continued pacing even in the unlikely event of a component failure. This is especially critical for the pacemaker-dependent patient. The Quantum's dimensions are 54 × 47 × 8 mm. It weighs 40 g and is powered by a 1.8 ampere hour lithium-iodine cell. The Quantum series pulse generators also incorporate the exclusive Inter-Lock electrode connection system, minimizing the need to handle loose screws and caps.

CyberLith Models 253–07 (unipolar) and 254–07 (bipolar). These pulse generators are multiprogrammable but do not include telemetry. They offer 15 programmable rates, 15 pulse widths, 7 sensitivities, and 3 modes. Their size is 51 × 47 × 11 mm, and they weigh 46 g. They are programmed by the same programmer as the Quantum series (Model 522–03 programmer).

Prima Models 235–01 (unipolar) and 236–02 (bipolar). These are small, nonprogrammable pacemakers that feature the exclusive Inter-Lock lead connection system. Their size is 50 × 47 × 8 mm, and they weigh 38 g.

These pulse generators incorporate a pulse-width stretching circuit that is activated as the battery voltage decreases during use. This feature assures relatively constant energy throughout the pulse generator's service life.

Pacemaker Characteristics

Pacemaker	Classification	Parameters	Salient Features
Cosmos Model 283–01	DDD, DVI, DVI[c], DOO, VDD, VVI, VVT, VOO, AAI, AAT, AOO, OOO, (multiprogrammable)	Mode, pacing rate, ventricular tracking limit, fallback rate, fallback deceleration, AV delay, nonphysiologic AV delay, atrial refractory period, atrial refractory extension, ventricular refractory period, ventricular blanking period, hysteresis, atrial pulse amplitude, ventricular pulse amplitude, atrial pulse width, ventricular pulse width, atrial sensitivity, ventricular sensitivity, telemetry	Dual unipolar configuration Pacemaker-mediated tachycardia controls: programmable atrial refractory period, programmable atrial refractory extension following PVC, automatic PMT termination algorithm Telemetered information: program register contents; measured pacing, lead system, and battery parameters; diagnostic register contents Upper rate responses: Wenckebach, fixed ratio block, variable rate fallback Available since March 1984

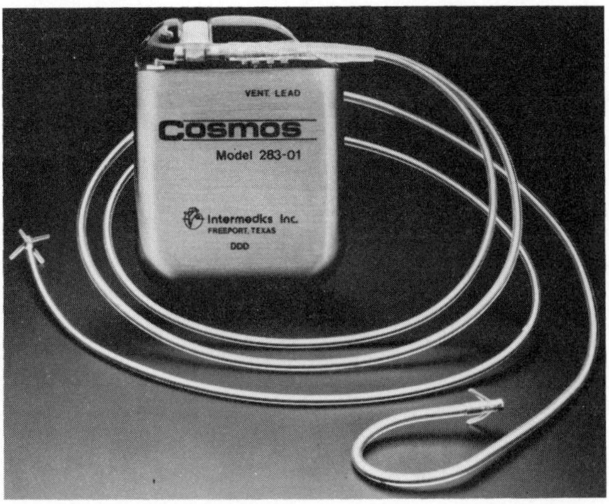

Table continued on following page

Pacemaker Characteristics *Continued*

Pacemaker	Classification	Parameters	Salient Features
Avius Model 263–01	DVI, DOO, VVI (multiprogrammable)	Mode, pacing rate, pulse width, sensitivity	Dual unipolar configuration, 11 mm thick, large battery capacity, telemetry: battery voltage and event markers

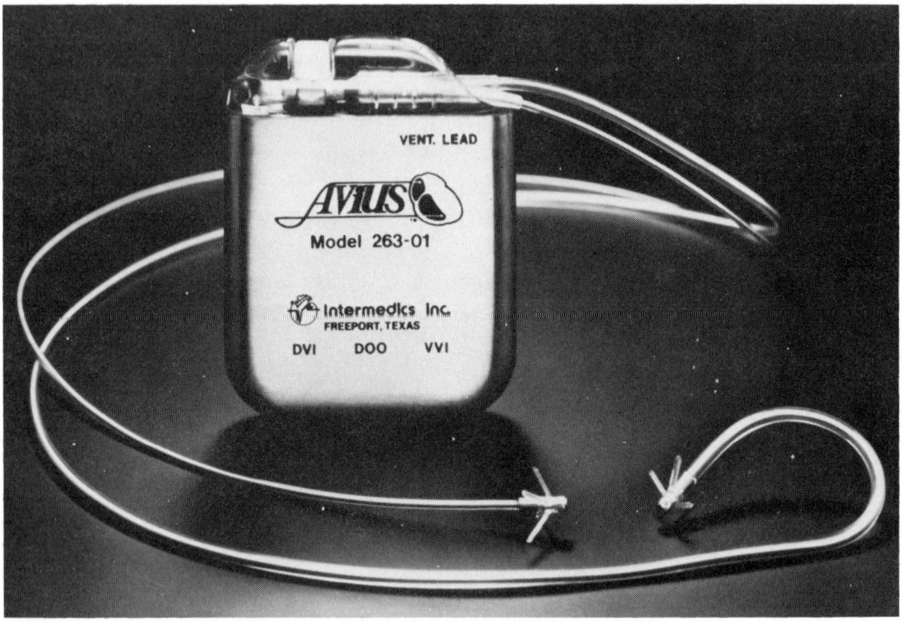

Pacemaker	Classification	Parameters	Salient Features
Quantum Model 253–19 Model 254–18 Model 254–20	VVI, VVT, VOO (multiprogrammable with telemetry)	Mode, rate, pulse width, pulse amplitude, sensitivity Telemetry supplies both programmed and actual measured values	Unipolar, bifurcated bipolar, in-line bipolar 54 × 47 × 8 mm thick, 40 g Exclusive Inter-Lock lead-connection system

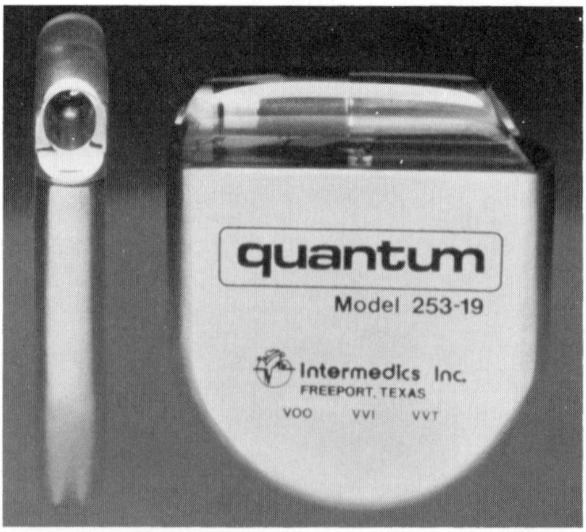

Pacemaker Characteristics *Continued*

Pacemaker	Classification	Parameters	Salient Features
CyberLith Model 253–07 Model 254–07	VVI, VVT, VOO (multiprogrammable)	Mode, rate, pulse width, sensitivity	Unipolar, bifurcated bipolar 54 × 47 × 11 mm, 49 g

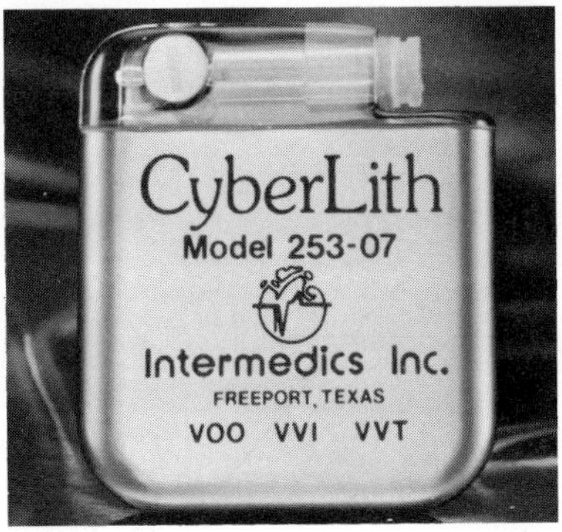

Pacemaker	Classification	Parameters	Salient Features
Prima model 235–01	VVI (nonprogrammable)	Fixed nominal values	Unipolar, bifurcated bipolar 50 × 47 × 8 mm, 38 g Exclusive Inter-Lock lead-connection system

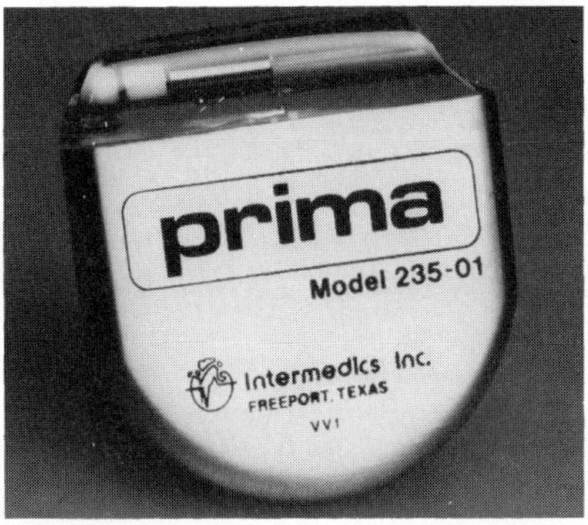

LEADS

Intermedics offers a variety of leads in both silicone rubber and polyurethane, for active and passive fixation, myocardial and endocardial placement, atrial and ventricular stimulation, and unipolar and bipolar modes. Most Intermedics leads feature a universal (5 mm/6 mm) connector, integral suture sleeve, and stylet funnel.

Lead Characteristics

Lead	Description	Salient Features
476–01	Endocardial bipolar, tined, silicone rubber 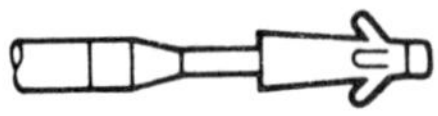	Bifurcated connector
484–01	Endocardial bipolar, tined, silicone rubber 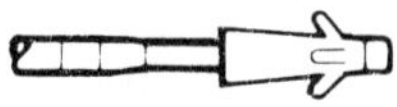	In-line connector
471–07/09	Myocardial sutureless, silicone rubber 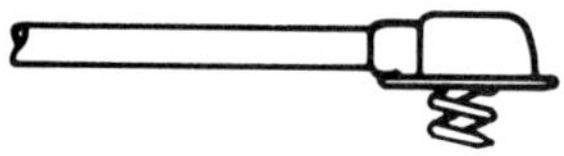 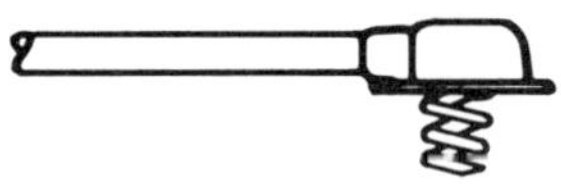	Universal connector available in 2 turn (07) or 3 turn (09)
487–05	Endocardial unipolar, tined, silicone rubber, ring tip 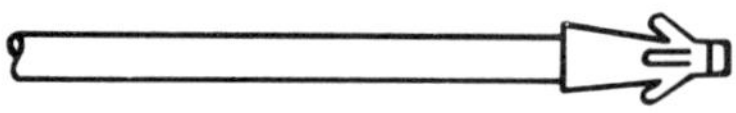	Universal connector, body diameter 6 French thick
479–01	Active fixation (screw-in), unipolar, polyurethane 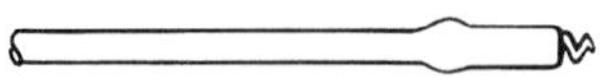	Universal connector, fixating coil electrically isolated from ring electrode
483–03/04	Endocardial unipolar, atrial J, tined, polyurethane, ring tip 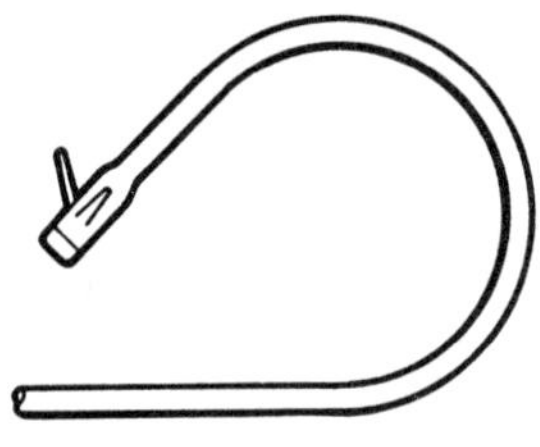 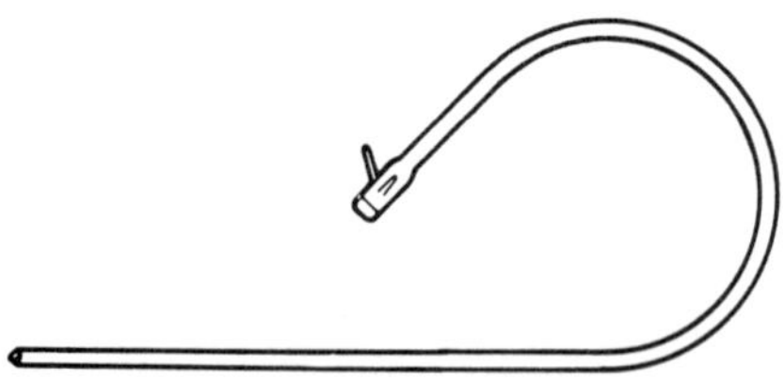	Universal connector, available in small J (03) or large J (04)

Lead Characteristics *Continued*

Lead	Description	Salient Features
493–03	Endocardial unipolar, tined, polyurethane, ring tip 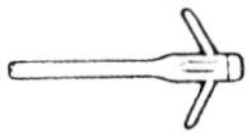	Universal connector
476–03	Endocardial bipolar, tined, polyurethane, ring tip 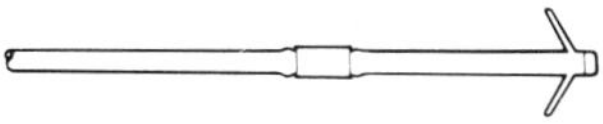	Universal bifurcated connector
480–01	Active fixation (screw-in), bipolar, polyurethane 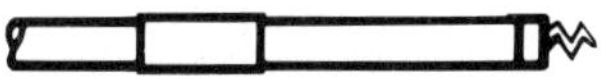	In-line connector, fixating coil electrically isolated from ring electrode
486–01	Endocardial bipolar, tined, polyurethane, ring tip 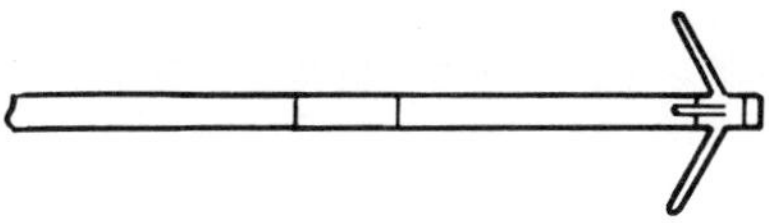	In-line connector
490–01	Endocardial bipolar, atrial J, tined, polyurethane 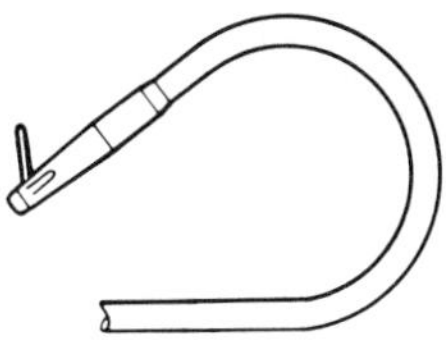	Universal bifurcated connector
492–01	Endocardial bipolar, atrial J, tined, polyurethane 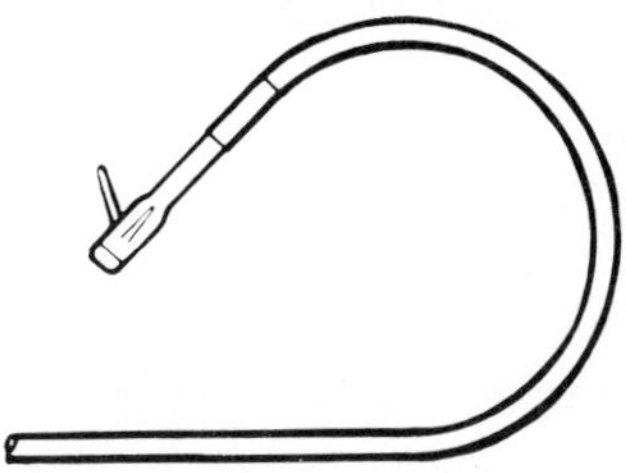	In-line connector
473–03	Epicardial suture-on, polyurethane 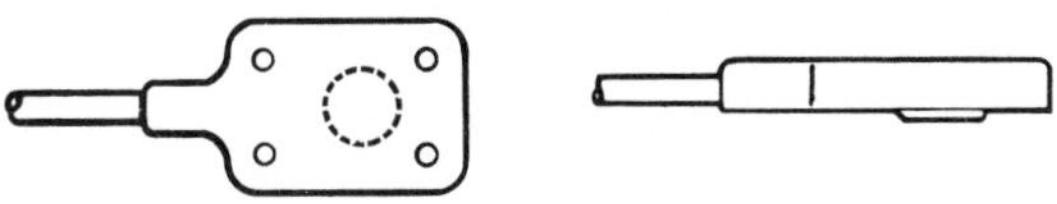	Universal connector

MEDTRONIC, INC.

Two Neshaminy Interplex
Suite 204
Trevose, Pennsylvania 19047
215-245-7880

INTRODUCTION

Medtronic is the world's leading producer of implantable medical devices. The company designs, manufactures, and markets heart pacemaker systems, mechanical heart valves and instrumentation for medical diagnosis and monitoring. Service operations include patient monitoring and physician education.

Medtronic employs approximately 5000 men and women around the world and does business in over 75 countries. International production facilities are located in Brazil, Canada, France, and The Netherlands. United States plants are located in Arizona, Colorado, Massachusetts, Michigan, Minnesota, and Puerto Rico. World headquarters are in suburban Minneapolis.

Medtronic was established as a partnership in 1949 and was incorporated in Minnesota in 1957.

PULSE GENERATORS

Versatrax Model 7000. This is a versatile dual-chamber pacemaker that can be programmed to pace in the AV universal (DDD), AV sequential (DVI), or ventricular-inhibited VVI mode.

In the universal mode, Versatrax combines AV sequential pacing (DVI) with atrial synchronous (VDD) pacing. If a patient's atrial rate is above the programmed lower rate, the ventricle will synchronize to the atrial rate either spontaneously or by paced stimuli. If a patient's atrial rate is below the programmed lower rate, the atrium will be paced at the lower rate and the ventricle will synchronize to the atrial rate either spontaneously or by paced stimuli.

A wide range of programmable parameters and modes makes it possible to accommodate a variety of patient needs. Versatrax has a longevity of 8 years.

Versatrax II Model 7000A. This is a smaller, lighter-weight version of the Versatrax Model 7000. In addition to the proven operational features of Versatrax, Versatrax II has an atrial refractory period that has been extended from 155 msec to 235 msec. Additionally, this atrial refractory period automatically extends to 340 msec following a PVC, for prevention of sensing retrograde conduction after PVCs.

Versatrax II can be programmed to pace in the AV universal (DDD), AV sequential (DVI), or ventricular-inhibited (VVI) mode.

Byrel-SX Model 5993SX. This is a multiprogrammable, AV sequential pacemaker that incorporates a noncommitted pacing system. The Byrel-SX Model 5993SX has the following programmable parameters: mode (DVI or VVI), rate, AV interval, atrial pulse width, ventricular pulse width, and ventricular sensitivity.

Spectrax-SXT Model 8420. This is a multiprogrammable, single-chamber pacemaker that incorporates telemetric functions. The Spectrax-SXT has the following programmable parameters: temporary or permanent settings, mode (asynchronous, synchronous, R- or P-wave inhibited/demand) rate, pulse width, amplitude, sensitivity, refractory period, and hysteresis. Telemetry to external programmers conveys the following information: programmed parameters, program confirmation, battery status and model number, and an endocardial electrogram.

Spectrax-SX Model 5984. This is a multiprogrammable, single-chamber pacemaker. It has the following programmable parameters: temporary or permanent settings, mode (asynchronous, synchronous, R- or P-wave inhibited/demand), rate, pulse width, amplitude, sensitivity, refractory period, and hysteresis.

Models 5998R and 5998T. This rapid atrial stimulation system consists of an implantable receiver (Model 5998R) and an external radio-frequency transmitter (Model 5998T). The patient uses the transmitter to initiate burst pacing for termination of episodes of supraventricular tachycardia. The range of burst pacing is from 50 to 400 ppm and is adjustable by the physician.

Enertrax Model 7100. This pacemaker is an atrial synchronous, ventricular-inhibited (VDD) device that can be programmed to the VVI mode. In addition to programmable mode, the Enertrax has the following programmable parameters: lower or backup pacing rate, AV delay, upper tracking rate, rate hysteresis (VVI only), atrial sensitivity, ventricular pulse width and amplitude, ventricular sensitivity, auto-threshold measurement, and temporary program settings.

The Enertrax Model 7100 offered telemetric communication with external programmers and recorders. The following information can be obtained via telemetry: programmed parameters, battery status and model number, intracardiac ventricular electrogram, and marker channel. This pacer is no longer manufactured.

Pacemaker Characteristics

Pacemaker	Classification	Parameters	Salient Features
Symbios Model 7005/7006 (unipolar/bipolar)	DDD, DVI, VVI, DOO, AOO, VOO (multiprogrammable)	Lower rate, AV delay, upper rate, pulse width (A&V), amplitude (A&V), sensitivity (A&V), atrial refractory	Bipolar or unipolar Bidirectional telemetry of programming and parameters Intracavitary electrograms (A&V) Wenckebach upper rate response Diagnostic telemetry marker channel to aid in interpretation of device operation Threshold margin test to determine loss of capture (A&V) Ventricular safety pacing (on/off) Programmable atrial refractory period with automatic extension after PVC Temporary memory Inhibit mode Cancel magnet mode 33-ml volume, 10 mm thick, 5–6 year life Projected market availability—Spring 1984
Symbios Model 7008 (bipolar)	DOD, DVI, VVI, DOO, AOO, VOO Tachycardia response (multiprogrammable)	Same as 7005/7006, atrial burst, dual demand	Same features as 7005/7006 Automatic atrial burst capability Automatic underdrive pacing AV or V Projected market availability—late 1984
Versatrax II Model 7000A	DDD, DVI, VII, DOO, VOO	Lower rate, AV delay, upper rate, sensitivity (A&V), pulse width (A&V)	Wenckebach upper rate response Automatic atrial refractory extension to 340 msec Threshold margin test to determine loss of capture (A&V) Inhibit mode period 12-msec blanking period Ventricular safety period Anti-Stim insulative coating Constant energy throughout service life (A&V) 23-ml volume, 52 g, 10 mm thick

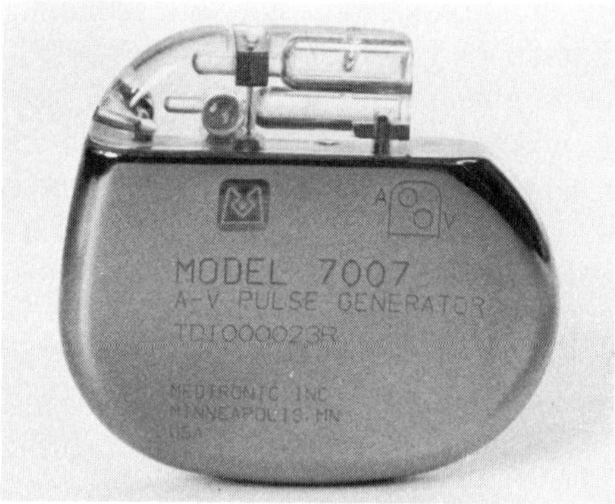

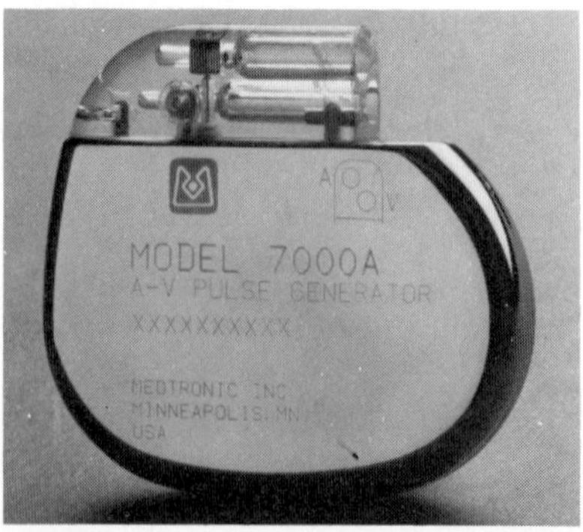

Pacemaker Characteristics *Continued*

Pacemaker	Classification	Parameters	Salient Features
Byrel-SX Model 5993SX	DVI, VVI, DOO, VOO	Rate, AV delay, pulse width (A&V), sensitivity (V)	Noncommitted AV pacing Ventricular safety pacing Threshold margin test to determine loss of capture (A&V) Inhibit mode 12-msec blanking period Anti-Stim insulative coating Constant energy throughout service life 23-ml volume, 52 g, 10 mm thick

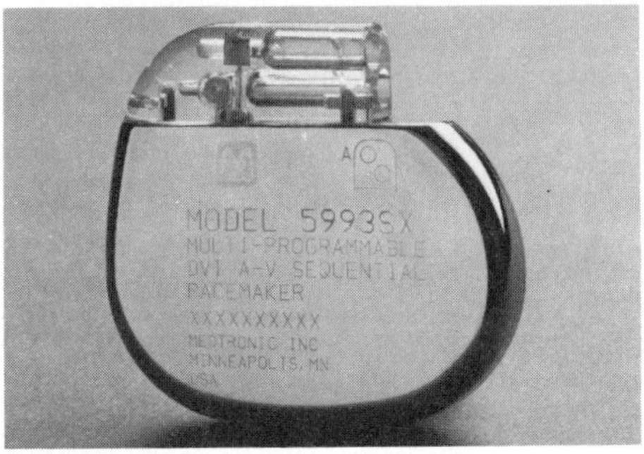

Pacemaker	Classification	Parameters	Salient Features
Spectrax-SXT Models 8420, 8422, and 8423	VVI, AAI, VOO, AOO, VVT, AAT	Rate, pulse, width, sensitivity, refractory period, hysteresis, amplitude	Bidirectional telemetry of programming and parameters Intracavitary electrogram Threshold margin test to determine loss of capture Inhibit mode Permanent & temporary programming Rates 30 to 400 ppm

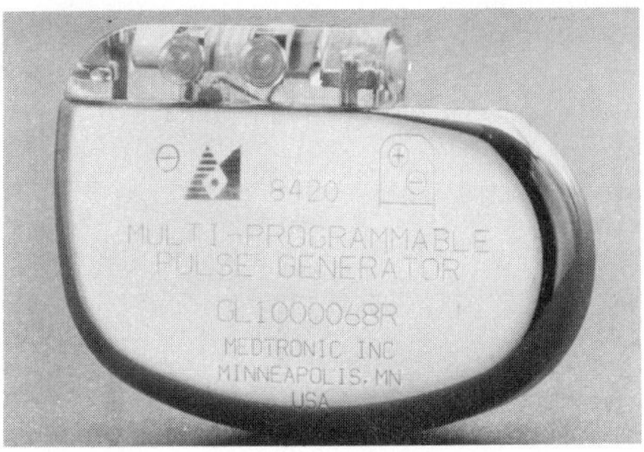

Pacemaker	Classification	Parameters	Salient Features
Spectrax-SX Models 5984, 5984LP, and 5985	VVI, AAI, VVT, AAT, VOO, AOO	Rate, pulse width, sensitivity, refractory period, hysteresis, amplitude	Same as Spectrax-SXT but no telemetry

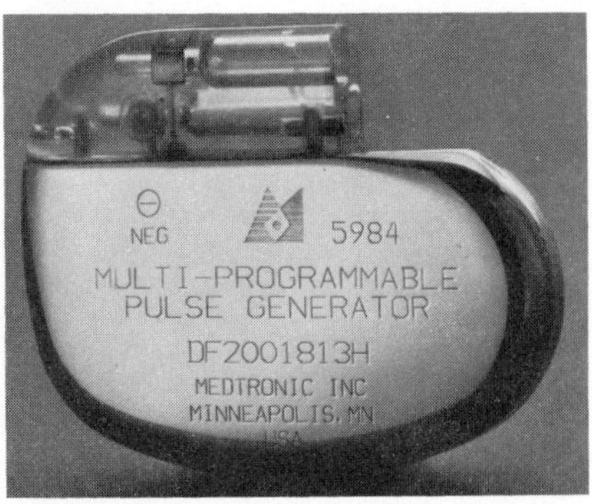

Table continued on following page

Pacemaker Characteristics *Continued*

Pacemaker	Classification	Parameters	Salient Features
Spectrax-SXHT Models 5976 and 5977	Same	Same	Same, but no telemetry 7.1-V full amplitude, 5.0-V half amplitude
Rapid Atrial Stimulator Models 5998R and 5998T	Radio-frequency	Rate	Patient-held transmitter allows implanted receiver to terminate supraventricular tachycardia with burst pacing (30–400 ppm)

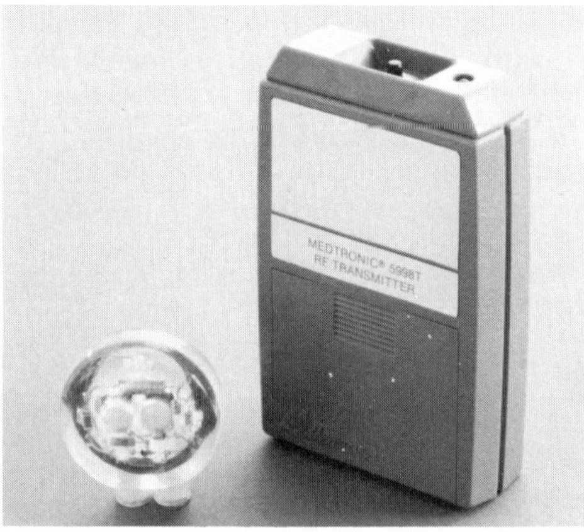

LEADS

Models 6971 and 6972. These are tined ventricular pacing leads with urethane insulation and coaxial conductor construction. Model 6972 (bipolar) and Model 6971 (unipolar) leads both have low dislodgement rates.

Model 4002. This bipolar ventricular pacing lead offers the same construction and handling techniques as are found in the urethane models 6971 and 6972. Model 4002 has an in-line, low-profile bipolar connector, making it suitable for use with Spectrax pacemakers with low-profile bipolar connectors.

Model 6957. This endocardial screw-in lead has a unique helix-type electrode that allows the physician to lodge the lead at any of several locations within the heart. The lead can be used for either atrial or ventricular applications and has proved useful in those cases in which recurrent dislodgement is a problem. The helix electrode can be extended or retracted by the physician for positioning or repositioning during or after threshold testing.

Model 6957J. This J-shaped urethane endocardial screw-in lead for atrial use has many of the same handling features of Model 6957. The J shape aids in placement in the atrial appendage. The extendable helix electrode aids in fixation in truncated appendages, the atrial septum, or the lateral wall.

Model 4951. This epicardial lead is suitable for atrial or ventricular application. The barbed electrode tip achieves fixation in thin tissue, with a minimum of trauma. A low-profile, lightweight electrode head reduces the chance of pericardial rub or pericarditis. An attached Dacron mesh provides fibrous ingrowth for chronic fixation away from the stimulation electrode.

Model 6880. This temporary cardioversion lead is a tripolar lead with four electrodes. Design of the lead is such that when lodged in the right ventricular apex, the ventricular electrode pair lie deep within the right ventricle and the proximal pair lie in the superior vena cava. The lead is designed to sense and cardiovert/defibrillate tachyarrhythmias. The lead can also be used for ventricular demand pacing.

Lead Characteristics

Lead	Description	Salient Features
6971	Ventricular passive fixation, unipolar transvenous	Small, flexible tines Urethane insulator DBS conductor (nickel alloy in a matrix of silver) 4.6-French body 8-French tip

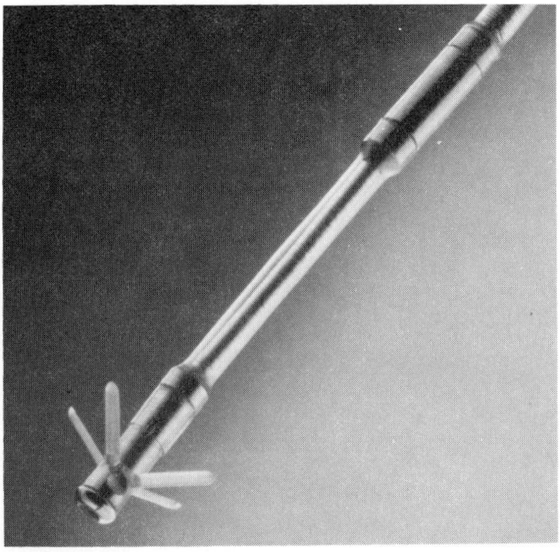

Table continued on following page

Lead Characteristics *Continued*

Lead	Description	Salient Features
4002	Ventricular passive fixation, bipolar transvenous	In-line bipolar connector (instead of bifurcated)

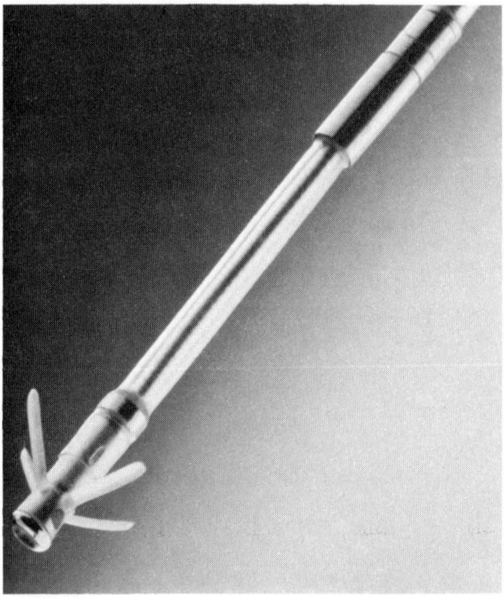

Lead	Description	Salient Features
6957	Atrial or ventricular active fixation, unipolar, transvenous	Helix manually extended or retracted Problem solver for truncated appendages or other anomalies 2-mm helix extension

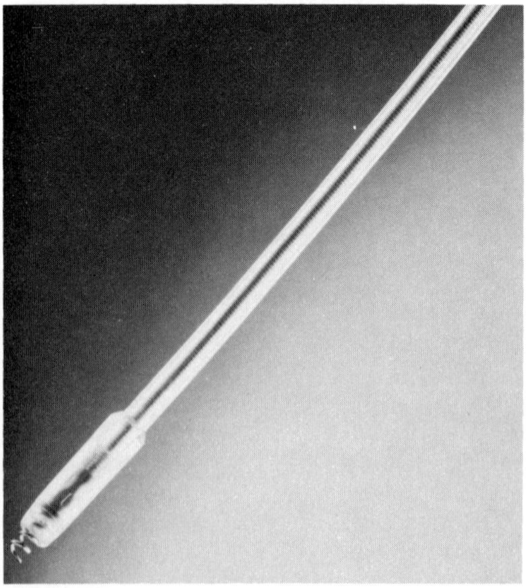

Lead Characteristics *Continued*

Lead	Description	Salient Features
6957J	Atrial active fixation, unipolar, transvenous	Similar to 6957 except has preformed J shape 1.5-mm helix extension
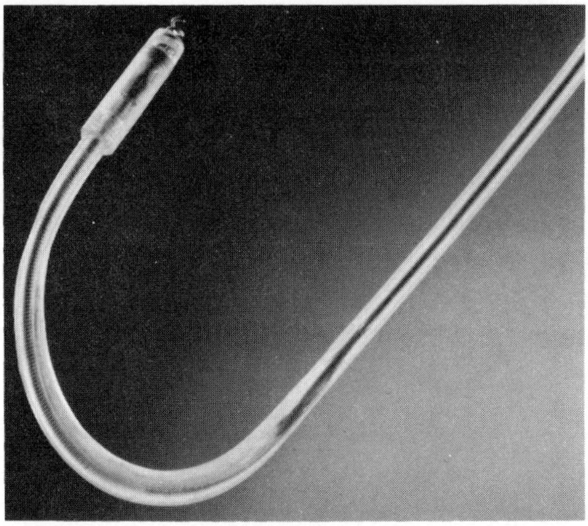		
6993	Atrial passive fixation, unipolar, transvenous	Preformed J shape with memory coil Canted tip Small, flexible tines
6990U	Atrial passive fixation, bipolar, transvenous	Coaxial construction Bipolar version of 6993
4502	Same as 6990U	In-line bipolar connector (instead of bifurcated)
4951	Active fixation, unipolar, epicardial	Low profile, lightweight Suitable for thin-walled atria
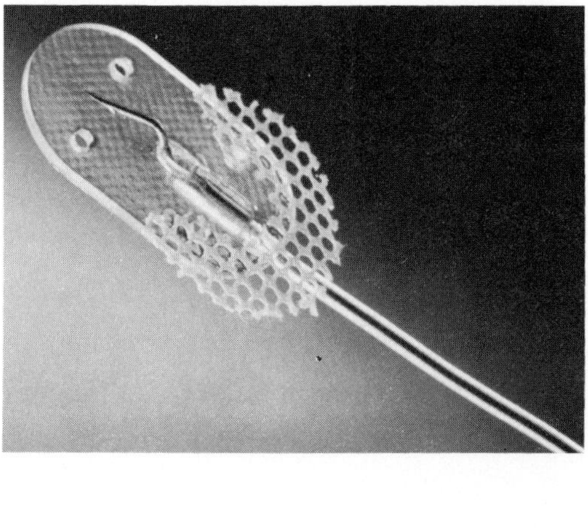		

Table continued on following page

Lead Characteristics *Continued*

Lead	Description	Salient Features
6880	Temporary cardioversion lead, tripolar, transvenous	10 French Designed to sense and cardiovert/defibrillate tachyarrhythmias

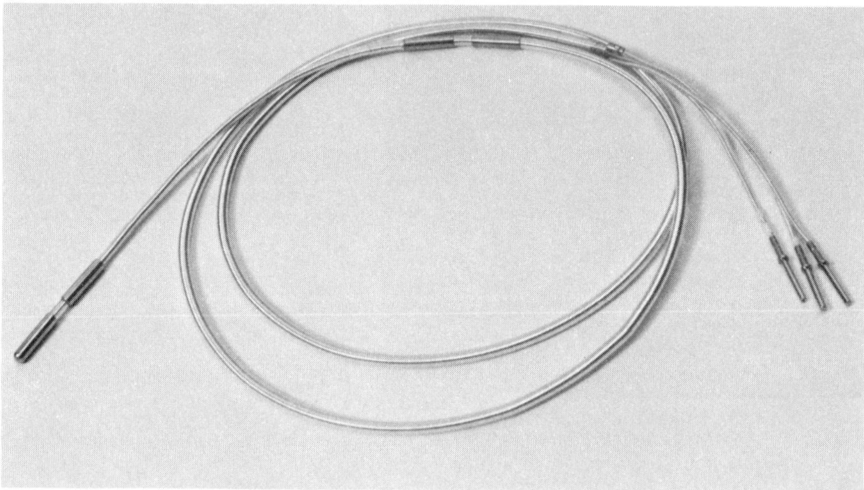

Lead	Description	Salient Features
4011	Unipolar ventricular target tip, passive fixation, transvenous lead	Low threshold Voltage threshold ⅓ conventional ring tip
4511	Unipolar atrial	same as 4011
4012	Bipolar ventricular	same as 4011
4512	Bipolar atrial	same as 4011

PACESETTER SYSTEMS, INC.

12884 Bradley Avenue
Sylmar, California 91342
818-362-6822

INTRODUCTION

In 1969, Alfred E. Mann, President of Spectrolab and Heliotek Divisions of Textron, Inc., was asked by The Applied Physics Laboratory of Johns Hopkins University to develop and produce a rechargeable pacemaker. The first commercial model became available in 1973, with a projected probable life exceeding 70 years. Already the first rechargeable pacemaker had a telemetry feature, unique in the early seventies. The first human implant of the new system took place in 1973 in a patient still living today.

When lithium-iodine batteries were developed, Pacesetter quickly transformed the advance technology that served the rechargeable system into lithium-powered units and entered the market with a lithium-iodine–battery-powered pulse generator in 1976.

Pacesetter's next advance was a programmable pacing system—the Programalith series—designed in 1979. This was the first multiprogrammable pulse generator with bidirectional telemetry, permitting the interrogation of the pacer for lead impedance, battery impedance, and battery current. This feature allows the interrogation and programming of rate, amplitude, pulse width, sensitivity, refractory period, and hysteresis. It also provides a permanent, printed record. The reliability of the Programalith is the highest in the pacemaker industry (Table 1). Since its introduction in 1979, this device has demonstrated a reliability of 98.79 percent (Table 2).

PULSE GENERATORS

Pacesetter's currently available models combine small size, longevity, and reliability with advanced programming and telemetry capability. In addition to the discontinued but still functioning Models 221, 221-A, 222, and 222-A, Pacesetter currently offers the following models:

Programalith II (Models 225 and 226). Since it was introduced in 1981, Programalith II has achieved recognition as a very reliable pulse generator. Table 3 shows its survival in the first 14 months after its introduction.

Table 1. Model Actuarial Survival (40 or More Units)*

Model	Number	12 Months	24 Months	36 Months	48 Months	60 Months	72 Months	84 Months	96 Months	110 Months
Medtronic										
8423	138	100% (22 mo)								
Lil										
Pacesetter										
221	138	100%	100%	100%	100%					
Lil										
Siemens-Elema										
668	58	100%	100% (30 mo)							
Lil										
Cordis										
184A	58	100%	100%	98.2%	96.2%	96.2%	93.3%	89.5%	89.5%	
238				±3.6%	±5.2%	±5.2%	±7.5%	±10.2%	±10.2%	
Pu										

*As of June, 1983. Source available from the authors, Pacesetter Systems, Inc., 12884 Bradley Avenue, Sylmar, CA 91342.

Table 2. Programalith Series: 47-Month Survival

Age in Months	Number of Units	New Units	Withdrawals		Exposed Units	Fraction Failed	Fraction Survival	Achieved Cumulative Survival
			In Spec	*Out Spec*				
0–2	36109	5450	129	56	33384	0.0017	0.9983	0.9983
3–5	30659	3428	56	14	28945	0.0005	0.9995	0.9978
6–8	27231	3056	46	7	25703	0.0003	0.9997	0.9975
9–11	24175	3168	29	11	22591	0.0005	0.9995	0.9970
12–14	21007	3620	25	4	19197	0.0002	0.9998	0.9968
15–17	17387	3243	22	3	15766	0.0002	0.9998	0.9966
18–20	14145	3042	13	3	12624	0.0002	0.9998	0.9964
21–23	11103	2646	6	5	9780	0.0005	0.9995	0.9959
24–26	8457	2414	7	2	7250	0.0003	0.9997	0.9956
27–29	6043	1977	3	0	5055	0.0000	1.0000	0.9956
30–32	4066	1368	2	2	3382	0.0006	0.9994	0.9950
33–35	2698	1123	3	1	2137	0.0005	0.9995	0.9945
36–38	1575	798	1	3	1176	0.0026	0.9974	0.9919
39–41	777	582	2	2	486	0.0041	0.9959	0.9879
42–44	95	171	0	0	110	0.0000	1.0000	0.9879
45–47	24	24	0	0	12	0.0000	1.0000	0.9879

*As of June, 1983. Source and data available from the authors, Pacesetter Systems, Inc., 12884 Bradley Avenue, Sylmar, CA 91342.

Table 3. Programalith II Series: Survival During First 14 Months

Age in Months	Number of Units	New Units	Withdrawals		Exposed Units	Fraction Failed	Fraction Survival	Achieved Cumulative Survival
			In Spec	*Out Spec*				
0–2	9411	3515	30	16	7654	0.0021	0.9979	0.9979
3–5	5896	2246	10	6	4773	0.0013	0.9987	0.9966
6–8	3650	1851	1	0	2725	0.0000	1.0000	0.9966
9–11	1799	1408	3	0	1095	0.0000	1.0000	0.9966
12–14	391	391	0	0	196	0.0000	1.0000	0.9966

Programalith III (Models 241 and 242). Pacesetter's Programalith III is a lithium-iodine–battery-powered, implantable pulse generator that can be interrogated. It is available in unipolar (241) and bipolar (242) models. Depending on the specific model, a number of parameters may be programmed or interrogated.

These small, lightweight, hermetically sealed pacemakers are designed to sense cardiac depolarization signals and deliver pacing impulses only when the patient's intrinsic rate falls below the programmed rate of the pulse generator.

For those patients in whom fine tuning of pulse generator parameters is indicated, Programalith III may be noninvasively programmed to modify its performance characteristics. At the time of implantation, or any time thereafter, an external programming system may be used to communicate with the pulse generator by means of pulsed radio-frequency signals in conjunction with a magnetic field.

Physicians will probably find Programalith III's thinness and light weight to be its most impressive features. It weighs only 35 g and is the thinnest (8 mm) of all the advanced pulse generators. Combined with its projected longevity, Programalith III is the pacer of choice for implants into children and thin, elderly patients.

AFP Models 261 and 262. These two new pacers are the first in Pacesetter's advanced function pacing (AFP) series. At the heart of the system is an expanded bidirectional telemetry capability coupled with greatly increased control over pacing parameters and modes of operation. Seven modes are available, along with rates that can be programmed in 1-ppm steps from 45 to 108 and in 2-ppm steps from 108 to 118. Sixteen choices each for pulse amplitude, pulse width, and sensitivity are programmed into this lightweight pacer. Four different refractory periods for either ventricular or atrial chambers are possible. The important difference between these AFP pacers and earlier ones is the ability to program triggered modes (VVT and AAT) and nonsensing modes (VOO and AOO).

None of the parameters of Models 261 and 262 will vary significantly from the nominal values as the battery impedance increases and the cell voltage decreases with time. For this reason, the performance characteristics of these pacemakers are exceptionally stable. The demand pacing rate, sensitivity, refractory period, and hysteresis are all independent of time, battery impedance, temperature, and load.

AFP Model 275. This is Pacesetter's first pulse generator that has dual-chamber sensing and can maintain AV synchrony in the presence of intrinsic atrial activity. In this model it is possible to program AV delay to optimize hemodynamics. Model 275 weighs 5 g and is 10 mm thick. It features a programmable maximum tracking rate (MTR). MTR is the maximum atrial rate that can be tracked by the pacemaker with a 1:1 ventricular response. It is particularly important to program the MTR for elderly patients with extensive heart disease or current ventricular tachyarrhythmias. In Model 275, when the rate is programmed to between 45 and 80 ppm, MTR will be between 90 and

150 ppm. At rates of 81 to 100 the MTR is between 110 and 150 ppm, and above 110 ppm the MTR will be 130 to 150 ppm. Both AV delay and MTR will operate only in the VDD mode. Model 275 has all the programmable parameters and the same number of choices as AFP Models 261 and 262, described above.

AFP Model 283. This is Pacesetter's most advanced dual-chamber pulse generator. It has 13 modes of operation, including DVI, DDI, DDD, and DDX. In many patients, a major limitation of the DVI mode is its lack of atrial sensing. Atrial competition, resulting in asynchronous atrial pacing, may induce competing rhythms. The DDD mode, which provides pacing and sensing in the atrium and the ventricle, gives a physiologic response to varying intrinsic atrial and ventricular activity and is therefore designed into the programming of the AFP Model 283 pulse generator.

The second major innovation of Model 283 is DDX. The timing diagram and function of this mode are identical to the previously described DDD mode except for the response to premature ventricular activity. When a PVC (a sensed ventricular event without a preceding atrial event) is detected during the ventricular alert period, both pacer channels will be inhibited and the pacer timing will reset to the end of AV delay (beginning of atrial escape interval). This response is identical to the DDD response. However, with the DDX mode, the atrial channel sensing will be turned off for one entire pacer cycle following PVC detection. This refinement of the DDD mode provides automatic conversion to the DVI mode following a PVC, resulting in protection from pacer-mediated tachycardias that are caused by retrograde conduction.

When the ATP pulse generators are employed in the DVI, DDI, DDD, and DDX modes, a period in which no sensing takes place (blanking period) will momentarily occur in the ventricular sensing circuit coincident with any atrial output pulse. The blanking period is necessary to prevent the detection of this pulse by the ventricular channel, resulting in arrest of the pulse generator's timing. In Model 283, the blanking period is programmable to 13, 25, 38, or 50 msec. In addition to the above innovations, to satisfy every clinical need Model 283 has the same programmable parameters and the great choice of values as the other pulse generators described above, including an atrial refractory period that may be programmed for as much as 550 msec (as with AFP Model 275). It has advanced telemetry (measured and programmed data) and ECG.

Pacemaker Characteristics

Pacemaker	Classification	Parameters	Salient Features
Programalith AV Model 223 (dual-unipolar)	VOO, VVI, VVT, DVI Committed dual-chamber pacing 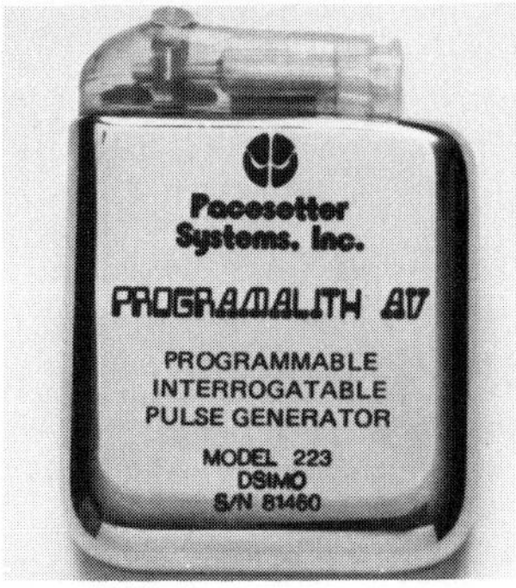 	Rate, mode, pulse amplitude, pulse width, sensitivity, refractory period	Longevity > 5 years Programmed telemetry, measured telemetry
Programalith II Model 225 (unipolar) Model 226 (bipolar)	VVI/AAI 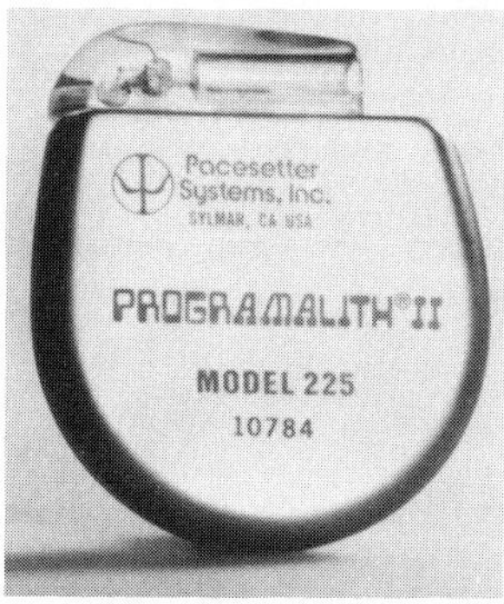 	Rate, pulse amplitude, pulse width, sensitivity, refractory period, hysteresis	11 mm thick Longevity > 8 years Programmed telemetry, measured telemetry
Programalith III Model 241 (unipolar) Model 242 (bipolar)	VVI/AAI 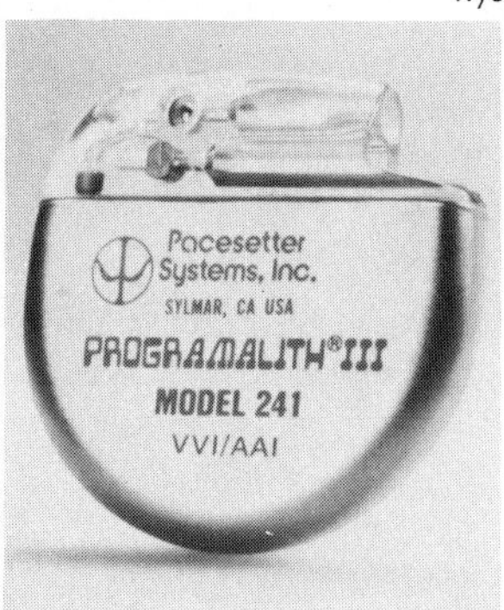 	Rate, pulse amplitude, pulse width, sensitivity, refractory period, hysteresis	Longevity > 9 years Programmed telemetry and measured telemetry 8 mm thick, 35 g High-output capability

Table continued on following page

Pacemaker Characteristics *Continued*

Pacemaker	Classification	Parameters	Salient Features
AFP Model 261 (unipolar) Model 262 (bipolar)	VVI, AAI, VVT, AAT, VOO, AOO, off 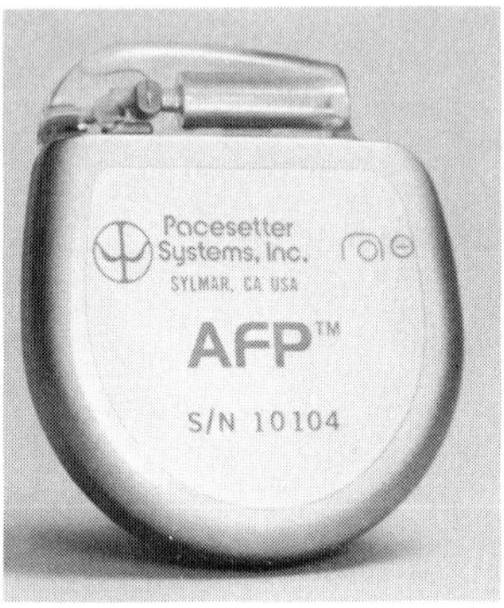 	Rate, mode, pulse amplitude, pulse width, sensitivity, refractory period, hysteresis, runaway limit	Longevity > 12 years Programmed telemetry, measured and stored data High-output capability Intracardiac electrogram Threshold tests 10 mm thick, 50 g
AFP Model 275 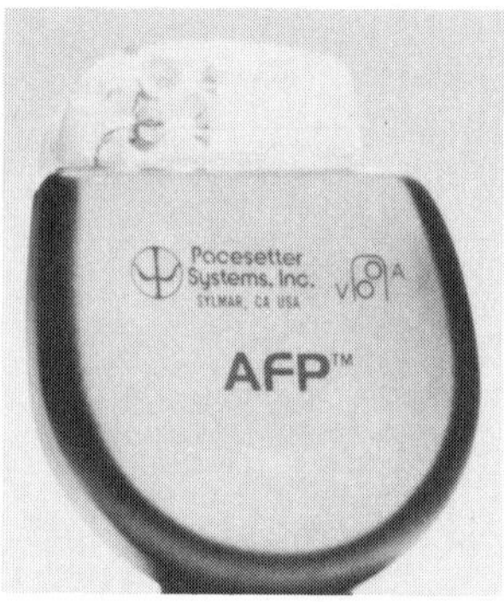 	VDD, VVI, VVT, VOO, off	Rate, mode, ventricular pulse amplitude and width, ventricular and atrial sensitivity and refractory period, hysteresis, AV delay, maximum tracking rate	Longevity > 11 years Programmed telemetry, measured and stored data Intracardiac electrogram (A and V) Magnet on/off High-output capability 10 mm thick, 50 g
AFP Model 283 (unipolar) 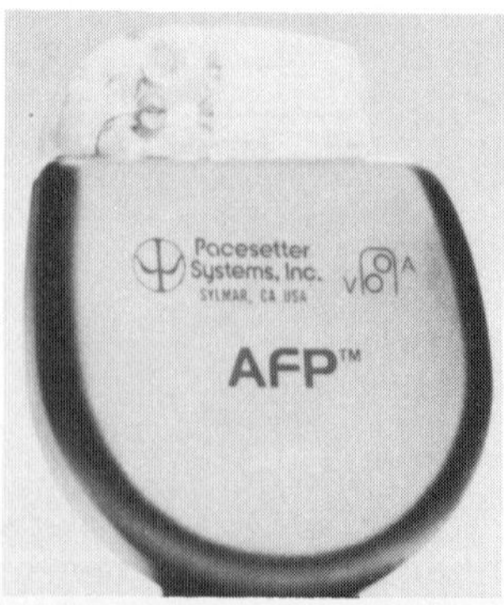 	DDD, DVI, VDD, DOO, VVI, VVT, VVO, AAI, AAT, AOO, DDX (DDD with PVC detector on), off	Rate, mode, ventricular and atrial pulse amplitude and width, ventricular and atrial sensitivity and refractory period, AV delay, hysteresis or stand-by rate, maximum tracking rate, ventricular blanking period following an atrial pulse	Longevity > 8 years Programmed telemetry, measured and stored data Intracardiac electrograms Magnet on/off Threshold tests High-output capability 10 mm thick, 50 g

Pacemaker Characteristics *Continued*

Pacemaker	Classification	Parameters	Salient Features
Coats Pacesetter Vivalith II Model 301 (unipolar)	VVI	Nonprogrammable Basic rate: 71 Pulse duration: 0.52 ± 0.04 msec Sensitivity: 2.0 ± 0.4 mv Pulse amplitude: 4.7 V Maximum Pulse Amplitude: 5.0 V Magnet test rate: 78 ± 2 PPM Pacing & sensing refractory period: 340 ± 30 msec	Longevity > 8 years Weight 45 g, 9 mm thick 5-mm leads

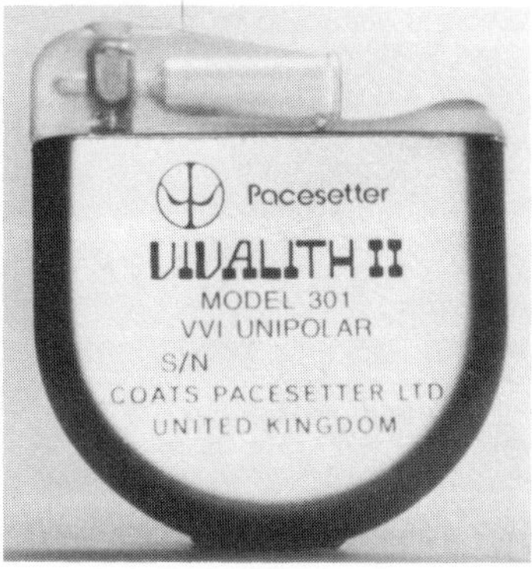

Lead Characteristics

Lead	Description	Salient Features
815/816	8.0/10.0 French, platinum iridium blunt-tip electrode	Unifilar 815: unipolar 816: bipolar Pacepath (silicone)

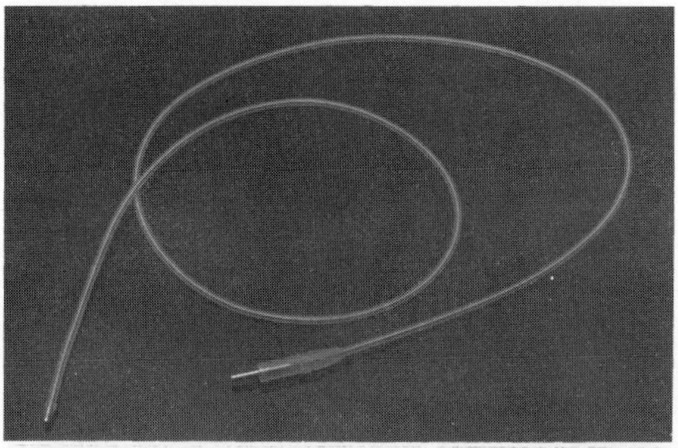

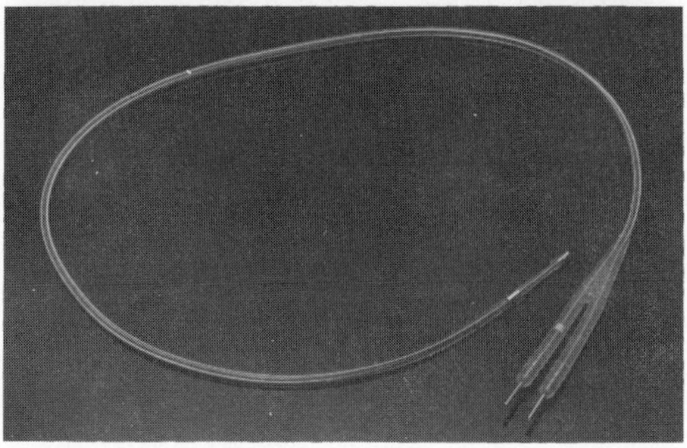

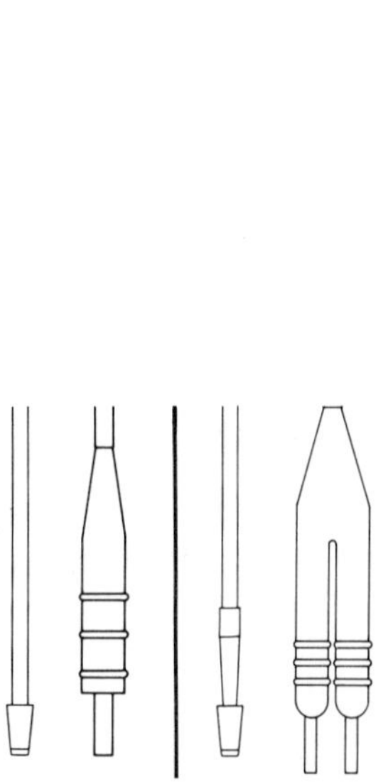

Table continued on following page

Lead Characteristics *Continued*

Lead	Description	Salient Features
818/819	6.8/10.0 French, platinum iridium blunt-tip electrode	Unifilar 818: unipolar 819: bipolar Pacepath (silicone)

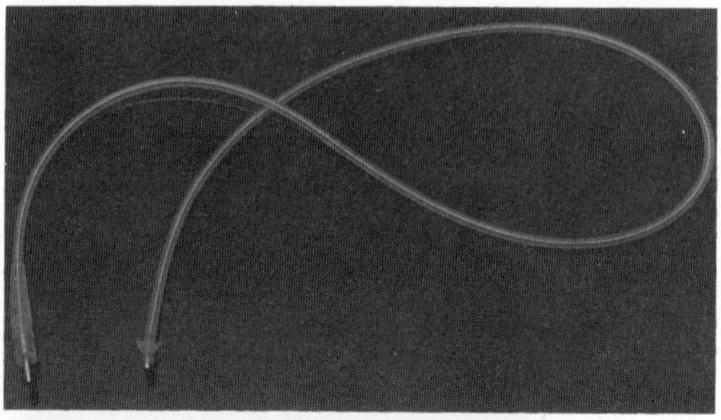

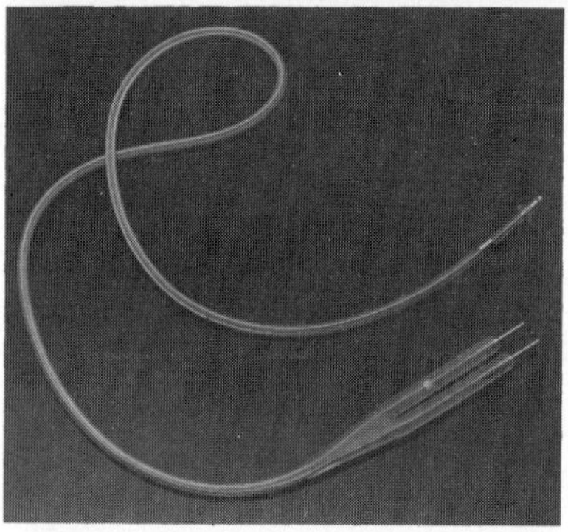

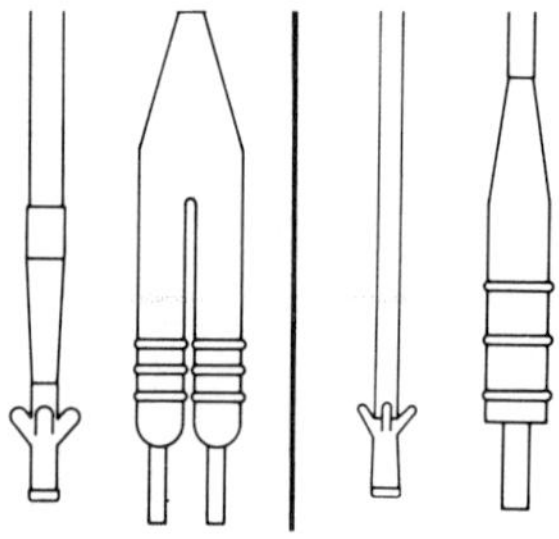

Lead	Description	Salient Features
829	5.3 French, platinum iridium ring-tip electrode	Unipolar, tined, atrial J High performance (silicone)

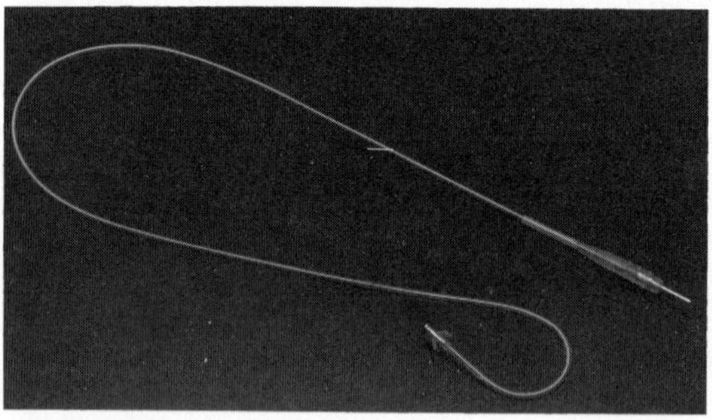

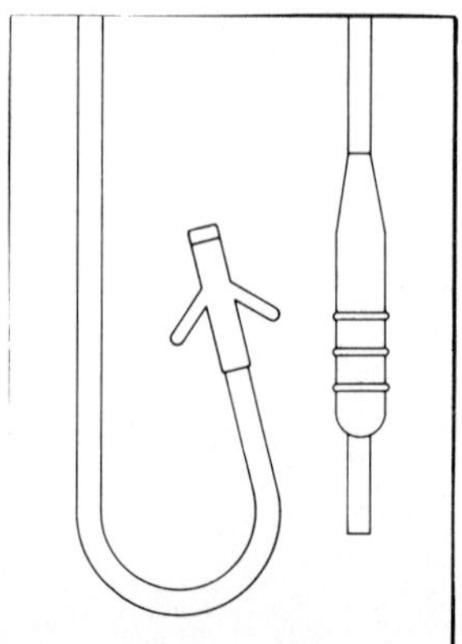

Lead Characteristics *Continued*

Lead	Description	Salient Features
850	5.0 French, platinum iridium ring-tip electrode	Bipolar, ventricular, tined, coaxial High performance (silicone)

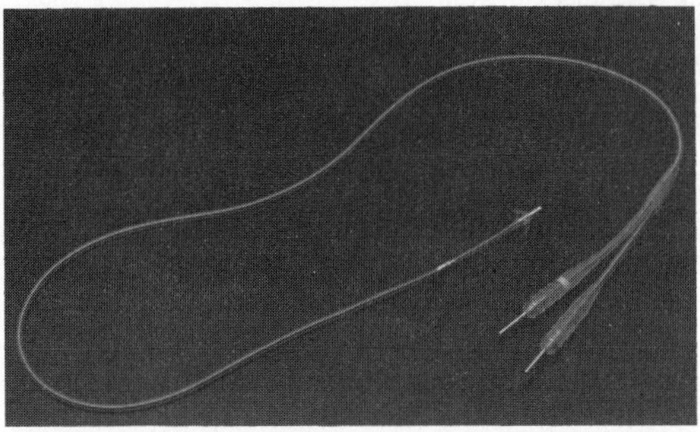

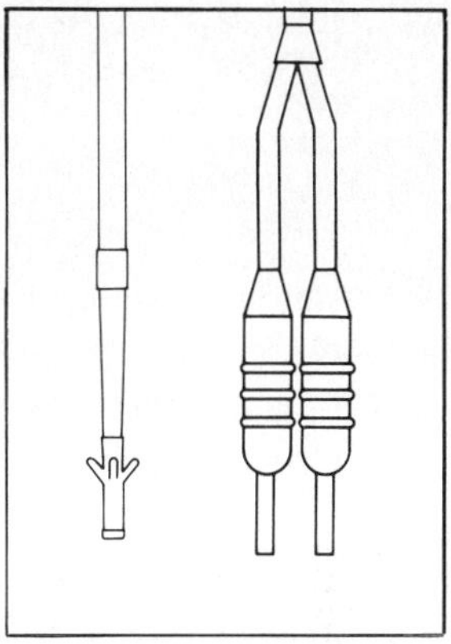

Lead	Description	Salient Features
851/853	4.5/5.3 French, platinum iridium ring-tip electrode	Unipolar, tined 851: ventricular 853: atrial J Fast-Pass (silicone)

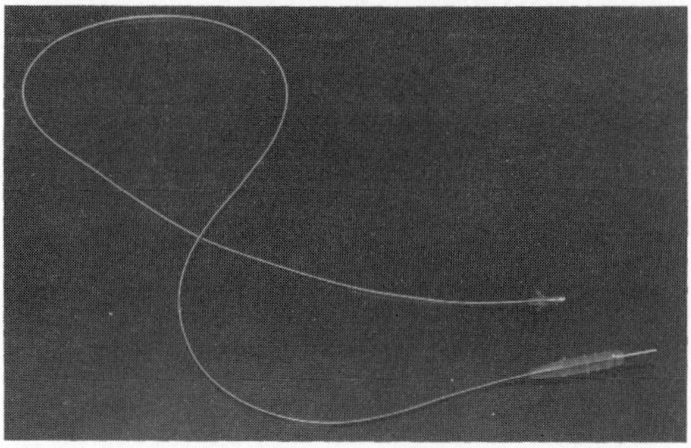

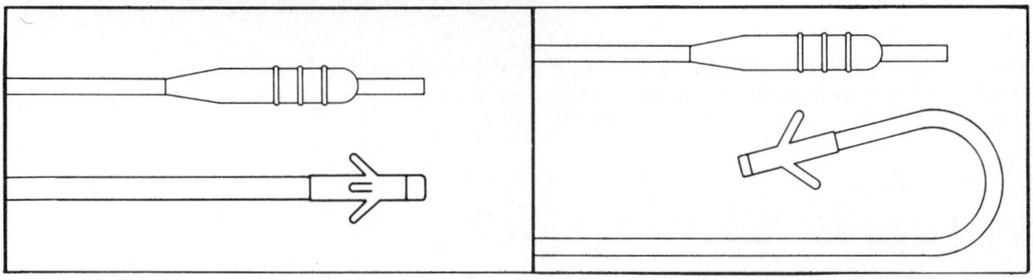

Table continued on following page

Lead Characteristics *Continued*

Lead	Description	Salient Features
866/869	4.5/3.8 French, platinum iridium ring-tip electrode	866: bipolar, ventricular, tined, multifilar 869: unipolar, atrial J, tined, trifilar Permathane (polyurethane)

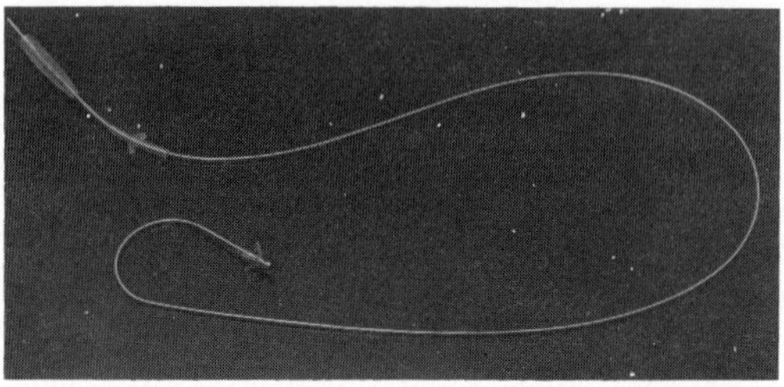

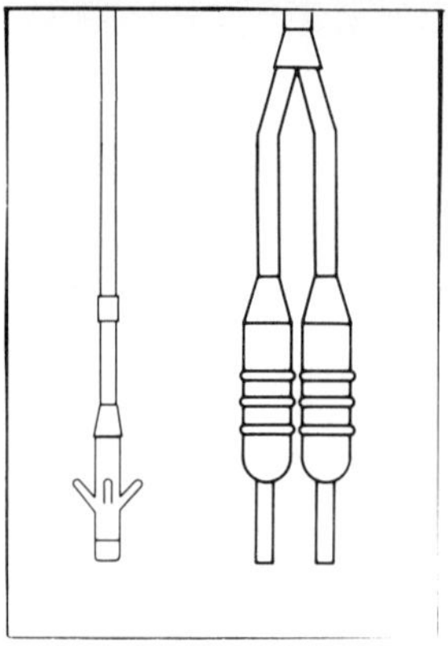

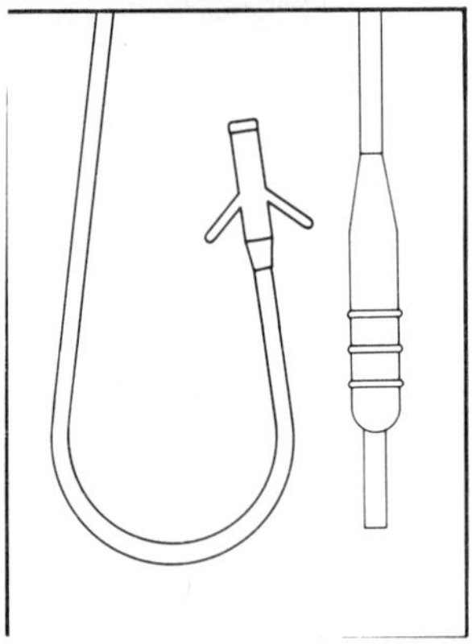

Lead and Pacer Compatibility Chart

Pacer	Pacepath Leads		High Performance Leads		Fast-Pass Leads		Permathane Leads	
	Wedge	*Tine*	*Atrial*	*Ventricular*	*Atrial*	*Ventricular*	*Atrial*	*Ventricular*
223	N/A	825	829	841	853	851	869	865
225	815	819	N/A	833	N/A	N/A	N/A	867
226	816	818 or 820*	N/A	850	N/A	N/A	N/A	866
241	N/A	825	N/A	841	N/A	851	N/A	865
242	816	818 or 820*	N/A	850	N/A	N/A	N/A	866
261	815	819	N/A	833	N/A	N/A	N/A	867
262	816	818 or 820*	N/A	850	N/A	N/A	N/A	866
275	N/A	825	829	841	853	851	869	865
283	N/A	825	829	841	853	851	869	865
C-P† 301	815	819	N/A	833	N/A	N/A	N/A	867

*Lead 818 accepts 2 stylets; lead 820 accepts 1 stylet.
†Coates-pacesetter.

SIEMENS-ELEMA

528 Viscount Road
Yardley, Pennsylvania 19067
215-343-2283

INTRODUCTION

On October 8, 1958, the first internal pacemaker was implanted in Stockholm, Sweden. The recipient, Mr. Arne Larsson, is still alive after 25 years of cardiac pacing.

Dr. Rune Elmqvist of Siemens-Elema (then Elema-Schonander) designed the first implantable pulse generator, which was implanted by Professor Ake Senning.

During these first 25 years of cardiac pacing Siemens-Elema has been a leader in developing reliable pulse generators and leads.

The company's headquarters are located in Solna, Sweden, and its products are distributed worldwide, mainly by Siemens offices.

PULSE GENERATORS

The past 25 years have seen the development of many types of pacing devices—from a constant fixed-rate pacemaker used in the treatment of bradycardia, to QRS-inhibited pacers, dual-chamber pacers, and multiprogrammable pacemakers in which rates and other electrical settings can easily be changed without surgery.

The following models are currently available from Siemens-Elema:

Model 674. This device, currently under clinical evaluation in the USA, is a unipolar, multiprogrammable, dual-chamber pacemaker. The risk of pacemaker-mediated tachycardias is substantially reduced by self-adapting refractory periods. The atrial and ventricular stimulation thresholds can easily be measured by the unique VARIO function activated by an ordinary test magnet.

To ensure the best possible ventricular filling, different AV intervals are used to equalize the duration of sensed and paced atrial events. The expected longevity is 7 years (DDD mode, 5 V both chambers, .75-msec pulse duration, 100 per cent pacing).

Model 668. This unipolar or bipolar multiprogrammable VVI pacemaker can also be used as a AAI pacemaker. Expected longevity at standard parameter settings is 11 years.

Model 678. This is essentially the same pacemaker as the 668. The 678 has a smaller battery than the 668, is a smaller size, and weighs only 39 g. The 10-V output is not available in the 678. Expected longevity is 5.5 years at standard program. With 2.5-V output the longevity is increased to approximately 13 years.

Model 718 Dialog. The Dialog is basically similar to the 668. The telemetry functions give parameter settings, mode identification, serial number, and date of last programming, as well as paced-event counter, tachycardia/interference counter, and intracardiac electrogram.

Programmer P 700. This pacemaker is fitted with a serial computer interface based on the RS232C. The P 700 can be easily connected with and give information to any computer configuration having serial data input in accordance with the same standard.

Pacemaker Characteristics

Pacemaker	Parameters	Features
Model 674	Mode, rate, P-wave hysteresis, highest synchronous rate, atrial amplitude, atrial pulse duration, atrial sensitivity, atrial refractory period, atrial VARIO function, AV interval, ventricular pulse duration, ventricular VARIO function	VARIO function for noninvasive measuring of atrial and ventricular voltage thresholds Different paced and sensed AV intervals to provide equal ventricular filling time Programmable atrial refractory periods and full atrial refractory period after PVC to protect against pacemaker-mediated tachycardias Long projected service life—7 years

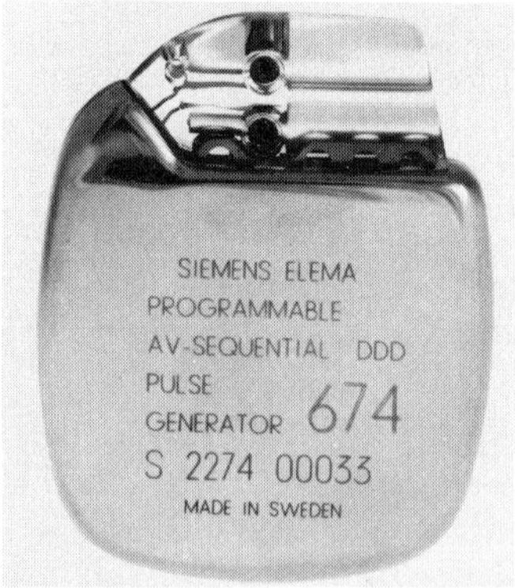

Pacemaker Characteristics *Continued*

Pacemaker	Parameters	Features
Model 668	Pulse duration, pulse amplitude, basic rate, sensitivity, refractory period, hysteresis, VARIO	Can be used as a VVI or AAI generator 10-V output for high thresholds 2.5-V for energy savings VARIO to check the safety margin Dual and distinct replacement criteria

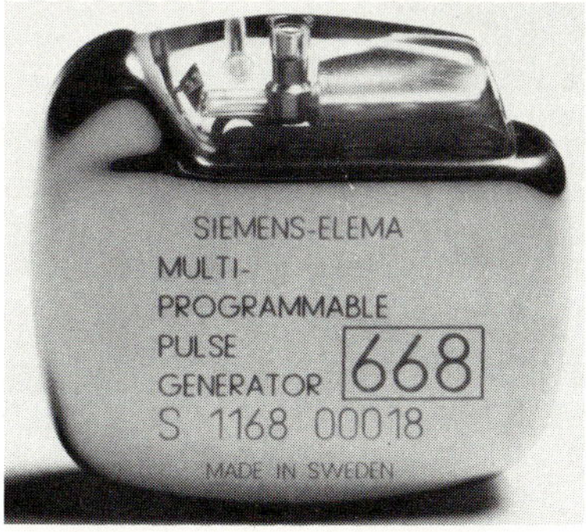

Pacemaker	Parameters	Features
Model 678	Pulse duration, amplitude, rate, sensitivity, refractory period, hysteresis, VARIO	Small size, 39 g 2.5-V output for increased longevity VARIO to check the safety margin.

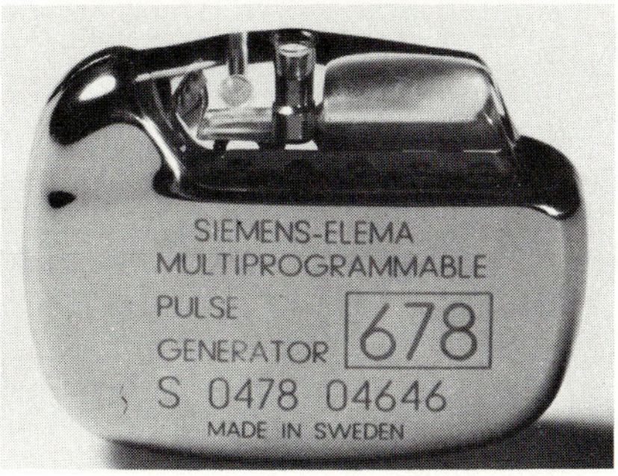

Pacemaker	Parameters	Features
Model 718 Dialog	Model, rate, amplitude, pulse duration, sensitivity, refractory period, hysteresis, VARIO	All of the Model 668 features plus telemetric information on the following: intracardiac electrogram, pacemaker model and serial number, program settings, lead impedance, battery status, detection and recording of tachycardia, number of paced events, date of last programming

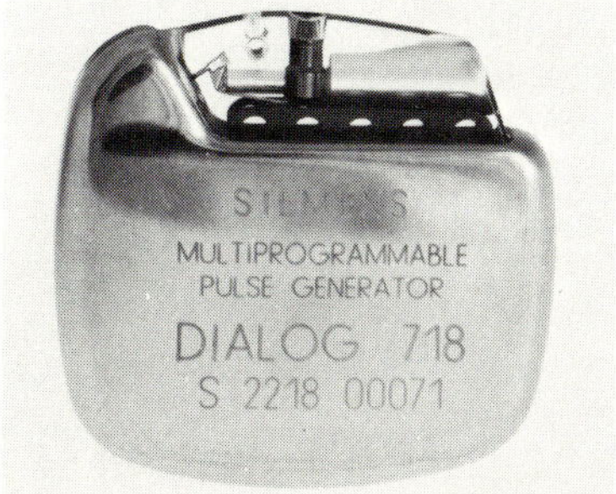

Pacemaker	Parameters	Features
Model 688	Pulse duration, pulse amplitude, basic rate, sensitivity, refractory period, hysteresis, VARIO	Similar to Model 668; to replace 668 in the near future 9 mm thickness Weight of less than 39 g

LEADS

Most of the complications that occur in pacemaker therapy today are in one way or another related to the pacing lead.

Siemens-Elema has developed what may prove to be the solution to many complications such as exit blocks and sensing difficulties: the vitreous carbon tip lead. Thanks to this lead tip, it is now possible to increase the total service life of programmable pulse generators by reducing pulse duration or amplitude without the risk of exit blocks.

Lead Characteristics

Lead	Description	Features
411S	Unipolar carbon tip lead with flange 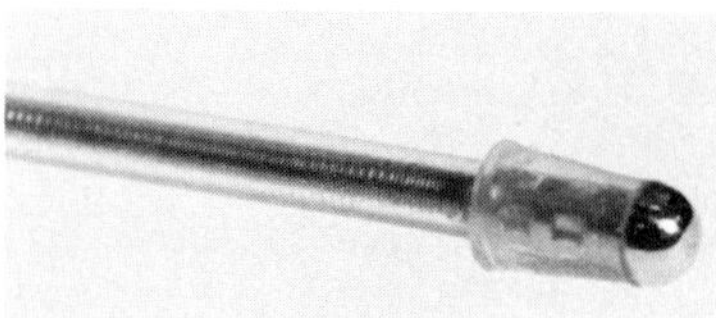	Organic, inert material with low fibrolytic growth Low polarization voltage Low acute and chronic threshold
412S	Unipolar carbon tip lead with tines 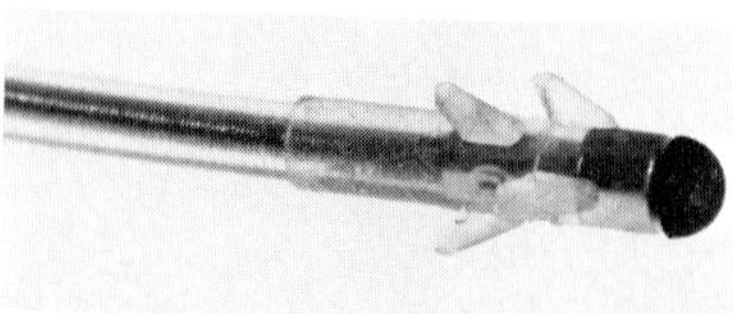	With the VARIO function measuring the safety margin, low-output programming can be used, prolonging the lifetime of the system
404B	Bipolar carbon tip lead with tines 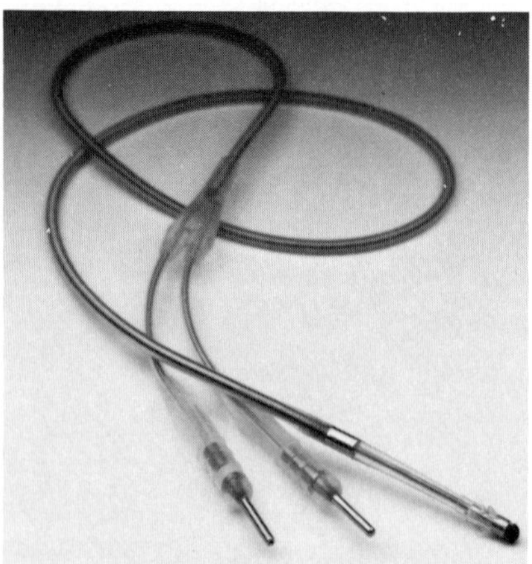	Same as 412S

Lead Characteristics *Continued*

Lead	Description	Features
402S	Endocardial screw-in lead with Elgiloy tip	For active atrial or ventricular fixation

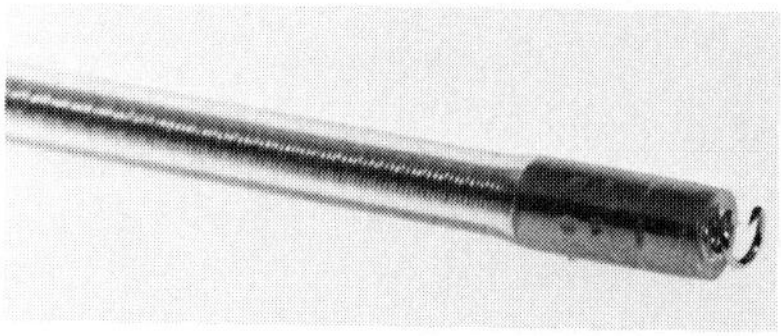

Lead	Description	Features
401S	Myocardial screw-in lead with platinum tip	For active myocardial fixation

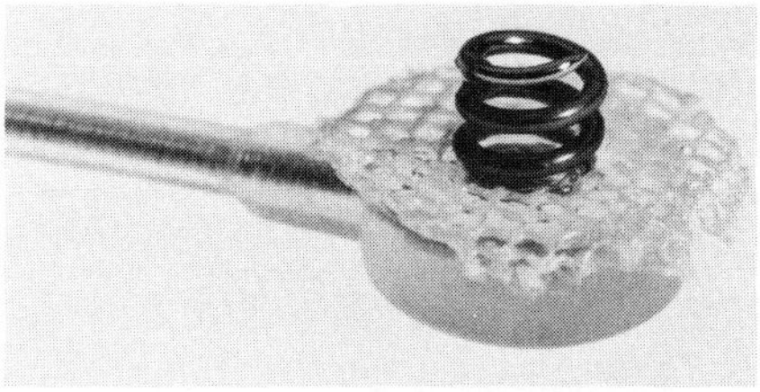

TELECTRONICS

101 Inverness Drive East
Englewood, Colorado 80112
303-779-4670

INTRODUCTION

The TELECTRONICS involvement with cardiac pacing has gone far beyond the simple requirement of manufacturing reliable pacing systems. Indeed, TELECTRONICS has pioneered many pacing developments which are today industry standards. From the first TELECTRONICS pacemaker implanted in 1962, innovations have included the clinical proving and use of a 0.5mS pacing pulse (1964); the first use of titanium as an encapsulation material (1969); the first use of integrated circuitry (1969); the first use of hermetically sealed encapsulations (1971); and the first use of silicone elastomer as a coating (1973). TELECTRONICS was at the leading edge of the use of lithium cells (1974), the use of programmable pacing (1979), the development of the thinnest commercial pacemaker (1980), and the use of dual chamber pacing (1981).

As pacing involves electrode leads a well as the pulse generator, TELECTRONICS has continued its development in this area also, the LASERPOR porous tip electrode lead being a fine example.

Reliable innovation, a TELECTRONICS theme of the last 20 years, will continue for the future.

Pacemaker Characteristics

<table>
<tr><th>Pacemaker</th><th>Classification</th><th>Parameters</th><th>Salient Features</th></tr>
<tr><td>Pasar* 4171 (bipolar)

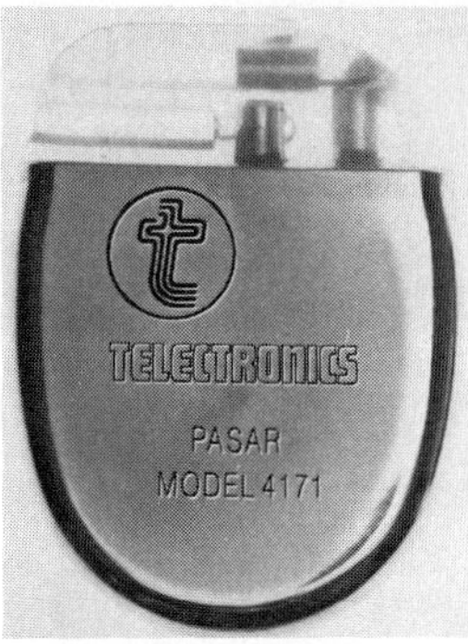
</td><td>Synchronized
Scanning burst bradycardia control</td><td>Number of pulses, burst status, initial delay, coupled delay, tachycardia detection rate
Pulse width, sensitivity, standby pacing</td><td>Synchronized burst—synchronizes off fifth cycle of tachycardia
Scanning—seeks the termination window
Memory function—stores the intervals that last terminated the tachycardia
Wide range of tachycardia detection rates—110–200
Automatic—requires no patient interface
Easy noninvasive testing</td></tr>
<tr><td>Optima 147/247 (unipolar)

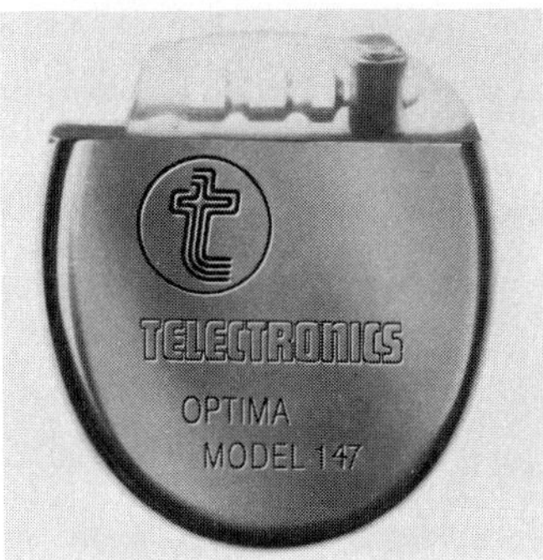
</td><td>VVI (nonprogrammable)</td><td></td><td>Unipolar configuration accepts Cordis or Medtronic connector sizes
Excellent reliability
10-year longevity
9 mm thick
Elliptical shape
Silicone elastomer coating</td></tr>
<tr><td>174/274

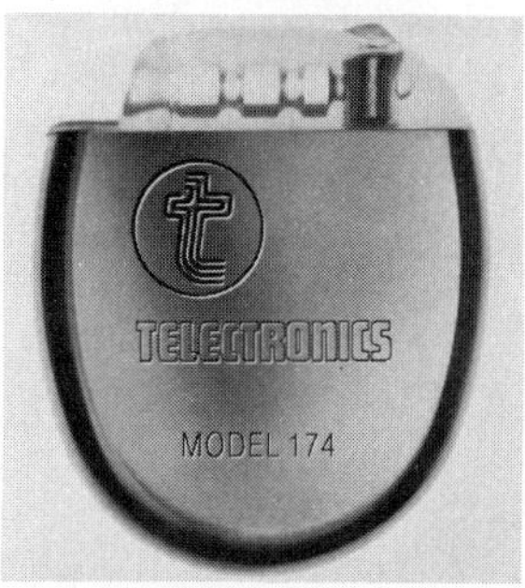

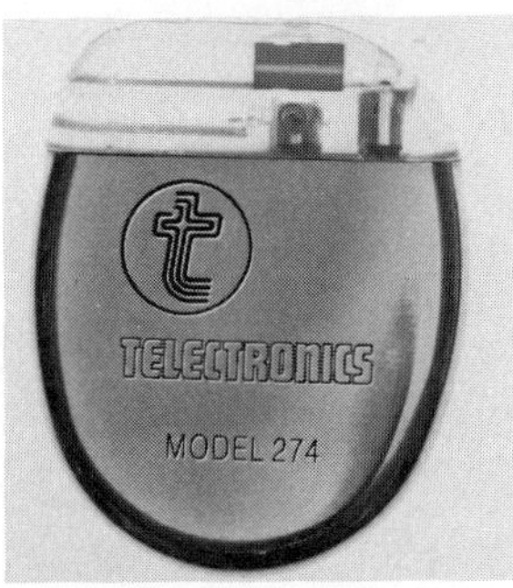
</td><td>VVI (multiprogrammable)</td><td>Rate (8), pulse amplitude (2), pulse width (4), sensitivity (2)</td><td>Unipolar or bipolar configuration
Inexpensive, multiprogrammable
8-year longevity
Excellent reliability
Unipolar silicone elastomer coating
83 μJ output available
Simple hand-held programmer
Elliptical shape</td></tr>
</table>

*Clinical investigation device of 1984.

Table continued on following page

Pacemaker Characteristics *Continued*

Pacemaker	Classification	Parameters	Salient Features
Optima MP 155/255	VVI, AAI, AOO, AOO (multiprogrammable)	Mode (2), rate (22), pulse amplitude (3), pulse width (4), sensitivity (4), refractory period (3), hysteresis (3)	Universal connector (unipolar accepts Cordis and Medtronic size connectors) 9 mm thick Hand-held programmer Unipolar silicone elastomer coating Elliptical shape Available in unipolar or bipolar configuration Long life of 11 years at standard settings Excellent reliability
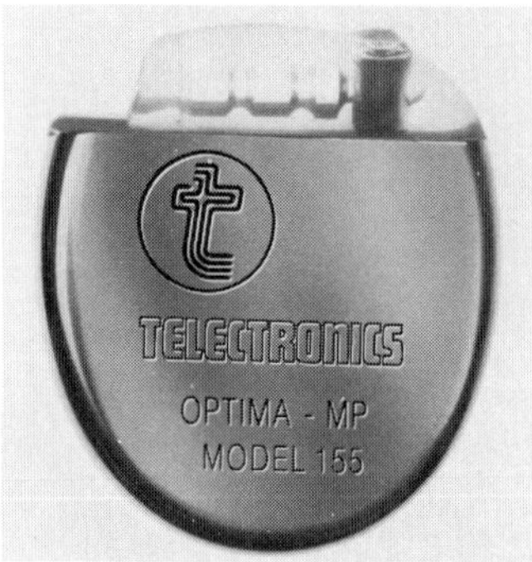	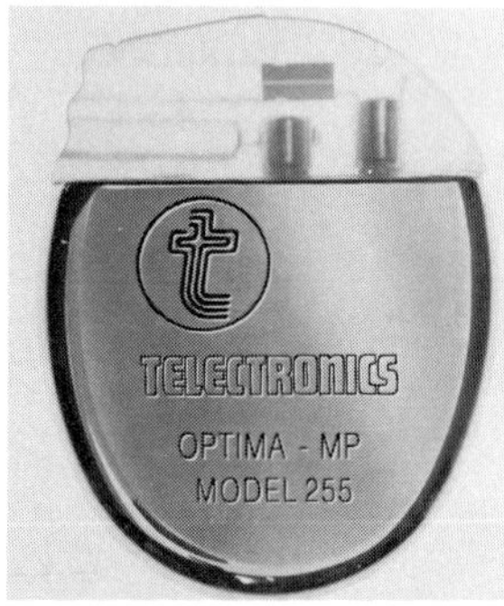		
Optima MPT 5281/5282	VVI, AAI, VOO, AOO (multiprogrammable)	Mode (2), rate (26), pulse amplitude (3), pulse width (4), sensitivity (7), refractory period (3), hysteresis (3)	Telemetry features provide program parameters, intracardiac electrogram, lead and cell impedance, percent of pacing, program counter, program confirmation, model and serial number identification Universal connector (unipolar accepts Cordis and Medtronic connector sizes 10 mm thick 10 V output, none higher Available in unipolar or bipolar configuration Long life of 11 years at standard settings Programmable automatic threshold test Atrial or ventricular applications Unipolar silicone elastomer coating Hand-held programmer Elliptical shape
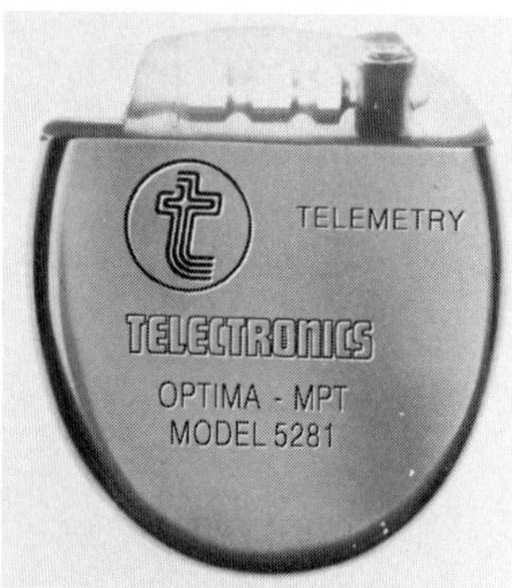	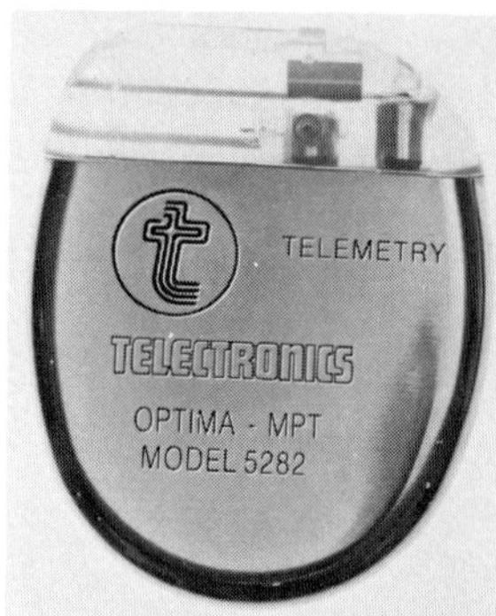		

Pacemaker Characteristics *Continued*

Pacemaker	Classification	Parameters	Salient Features
Autima II 2291 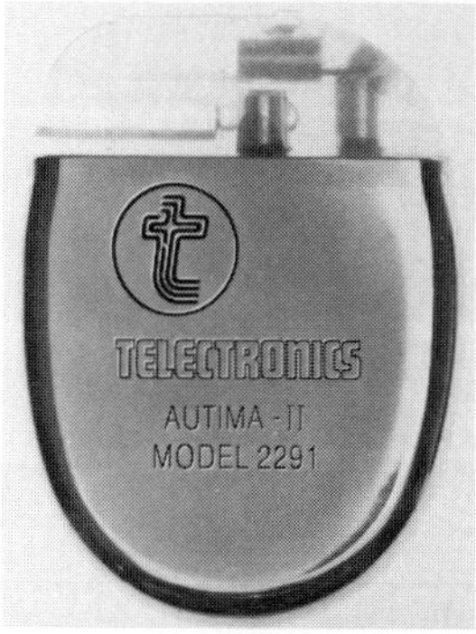 	DDD, VDD, DVI, VVI, DOO, VOO (multiprogrammable)	Mode (6), standby rate (8), maximum tracking rate (4), atrial sensitivity (2), ventricular sensitivity (2), atrial pulse width (4), ventricular pulse width (4), postventricular atrial refractory period (PVARP) (4)	Programmable PVARP to reduce possibility of pacemaker-mediated tachycardia (PMT) Noncommitted ventricular output Dual unipolar 25-msec blanking Programming confirmation Programmable maximum rate response; Wenckebach or 2:1 block 7 years minimum longevity 6-mm Ventricle terminal Programming printout from Universal printer Modified elliptical shape Silicone elastomer coating
Autima 2251 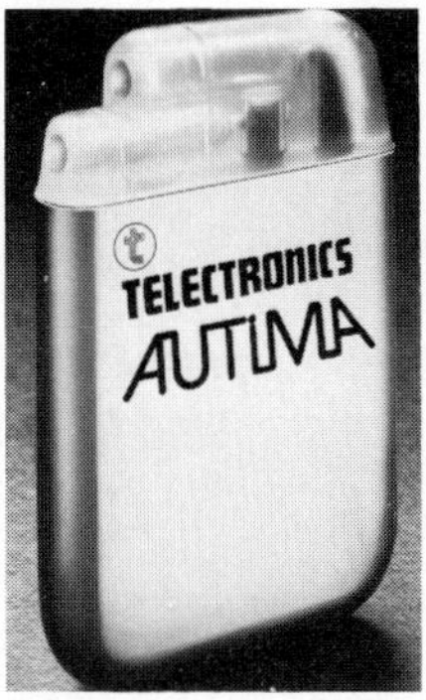 	DDD, VDD, DVI, VVI, DOO, VOO (multiprogrammable)	Mode (6), standby rate (8), AV delay (7), maximum tracking rate (3), atrial sensitivity (2)	US market released Feb. 1983 Adjustable PVARP to control PMT Dual unipolar 25-msec blanking Noncommitted Ventricular output Wenckebach high-rate response Silicone elastomer coating

Lead Characteristics

Lead	Description	Salient Features
241	Atrial J, unipolar, passive fixation, endocardial	Trailing tines Polyurethane 9 French tip diameter Porous tip

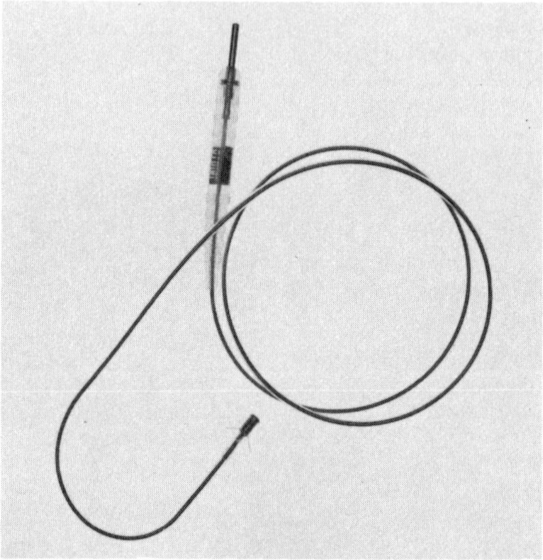

Lead	Description	Salient Features
240	Ventricular, unipolar passive fixation, endocardial	Trailing tines Polyurethane 9 French tip diameter Porous tip

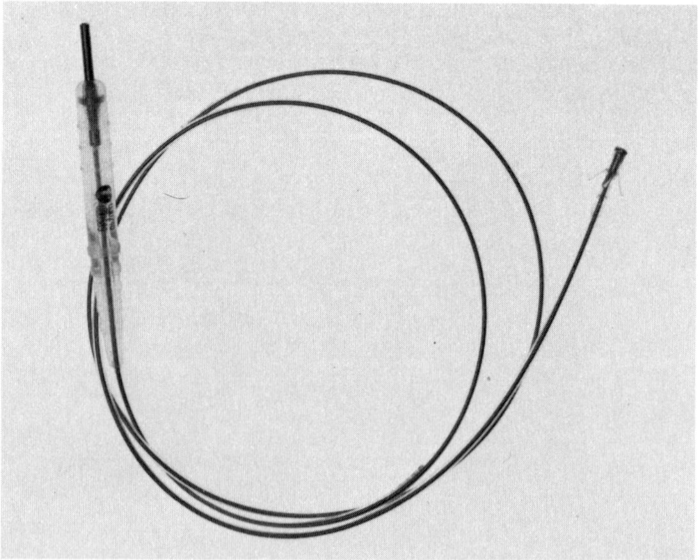

Lead Characteristics *Continued*

Lead	Description	Salient Features
236	Ventricular, unipolar passive fixation, endocardial	Trailing tines Polyurethane 9 French tip diameter Porous tip

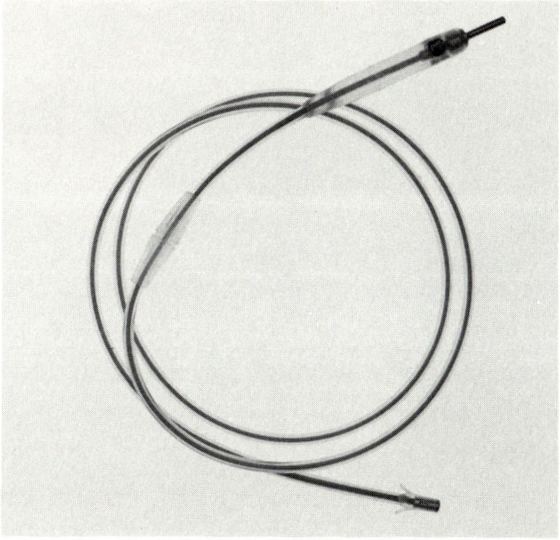

Lead	Description	Salient Features
171	Intramyocardial sutured, active fixation, unipolar	Silastic 2.1 mm body diameter 50 cm long

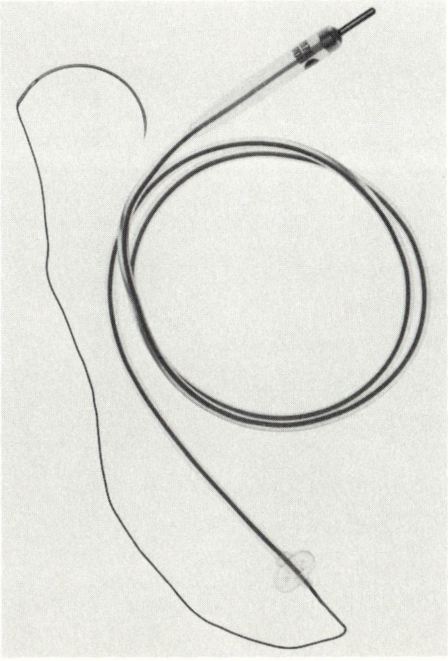

INDEX

Note: Numbers in *italics* refer to illustrations; numbers followed by t indicate tables.

Abscess, of conduction system, 26–27
Action potential, cathodal and anodal stimulation and, *33*
  upstroke velocity of, membrane potential and, 32, *33*
AFP Model 261 and 262, 319, 322t
AFP Model 275, 319–320, 322t
AFP Model 283, 320, 322t
Afterpotential sensing, in sensing failure, 171
AID, 250–251, *251*, 257
Air embolism, with transvenous approach, 162
Amyloidosis, of conduction system, 26, *26*
Angina pectoris, induced by atrial pacing, 64–67
Anodal stimulation, action potential induction and, *33*
Anterior septal artery, origin and course of, 16
Antitachycardia pacemaker, 243–258
  available types of, 254–258. See also individual types.
  criteria for selection of, 253–254
  manual vs automatic, 253–254
  nursing care with, 213–214
  reentrant arrhythmia termination with, 243
  tachycardia amelioration by, 245–246
    continuous overdrive pacing in, 245–246
    paired and coupled pacing in, 246, *246*
  tachycardia prevention by, 244–245
    dual site stimulation in, 245
    overdrive suppression in, 244–245, *245*
    rate support in, 244, *244*
  tachycardia termination by, 246–253
    burst pacing in, 249–250, *249–250*
    cardioversion and defibrillation in, 250–253, *251–252*
    double scanning extrastimuli in, 248, *249*
    overdrive pacing in, 249–250, *249–250*
    timed stimuli in, 246–249, *247–249*
    underdrive pacing in, *247*, 247–248
    upside-down demand pacing in, 248, *248*
Archos 06 pacemaker, 266, 268t
Arrhythmia, with normal pacer function, criteria for telephone reporting of, 186t–187t
ASVIP pacemaker, prevention of ventricular arrhythmia by, 241
Atrial competition, DVI pacemaker and, 238, *238*
Atrial fibrillation, DVI pacemaker and, 238, *239*
Atrial hexagonal loop electrode, 97
Atrial leads, cumulative actuarial survival of, 223, *225*
  threshold and amplitude characteristics of, 223–224, *225*
Atrial pacing, exercise testing vs, 66
  in coronary artery disease, 64–67
  in normal subjects, 60–64, *63*, 63t–64t
  myocardial blood flow and, 67–71, 69t
  overdrive, ventricular tachycardia and, 89, *89*
  surgical technique in, 111–112
  temporary cardiac, catheter position in, 96–97
Atrial synchronous pacemaker, function and selection of, 229–231, *230*
Atrial systole, oxygen consumption and, 222–223
Atrioventricular block, acquired, permanent pacing in, 79–80
  after open-heart surgery, 134–135, *135*
  causes of, 21
  complete, causes and symptoms of, 80
  congenital, in children, 129
    permanent pacing in, 80–81
  second-degree, progressive, in children, 130
  surgical, in children, 126–128
  temporary pacing for, 87–88
  third-degree, acquired, chronic, nonsurgical, in children, 129–130
Atrioventricular node, 14–15
  blood supply to, 15
  histologic identification of, 14
  left and right bundle branches of, 14
  location of, 14

Atrioventricular node (*Continued*)
obtaining material for examination of, 17, *17–19*
Atrioventricular pacing, surgical technique in, 113–115, *114*
Atrioventricular sequential pacemaker, 92, *94*
function and selection of, 228–229, *228–229*
radiographic evaluation of, *147*
Autima 2251, 335t
Autima II 2291, 335t
AVflex pacemaker, 281t
Avius Model 263–01, 299, 302t

Battery failure, radiographic evaluation of, 156
Biotronik, 265–270
lead systems of, 270, 270t
pulse generators of, 265–266, 267t–269t. See also individual types.
Bipolar electrogram, sensing circuit and, 50–52, *51*
Bipolar recording system, advantages and disadvantages of, 55–56
Brachial plexus injury, with transvenous approach, 162
Brachial vein, in temporary pacing, 95
Bradyarrhythmia, after open-heart surgery, 134–136
temporary cardiac pacing and, 86–89, *88*
Brownlee code, *227*
for atrial synchronous pacemaker, *230*
for AV sequential pacemaker, *228*
for fully automatic pacing, *232*
Bundle of His, identification of, *17–19*
Burst pacing, 249–250, *249–250*
Byrel-SX Model 5993SX, 307, 309t

Calcification, of conduction system, 21–22, *22*
Cardiac Pacemakers, Inc., 271–274
lead systems of, 274t
pulse generators of, 272t–274t
Cardiac perforation, nonpacing in, 165
in temporary cardiac pacing, 102, *103*
radiographic evaluation of, 151–153, *155*
Cardiac skeleton, sclerosis of left side of, 21
Cardio–Pace Medical, 275–276
lead systems of, 276
pulse generators of, 275, 276t
Cardioversion, transvenous, 251–253, *252*
Carotid hypersensitivity syndrome, DVI pacemaker and, 234
Carotid sinus syndrome, hypersensitive, in children, 130–131
Catheters, bipolar vs unipolar, 200
Cathodal stimulation, action potential induction and, *33*
Cephalic vein, in permanent pacing, 108–109, *110*
Charge threshold, 35
clinical implications of, 47
Children, congenital heart block in, 129
hypersensitive carotid sinus syndrome in, 130–131
permanent cardiac pacing in, 123–126
epicardial approach for, 124–126, *124–128*
battery pack placement in, 125–126, *127*
Medtronic harpoon lead in, 125, *126*
screw-in and post-type leads in, 125, *125*
Teletronic lead in, 125, *126*
indications for, 123, 123t
transvenous approach for, 123
refractory tachyarrhythmias in, 131
second-degree AV block in, progressive, 130
sick sinus syndrome in, 130
surgical AV block in, 126–128
temporary cardiac pacing in, 120–122
epicardial approach for, 121–122
atrial wire placement in, 122, *124*
ventricular wire placement in, 122
esophageal approach for, 121
indications for, 120
transcutaneous approach for, 122
transthoracic approach for, 121
transvenous approach for, 120–121
third-degree AV block in, acquired, chronic, nonsurgical, 129–130
Circumflex artery, left, origin and course of, 16
Clot formation along electrode, 158
Coats Pacesetter Vivalith II Model 301, 323t
Conduction system, 12–16
abscess of, 26–27
amyloidosis of, 26, *26*
atrioventricular node, 14–15
blood supply to, 15–16
calcification of, 21–22, *22*
congenital disorders of, 20
endocardial fibroelastosis of, 26
fibrosis of, 23
frequent disease processes of, 20–21
hemorrhage of, 24–25, *25*
less frequent disease processes of, 21
myocardial infarction of, 23–24, *24*
myocarditis of, 25–26
pathologic changes in, 20–27
sinoatrial node in, 12–14
Constant-current constant-voltage generator, 39, *40*
Constant-current source generator, 37–39, *38*
Constant-voltage source generator, *39*, 39–41
Cook Pacemaker Corp., 277–283
lead systems of, 282(t)–283(t)
pulse generators of, 277–281, 278(t)–281(t)
Coratomic, 284–287
conventional pacemakers of, 285, 287t
multiprogrammable pacemakers of, 284–285, 286t
pacing electrodes of, 287, *287*
Cordis, 288–294
lead systems of, 292, 292t–294t
pulse generators of, 288, 289t–292t

Cordis 184A, actuarial survival months of, 316t
Cordis Omni-Orthocor, 247, 248, 255
Cordis Sequicor, upper rate behavior with, 242
Coronary artery, right, origin and course of, 16
Coronary artery disease, atrial pacing in, 64–67
  hemodynamic data at rest and during pacing in, 67, 68t, *69–71*
  hemodynamic data during exercise in, 67, 69t
Coronary sinus pacing, 72
  in normal subjects, 62–64, *63*, 63t–64t
  radiographic evaluation of, 149, *150*
  surgical technique in, 113
Cosmos Bipolar Model 284–02, 300
Cosmos Model 283–01, 299–300, 301t
CPI Delta, 273t
CPI MICROTHIN P2 Models 0523 and 0623, 273t
CPI P5 Models 0530 and 0630, 273t
CPI Ultra I Models 0531 and 0631, 272t
CPI Ultra II Model 0910, 272t
Current amplitude, overpotential amplitude and, 42, *42*
Current density, overpotential amplitude and, 42, *43*
Current threshold, 30–34, *30–34*
  cathodal and anodal stimulation and, 31–32, *33*
  clinical implications of, 46–47, 46t
  electrode size and position and, 31, *32*
  factors influencing, 35–36
  intracellular ion concentration and, 36
  strength-duration curve for, 30, *31*
  strength-interval curve and, 32, *34*
  sympathetic tone and, 35–36
  timing of current delivery and, 32, *33*
CyberLith Models 253–07 and 254–07, 301, 303t

DDD pacemaker, function and selection of, 231–232, *232*
  function of, *191*
  loss of atrial sensing with, 242, *242*
  programming combinations for, 237, *237*
  telemetry printout from, 224, *226*
Defibrillation, with permanent pacemaker, 211
Demand pacemaker, historical development of, 9
Diaphragmatic muscle stimulation, in sensing failure, 172
Diplos 03 pacemaker, 265–266, 267t
Diplos 04 pacemaker, 266, 269t
Direct cardiac stimulation, history of, 5–10
  electrodes in, 6–7
  energy sources in, 8
  pacemaker rhythmicity in, 8–10
  rising threshold in, 5–6
  temporary pacing in, 7
Dual-chamber pacemaker. See also individual types.
Dual-chamber pacemaker (*Continued*)
  complications of, 236–242
  value of, hemodynamic proof of, *233*, 233–235
Durapulse pulse generator, 272t
DVI pacemaker, advantages of, *233*, 233–234
  atrial competition with, 238, *238*
  atrial fibrillation with, 238, *239*
  carotid hypersensitivity syndrome and, 234
  committed vs noncommitted, 228–229, *229*
  function and selection of, 228–229, *228–229*
  function of, *191–192*
  pseudo–pseudo fusion with, 229
  VVI vs, in sick sinus syndrome, 234

Eikos 04 pacemaker, 266, 268t
ELA Medical, 295–298
  pulse generators of, 295–296, 296t–297t
Electrical engineering, 36–57
Electrode, displaced or broken, radiography for, 151, *152–154*
  displacement of, 56
  history of development of, 6–7
  maturation of, 56
  surface area of, threshold current and, 31, *32*
    voltage threshold and, 34, *35*
  temporary epicardial, nursing management with, 195–197
Electrode catheter, balloon-tipped, *91*
  firm vs flexible, 90–92
  in temporary cardiac pacing, 90–92, *91–93*
  multipolar, 92, *93*
  transvenous, 90–92, *91*
  unipolar vs bipolar, 92
Electromagnetic interference, 211, 212t
  in sensing failure, 171
Electrophysiology of pacing, 29–58
Embolism, air, with transvenous approach, 162
Encor bipolar pervenous ventricular lead, 293t
Encor epicardial lead with porous-surfaced electrode, 294t
Encor linear bipolar pervenous J atrial lead, 293t
Encor pervenous active-fixation lead, 293t
Encor unipolar pervenous J atrial lead, 292t
Encor unipolar pervenous ventricular lead, 293t
Endocardial fibroelastosis, of conduction system, 26
Endocardial pacing, transvenous, screw-in J lead for, 112–113
Energy threshold, 35
  formula for, 45
Enertrax Model 7100, 307, 310t
Epicardial approach, in permanent pacing, in children, 124–126, *124–128*
  in temporary pacing, 121–122
Erosion, pacemaker, 172–173
Esophageal approach, in temporary pacing, in children, 121
Excitability, 29–30

Exercise testing, atrial pacing vs, 66
with fixed ventricular rate, 71
Exit block, nonpacing in, 166, *166*
External pacing, history of, 3–4

Femoral vein, in temporary pacing, 95–96
FH lead, 270t
Fibrosis, of conduction system, 23
Fixed-rate pacemaker, exercise testing with, 71
historical development of, 8–9
Flap coverage, 177–181
local skin flap for, 177–178, *178–179*
muscle flap for, 179–181, *180–181*
Focal motor seizure, 172
Follow-up, 182–194
criteria for pacemaker malfunction reporting in, 184t
criteria for reporting arrhythmias with normal pacer function in, 186t–187t
criteria for reporting symptoms with normal pacer function in, 185t
form for, *193*
for pacemakers, 182–194
frequency of, 185
Medicare schedule for, *193*
need for, 182–183
outpatient care for, 212–213
pacemaker clinic for, 183
rate change in, 183, 185
transtelephonic pacemaker analysis for, 183
Fully automatic pacemaker, function and selection of, 231–232, *232*

Gemini III Model 418A, 285t
Gemini Theta Model 415A, 285t

Heart rate, coronary hemodynamics and, 72
Hemodynamics of pacing, 59–75
Hemorrhage, of conduction system, 24–25, *25*
Hemothorax, with transvenous approach, 161
Hiccups, 172
right ventricular implants and, 116
High-sensitivity pacers, myopotentials and, 56
Hypersensitive carotid sinus syndrome, in children, 130–131
Hysteresis, *188*

I-2 lead, 270t
ICHD code, *227*
Identification, pacemaker, 211
Impedance, lead, implantation problems and, 46t, 47
load, of sensing circuit, 48–50, *49*

Impedance (*Continued*)
ohmic, 41–46, *42–43*
output, 41–46
polarization, 41–46, *42–43*
Indications, for cardiac pacing, 79–85
for permanent cardiac pacing, 79–82
acquired AV block as, 79–80
congenital AV block as, 80–81
physiologic pacing as, 82
sick sinus syndrome as, 81
tachyarrhythmia as, 81–82
for temporary cardiac pacing, 82–84, 86–90, 87t, *88–90*, 197, 198t
acute myocardial infarction as, 83–84
bradyarrhythmia as, 86–89, *88*
cardiac and noncardiac surgery as, 83
drug use and, 88–89
tachyarrhythmia as, 89, *89–90*
Infection, sensing failure in, 173
Input circuit. See *Sensing circuit.*
Intermedics, 299–305
lead systems of, 303, 304t–305t
pulse generators of, 299–301, 301t–303t
Intermedics Cyberlith, 254–255
Intermittent pacing, 167, 167t

J lead, screw-in, 112–113
Jugular vein, external, in permanent pacing, 109–110, *111*
in temporary pacing, 95
internal, in permanent pacing, 110–111

K-10 lead, 270t
Kalos 03 pacemaker, 266, 267t

L-40 Endo-Loc electrode, 283
Latissimus dorsi muscle flap, 180–181, *180–181*
Lead, Biotronik, 270, 270t
Cardiac Pacemakers, Inc., 274t
Cardio-Pace Medical, 276
Cook Pacemaker Corp., 282t–283t
Cordis, 292, 292t–294t
ELA Medical, 297–298, 298t
Intermedics, 303, 304t–305t
Medtronic, 310–311, 311t–314t
Pacesetter Systems, 323t–326t
Siemens-Elema, 330, 330t–331t
Teletronics, 336t–337t
Lead connection problems, 167–168
Lead dislodgement, 164–165
Lead fracture, nonpacing and, 167, 167t
pseudobreak in, 156, *157*
radiographic evaluation of, 154–156, *156*
tight sutures simulating, 156

Lead impedance, implantation problems and, 46t, 47
Lead insulation break, 165
Left bundle branch, identification of, *19*
location of, 14
Left ventricular performance, in normal subjects, 60–64, *63*, 63t–64t
Leukos 03 pacemaker, 266, 268t
Lithium battery, 188
Load impedance, of sensing circuit, 48–50, *49*
Long-term cardiac pacing, indications for, 6

Medrad Automatic Implantable Defibrillator (AID), 257
Medtronic, 306–314
lead systems of, 310–311, 311t–314t
pulse generators of, 306–314, 308t–310t
Medtronic (Model 5998) Radio-Frequency Pacemaker, 254
Medtronic 8423, actuarial survival months of, 316t
Medtronic harpoon lead, 125, *126*
Medtronic Interactive Tachycardia Terminating System, 248, 256
Medtronic Internal Cardioverter, 257–258
Membrane potential, action potential upstroke velocity and, 32, *33*
Mercury/zinc battery, 188
Microshocks, 196
Migration, pacemaker, 172–173
Multicor Gamma Model 337A, 287t
Multicor II, 287t
Multilith II, 296
Multilith Models 1140 and 2140, 295, 296t
Multilith Models 1141 and 2141, 296, 296t
Multiprogrammable pacemaker, Coratomic, 280–281, 282t
Muscle flap, 179–181, *180–181*
latissimus dorsi, 180–181, *180–181*
pectoralis major, 179, *180*
Muscle stimulation, in sensing failure, 172
$M\dot{V}O_2$, factors in, 59
Myocardial blood flow, atrial pacing and, 67–71, 69t
Myocardial infarction, acute, temporary pacing in, 83–84
of conduction system, 23–24, *24*
Myocardial ischemia, 60
Myocarditis, of conduction system, 25–26
Myopotential, high-sensitivity pacers and, 56
in sensing failure, 170–171

N lead, 270t
Neos 01 pacemaker, 266, 269t
New advances in cardiac pacemaking, 219–261. See also individual pacemakers.
Nomos 02 pacemaker, 266, 267t
Noncardiac surgery, temporary pacing in, 83
Nonpacing, 164–168, 164t
exit block in, 166, *166*
intermittent, 167, 167t
lack of capture or lack of current in, 164t
lead connection problems in, 167–168
lead dislodgement in, 164–165
lead fracture in, 167, 167t
lead insulation break in, 165
ventricular perforation in, 165
Normal pacer function, arrhythmia with, criteria for telephone reporting of, 186t–187t
symptoms with, 185t
Nuclear pacemaker, 188
Nursing management, 195–214
in permanent transvenous pacing, 204–214
antitachycardia pacemaker, 213–214
clinical assessment, 209
defibrillation, 211
discharge planning, 210–211
electromagnetic and radio-frequency interference, 211, 212t
outpatient care, 212–213
paced rhythm analysis, 209
paced rhythm feature identification, 209
pacemaker identification, 211
pacemaker laboratory, 206–207, 206t–207t
postoperative complications, 208–209
postoperative infection, 210
postoperative period, 207–212
preoperative period, 204–206
sample pacemaker laboratory record, 208t
written instructions at discharge, 211
in temporary epicardial pacing after open-heart surgery, 195–197
in temporary transvenous pacing, 197–204
catheters, 200
electrical hazards, 202–204
equipment, 199–201
external pulse generator, 200–201
immediate postoperative period, 201
insertion, 198–199
malfunctions, 202–204, 203t
patient preparation, 198
procedure, 201–202
stabilizing external pulse generator, 201–202

Ohmic impedance, 41–46, *42–43*
Open-heart surgery, 133–141
atrioventricular block after, 134–135, *135*
bradyarrhythmia after, 134–136
pacing complications after, 139
sinus node dysfunction after, 135–136
supraventricular tachyarrhythmia after, *136*, 136–137
tachyarrhythmia after, 136–138
temporary atrial pacing after, 138–139
temporary pacing after, 133–134, 134t

Open-heart surgery (*Continued*)
  temporary ventricular pacing after, 138, *139*
  ventricular tachycardia after, 137–138, *137–138*
Optima 147/247 and 174/274, 333t
Optima MP 155/255, 334t
Optima MPT 5281/5282, 334t
Output circuit, 36–37, *37*
Output impedance, 41–46
Ovalife C-101-P, 285, 286t
Ovalith-920, 285, 287t
Ovalith-920BP, 285, 287t
Overpotential amplitude, current amplitude and, 42, *42*
  current density and, 42, *43*
Oversensing, *170*, 170–171
Oxygen consumption, at rest and during exercise, 221–223

P cells, 13
P-wave sensing, in sensing failure, 171
Pacemaker clinic for follow-up, 183
Pacemaker codes, 224–228, *227*
  Brownlee code, *227*
  five-position ICHD code, *227*
Pacemaker identification, 211
  radiography for, *148*, 149–151
Pacemaker laboratory record, 208t
Pacemaker malfunction, criteria for telephone reporting of, 184t
Pacemaker migration or erosion, 172–173
Pacemaker syndrome, 174, 221, *222*
Pacemaker tray equipment, 207t
Pacemaker-mediated tachycardia, with VDD/DDD pacemaker, *239*, *239–240*, 239–241
Pacesetter 221, actuarial survival months of, 316t
Pacesetter Systems, 315–326
  lead systems of, 323t–326t
  pulse generators of, 315–320, 316t–318t, 321t–323t
Pacing circuit, 36–37, *37*
Pacing electrode, Coratomic, 283
Pasar Model 4171, 333t
Patient-activated pacemakers, 213–214
PBAF lead, 298, 298t
Pectoralis major muscle flap, 179, *180*
Perforation. See *Cardiac perforation.*
Permanent cardiac pacing, anterior thoracotomy in, 115–117, *116*
  atrial, 111–112
  atrioventricular, 113–115, *114*
  cephalic vein cutdown in, 108–109, *110*
  complications of, 160–176.
    intraoperative, 160–163
    postoperative, 163–174
    transthoracic, 163
    transvenous, 160–162
    troubleshooting categories for, 163, 164t
  external jugular cutdown in, 109–110, *111*
Permanent cardiac pacing (*Continued*)
  failure of, 164–168, 164t, 167t. See also *Non-pacing.*
  in children, 123–126
  indications for, 79–82
  internal jugular puncture in, 110–111
  sensing failure in, 168–174. See also *Sensing failure.*
  subclavian vein puncture in, 108, *109*
  surgical technique in, 106–119
  transmediastinal approach in, 117–118
  transthoracic approach in, 115–118
  transvenous, 106–115
    nursing management in, 204–214. See also under *Nursing management.*
  transvenous coronary sinus, 113
  transvenous endocardial, 112–113
  transxiphoid approach in, 117, *118*
Phrenic nerve injury, with transvenous approach, 162
Physiolith, 296, 297t
Physiologic pacemaker, historical development of, 9
Physiologic pacing, 220–224
  permanent pacing in, 82
  technical considerations in, 223–224, *224–225*
  theoretic considerations in, 220–223, *222*
PMAF lead, 297–298, 298t
PMCF lead, 298, 298t
Pneumothorax, radiographic evaluation of, 158, *158*
  with transvenous approach, 161
Polarization impedance, 41–46, *42–43*
Posterior descending artery, origin and course of, 16
Posterior septal artery, origin and course of, 16
Prima Models 253–01 and 236–02, 301, 303t
Programalith II Models 225 and 226, 315, 320, 321t
Programalith II series, 14-month survival of, 318t
Programalith III Models 241 and 242, 319, 321t
Programalith series, 47-month survival of, 317t
Pseudo–pseudo fusion, 229
Pulse generator. See also individual types.
  actuarial survival of, as function of power source, 223, *224*
  Biotronik, 265–266, 267t–269t
  Cardiac Pacemakers, Inc., 272t–274t
  Cardio-Pace Medical, 275, 276t
  Cook Pacemaker Corp., 277–278, 278t–281t
  Cordis, 288, 289t–291t
  ELA Medical, 295–296, 296t–297t
  external, 92, *93–94*, 200–201
    AV sequential, 92, *94*
    rapid pacing, 92, *94*
  failure of, 171
  historical development of, 8
  Intermedics, 299–301, 301t–303t
  Medtronic, 306–314, 308t–310t
  migration of, 151

Pulse generator (*Continued*)
  Pacesetter Systems, 315–320, 316t–318t, 321t–323t
  Siemens-Elema, 327–328, 328t–329t
  Teletronics, 333t–335t
  types of, 37–41, *38–40*

Quantum Models 253–19, 254–18, and 254–20, 300–301, 302t

R-wave polarities, 168, *168*
Radio-frequency interference, 212t
Radiographic evaluation of pacemakers, 145–159
  for battery failure, 156
  for cardiac perforation, 151–153, *155*
  for coronary sinus pacing, 149, *150*
  for lead fractures, 154–156, *156*
  for malpositioned leads, 151, *152–154*
  for pacemaker identification, *148*, 149–151
  for pneumothorax, 158, *158*
  for transthoracic pacing, *148*, 149
  for transvenous pacing, 145–149, *146–148*
  identification of complications with, 151–158
Rate difficulties, fast vs slow, 171–172
Recurrent laryngeal nerve injury, with transvenous approach, 162
Right bundle branch, identification of, *19*
  location of, 14

Screw-in J lead, 112–113
Sensing circuit, 48–57
  configuration and slew rate for, *52*, 52–53
  electrogram amplitude and, 50–52, *51*
  filtering characteristics of, 50
  frequency spectral analysis for, *53*, 53–54
  insulation break and, 50
  load impedance of, 48–50, *49*
Sensing failure, 168–174
  afterpotential sensing in, 171
  electromagnetic interference in, 171
  infection in, 173
  muscle stimulation in, 172
  myopotentials in, 170–171
  oversensing in, *170*, 170–171
  P-wave sensing in, 171
  pacemaker migration or erosion in, 172–173
  pulse generator failure in, 171
  R-wave polarities and, 168, *168*
  rate difficulty in, 171–172
  T-wave sensing in, 171
  undersensing as, 168–170, 169t
Sensing threshold, 48
Sequicor II Theta Model 233F, 286t
Sequicor III Model 233G, 286t
Sick sinus syndrome, DVI vs VVI pacing in, 234
  in children, 130
  permanent pacing in, 81

Siemens-Elema, 327–331
  lead systems of, 330, 330t–331t
  pulse generators of, 327–328, 328t–329t
Siemens-Elema Model 668, actuarial survival months of, 316t
Sinoatrial node, 12–14
  anterior internodal tract of, 13
  blood supply to, 15
  histologic identification of, 12–13
  location of, 12
  middle internodal tract of, 13
  obtaining material for examination of, 16
  P and T cells in, 13
  posterior internodal tract of, 13
Sinus node dysfunction, after open-heart surgery, 135–136
Skin flap, 177–178, *178–179*
Spectrax-SX Models 5984, 5998R, and 5998T, 307, 309t
Spectrax-SXT Model 8420, 307, 309t
Strength-duration curve, 30, *31*
Strength-interval curves, 32, *34*
Subclavian artery, puncture of, with transvenous approach, 162
Subclavian vein, in permanent pacing, 108, *109*
  in temporary pacing, 95
  thrombosis of, with transvenous approach, 162
Supraventricular tachycardia, after open-heart surgery, *136*, 136–137

T cells, 13
T-wave sensing, in sensing failure, 171
Tachyarrhythmia, after open-heart surgery, 136–138
  permanent pacing in, 81–82
  refractory, in children, 131
  temporary cardiac pacing and, 89, *89–90*
Tachycardia, antitachycardia pacing for, 243–258. See also *Antitachycardia pacing.*
  coronary hemodynamics and, 72–73
  pacemaker-mediated, with VDD/DDD pacemaker, *239*, *239–240*, 239–241
  supraventricular, after open-heart surgery, *136*, 136–137
  ventricular, 137–138, *137–138*
    atrial overdrive pacing in, 89, *89*
    rapid ventricular pacing in, 89, *90*
Telectronic permanent epicardial lead, 125, *126*
Telemetry printout, from DDD pacemaker, 224, *226*
Teletronics, 332–337
  lead systems of, 336t–337t
  pulse generators of, 333t–335t
Teletronics (Model 4151) Pasar, 255–256
Temporary cardiac pacing, 86–105
  atrial pacing with, 96–97
  brachial vein in, 95
  catheter perforation in, 102, *103*
  complications of, 102–104, *103*

Temporary cardiac pacing (*Continued*)
  dual-chamber, 100–101
  EKG monitoring during catheter insertion in, 98–100, *99–100*
  electrical hazards and, 101
  electrode catheter in, 90–92, *91–93*
  electrode configurations for, 92, *93*
  endocardial electrogram sensing in, 100
  equipment for, 90–92, *91–94*
  external pulse generator for, 92, *93–94*
  failure to sense with, 104
  femoral vein in, 95–96
  history of, 7
  in children, 120–122
  in open-heart surgery, 133–134, 134t
  inappropriate sensing with, 105
  indications for, 82–84, 86–90, 87t, *88–90*, 197, 198t
  infection in, 104
  insertion and placement of electrode catheter in, 97–101, *98–100*
  insertion site care in, 101
  jugular vein in, 95
  management of, 101–105
  mechanical stimulation of ventricle in, 102–104
  nonpacing or noncapture with, 104
  pacemaker threshold determination in, 100, *100*
  post-surgical myocardial, 96
  procedure for, 95–101
  subclavian vein in, 95
  techniques for, 90–101
  transthoracic approach in, 96
  transvenous, nursing management in, 197–204. See also under *Nursing management.*
    problems associated with, 203t
  troubleshooting malfunctions in, 104–105
  ventricular pacing with, 96
  ventricular vs atrial, 90
Temporary epicardial electrodes, nursing management with, 195–197
Thoracic duct injury, with transvenous approach, 161
Thoracotomy, anterior, in permanent cardiac pacing, 115–117, *116*
Threshold current. See *Current threshold.*
Threshold energy. See *Energy threshold*
Threshold voltage. See *Voltage threshold.*
Transcutaneous approach, in temporary pacing, in children, 122
Transmediastinal approach, in permanent cardiac pacing, 117–118
Transtelephonic pacemaker analysis, 183, 212–213
  criteria for reporting arrhythmias with normal pacer function in, 186t–187t
  criteria for reporting malfunction in, 184t
  criteria for reporting symptoms with normal pacer function in, 185t
Transthoracic approach, in permanent pacing, 115–118
Transthoracic approach (*Continued*)
  in temporary pacing, 96
    in children, 121
  intraoperative complications of, 163
  radiographic evaluation of, *148*, 149
Transvenous approach, in permanent pacing, in children, 123
  in temporary pacing, 120–121
  intraoperative complications of, 160–162
  radiographic evaluation of, 145–149, *146–148*
Transvenous cardioversion, 251–253, *252*
Transxiphoid approach, in permanent cardiac pacing, 117, *118*
Twiddler's syndrome, 151, *154*

Undersensing, 168–170, 169t
Unilith Models 7540 and 7542, 296, 297t
Unipolar electrogram, sensing circuit and, 50–52, *51*
Upper rate behavior, with VDD/DDD pacemaker, 241–242, *242*
Upside-down demand pacemaker, 248, *248*

VAT pacemaker, function of, *190*
VDD pacemaker, function and selection of, 229–231, *230*
  function of, *192*
  VVI vs, 234–235, *235–237*
VDD/DDD pacemaker, 234–235, *235–237*
  pacemaker-mediated tachycardia with, *239*, *239–240*, 239–241
  upper rate behavior with, 241–242, *242*
  ventricular arrhythmias with, 241, *241*
Ventricular arrhythmia, with VDD/DDD pacemaker, 241, *241*
Ventricular pacing, in normal subjects, 60–64, *63*, 63t–64t
  short-term and long-term effects of, 71–72
  temporary cardiac, catheter position in, 96
Ventricular tachycardia, after open-heart surgery, 137–138, *137–138*
  atrial overdrive pacing in, 89, *89*
  rapid ventricular pacing in, 89, *90*
VENTRIflex pacemaker, 276t
Versatrax Model 7000, 306
Versatrax II Model 7000A, 307, 308t
Voltage threshold, 30, 34, *35*
  clinical implications of, 46, 46t
VVI pacemaker, DVI vs, in sick sinus syndrome, 234
  function of, *188–190*
  VDD vs, 234–235, *235–237*

Y lead, 270t
YC lead, 270t
YR lead, 270t